PSYCHIATRY IN MEDICAL PRACTICE

THIRD EDITION

David Goldberg

Linda Gask

Richard Morriss

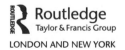

Routledge
Taylor & Francis Group

LONDON AND NEW YORK

First published in 1987 by Tavistock Publications
Reprinted in 1991 by Routledge
Second Edition published in 1994 by Routledge
Third edition published in 2008 by Routledge
27 Church Road, Hove, East Sussex BN3 2FA

Simultaneously published in the USA and Canada
by Routledge
270 Madison Avenue, New York, NY 10016

Routledge is an imprint of the Taylor & Francis Group, an Informa business

© 2008 David Goldberg, Linda Gask and Richard Morriss

Typeset in Palatino by Garfield Morgan, Swansea, West Glamorgan
Printed and bound in Great Britain by Bell & Bain Ltd, Glasgow
Cover design by Sandra Heath

This publication has been produced with paper manufactured to strict
environmental standards and with pulp derived from sustainable forests.

British Library Cataloguing in Publication Data
A catalogue record for this book is available from the British Library

Library of Congress Cataloging in Publication Data
Goldberg, David P.
  Psychiatry in medical practice / David Goldberg, Linda Gask and Richard
Morriss. – 3rd ed.
      p. ; cm.
  Includes bibliographical references and index.
  ISBN 978-0-415-42544-5 (pbk.)
  1. Psychiatry. I. Gask, Linda. II. Morriss, R. K. (Richard Keith), 1960- III. Title.
  [DNLM: 1. Mental Disorders. WM 140 G618p 2008]
  RC454.G588 2008
  616.89–dc22

                                                                          2007036630

ISBN 978-0-415-42544-5

CONTENTS

Contents

Contents

ILLUSTRATIONS

FIGURES

TABLES

BOXES

PREFACE TO THE THIRD EDITION

This edition sees two new editors – Professor Linda Gask from Manchester, and Professor Richard Morriss from Nottingham – and this has been the occasion of a complete revision of the book. We thank our previous editors, Professor Francis Creed and Dr Sidney Benjamin, and they will find some sections of their original text still surviving in our new text. In particular, Dr Benjamin's chapter on the mental states was found to require very little revision.

Many chapters have been completely re-written, and two completely new chapters have been introduced – on risk assessments, and on the mental health services. There have been major changes in medical education since our last edition in 1994, and we have introduced new sections on problem based learning and objective structured clinical examinations (OSCEs). Knowledge has also advanced since the last occasion, and new treatments are now available.

Although we have each written several chapters ourselves, we are very grateful to colleagues in specialized areas who have contributed additional text. Professor Bill Deakin has completely revised the section on drug treatments and ECT in the 'Treatment' chapter, and Professor Simon Gowers of Liverpool University has revised the section on eating disorders and the chapter entitled 'Childhood and adolescence'. Dr Sophie Anhoury and Dr Dene Robertson of the Institute of Psychiatry, King's College, London revised the chapter on learning disability, and Dr Gillian Stratford has re-written the chapter on sexual disorders. Professor Shon Lewis wrote the section on brain imaging, and Professors Alastair Burns and Dave Jolley the chapter on organic disorders and old age.

To all these contributors, we extend our profound thanks, but we must accept final responsibility for the opinions expressed throughout the book.

David Goldberg
Linda Gask
Richard Morriss

1   INTRODUCTION

This book sets out the knowledge you will need to enable you to understand and manage the common psychiatric disorders and psychological problems that you will encounter among your patients in your pre-specialist years. It contains everything you are likely to need for your Finals examination, and then some more. It does not pretend to be a textbook for psychiatrists, but it should provide a useful introduction to the subject even for those students who intend to enter psychiatry or general practice.

THE CLINICAL APPROACH TO THE PATIENT

We start by giving an account of those **interview techniques** that are necessary in order to evaluate the importance of psychological factors in the individual case. We distinguish between the brief, focused examinations that are appropriate in the general wards and the A&E Department, and the much more comprehensive examinations for in-patients in the psychiatric wards. Next comes a chapter on the **mental state examination**, followed by chapters dealing with **risk assessment**, and with the **classification, aetiology, assessment**, and **treatment** of psychiatric disorders, and this part concludes with a chapter explaining how you should set about the **formulation** of an individual patient's problems in the psychiatric setting.

The chapters in this first part are fundamental to understanding what goes on in a department of psychiatry and are also relevant to work in the general wards. They will help you to elicit data relevant to a proper understanding of a patient's psychological problems, and then go on to make appropriate plans for treatment and management.

SYNDROMES OF PSYCHIATRIC DISORDER

The second part of the book gives a general account of the more common syndromes of psychiatric disorder. We start with psychological disorders that commonly accompany **physical diseases**, and include sections on epilepsy and pain. We then start at the top of a *hierarchy* of psychiatric disorders: beginning with **organic brain syndromes**, going on to **schizophrenia**, and then considering **bipolar disorder**. The next two chapters deal with **internalizing disorders**, where people experience subjective distress, First comes a chapter on anxiety, depression and fear disorders, followed by somatic presentations of emotional distress. Next come the **externalizing disorders**, where abnormalities occur mainly in outwardly observable behaviour: misuse of alcohol and drugs, and eating disorders. We conclude this part with a chapter on **personality disorders**.

The disorders described in this part are defined in terms of **syndromes** or collections of symptoms that commonly occur together, and in this respect they are therefore fairly similar to illnesses you will already have come across in general medicine, such as migraine or asthma.

DISORDERS RELATED TO STAGES OF THE LIFE CYCLE

In the third part we will consider disorders that either take their onset at a particular stage of human development, or are peculiar to a stage of the life cycle. We start with **learning disability** since this group of disorders reflects problems arising at conception, during intra-uterine development, or from events during or shortly after birth. We then work our way through the life cycle with chapters on **disorders of childhood and adolescence** followed by **sexual and reproductive disorders**, and finally **disorders of older people**.

EPIDEMIOLOGY

We will be giving you figures for each illness in later chapters: here we consider overall rates for *any psychiatric diagnosis* in various populations. Between a quarter and one-third of the population can be expected to experience a period of mental ill-health in the course of a year, but some of these are self-limiting episodes for which care is not sought. Just over 20 per cent of the population will consult their family doctor with a mental disorder, and in 11 per cent the GP will make a formal psychiatric diagnosis. However, only about 2 per cent of the population are likely to be referred to the mental illness services, and most of these will be dealt with as out-patients.

If we consider consecutive attenders at general practitioners' surgeries, then somewhere between 25 and 35 per cent of them will meet research criteria for psychiatric illness. Figures for those admitted to medical wards of general hospitals are approximately similar: recent estimates range between 20 and 40 per cent. Most of these illnesses are states of anxiety or depression, and such disorders are usually an integral part of the various physical disorders for which help is being sought (see Chapters 11 and 12 for a fuller discussion). It is for this reason that an understanding of the assessment and management of psychiatric illness is an essential part of your medical training.

Females are at much greater risk for disorders characterized by depression and anxiety ('internalizing disorders'), and males have much higher rates for alcohol and drug disorders, and anti-social behaviour ('externalizing disorders') (see *Figure 1.1*).

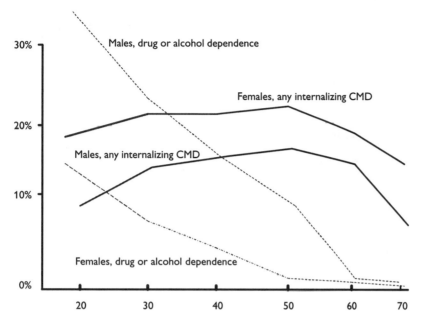

Figure 1.1 *Rates for any common mental disorder, and drug or alcohol dependence, by age and sex (ONS 2000, data for Great Britain)*

SKILLS TO BE ACQUIRED

With the help of this book and the opportunity to interview patients, you should aim to acquire the following skills between now and the time that you qualify:

1. The ability to **take a history** from a patient in such a way that you are able to assess the importance of psychological factors.
2. The ability to **make a short assessment of a patient's personality** and to distinguish it from illness.
3. The ability to **carry out a mental state examination** of a patient with a psychiatric illness, and the ability to assess dementia.
4. The ability to **adapt your interview techniques** to special types of clinical interview, for example brief focused interviews in primary care, on general wards or in A&E departments, interviews with children, with old people, with immigrants and those with communication problems.
5. The ability to **write a formulation** of a patient's illness.
6. The ability to **assess an episode of self-harm**.
7. The ability to **assess suicidal risk**.
8. The ability to **take a history from a relative**.

3

KNOWLEDGE OF MANAGEMENT PROCEDURES

By the time you qualify you should aim to acquire knowledge of the following management procedures. You should aim to cover most of them during your time in the department of psychiatry. It helps a great deal if you have actually seen them carried out, but there is no need for you to have done them yourself.

Medical procedures

1. The management of **alcohol withdrawal**.
2. The management of an **acutely psychotic** patient.
3. How to prescribe antidepressant medication
4. **Giving** electro-convulsive treatment (ECT).

Psychological procedures

1. (On the general wards)
   - How to break bad news.
   - Problem solving.
   - Talking to aggressive patients.
   - Talking to suicidal patients.
   - Helping the dying patient.
2. (In the paediatric department)
   - How to interview a child.
3. The management of violent behaviour in hospital settings.
4. Emergency procedures under the Mental Health Act.

PREVENTION OF MENTAL DISORDERS

It is customary to divide preventive activities into three types: **primary prevention**, which seeks to prevent a disorder occurring at all; **secondary prevention**, which seeks to bring early and effective treatment to those who have developed a disorder; and **tertiary prevention**, which seeks to reduce disability that has developed already.

Primary prevention includes measures to reduce psychosyndromes associated with head injury by seat belts and safer cars; health education to prevent AIDS by reducing promiscuous sexual contact or by use of appropriate contraceptive techniques; health education to provide clear guidance about safe levels of alcohol ingestion, measures to reduce sexual and physical abuse of children and to reinforce the desirability of providing children with a secure, caring environment and so reducing vulnerability to later anxiety and depression. There have been interesting preventive programmes in schools aimed at reducing both bullying and anti-social behaviour, and interventions to promote good parenting practices, which can be provided by psychologists, or brief interventions by family doctors. The arrival of computerized psychological treatments offers promise of much greater availability of preventive interventions.

Secondary prevention is best directed at high-risk groups: young widows, women who have experienced depressive symptoms in pregnancy, and young mothers at high risk of abusing their babies are examples. Post-natal depression can be reduced by visits from health visitors, and child abuse by arranging friendly follow-up visits by nurses.

Tertiary prevention can best be directed at those with mental disorders that will otherwise be long-term and will be associated with great disability: examples would be those with chronic psychosis and young adults with head injury.

PROBLEM BASED LEARNING

In clinical practice, problems, rather than mental or physical disorders, are presented by patients and their carers. The problem presented by the patient may be a symptom of one of a number of disorders and the doctor has to establish from other symptoms and other sources of information the most likely cause of the problem. The cause of the problem may be a mental disorder, but it may be unrelated to a mental disorder. While it is important to diagnose accurately the mental disorder, there are other features of a problem that are just as important such as the risk of death or serious injury to the person, or the best setting to treat the patient (e.g. hospital in-patient unit, hospital out-patient department, at home). Furthermore a patient may present with several new and ongoing problems that may or may not be related. For all these reasons, there is an increasingly widespread view that the teaching of medicine should start from the problems that patients present with rather than learning only about the major disorders patients can suffer from.

Problem based learning refers to the definition of learning goals from the problems that the patient presents with. The medical student lists the main problems that the patient may have and uses these problems to identify the potential disorders and other important related information to decide what to read and learn about. In this way problem based learning fulfils two aims that are not so readily captured in more traditional approaches to learning – to take a set of problems from the clinical setting and directly relate these to what the student needs to learn, and to define the most relevant and salient features of the case. A book such as this can be a source of information about the disorders a person might have and their management. However, it is important that the student does not only generate lists of individual mental and physical disorders that a patient might have from the problems they describe. The student needs to consider the person's problems in relation to their life situation, the effects the problem might have on other people, if the problem can be seen as a developmental or degenerative issue, and what effect the problem might have in relation to the public as a whole (the public health perspective).

Box 1.1 gives an example of a case to which a student has applied problem based learning. Note that a brief summary of the case capturing its salient features is used as the basis for setting learning objectives, otherwise each case will generate too many learning objectives and there will be a considerable amount of pointless repetition as the student moves from one case to the next. The italics indicate the words that the student has picked out and used to define a learning objective in the order that these words appear in the description of the case. The last sentence about the boy's sister and father coping poorly indicates that family issues are important. All of these topics can be found within this book, but the student may well wish to consult additional sources of information such as journal articles, books or official websites. There is often a considerable degree of overlap between the learning objectives, such as in this instance between depression and bereavement, attempted suicide and suicide risk, and the links might be indicated by drawing a line between the learning objectives if the student wishes.

Box 1.1 Problem based learning example

A *15-year-old* boy was assessed by a psychiatrist in the general medical ward after an *overdose* of paracetamol for which he was successfully medically treated. His *mother had died a year earlier* from cancer. He had been *drinking alcohol heavily*, became *low in mood*, *stopped school* and *planned his suicide*. His 9-year-old sister and father are also not coping well.

Problem list of learning objectives:

1. Adolescence – psychological issues
2. Attempted suicide – in the individual
3. Attempted suicide – as a public health problem
4. Bereavement – effects on the individual
5. Bereavement – effects on the family
6. Alcohol misuse – in the individual
7. Alcohol misuse – effects on the family
8. Alcohol misuse – as a public health problem
9. Depression – adolescence
10. School refusal
11. Suicide risk – assessment in the individual
12. Suicide in adolescence – epidemiology

HOW TO READ THIS BOOK

We have written the book in the order you should read it: Part 1 deals with fundamental aspects of the psychological approach to clinical problems. Try to read Chapters 2, 3 and 4 right away: although you can skip the remaining chapters in Part 1 until you have clerked your first patient. In particular, there is more information than you need to pass Finals in the chapter on 'Treatment': however, you will need this information to manage common psychological disorders adequately – so we make no apologies for the surplus!

As soon as you have interviewed a patient with a particular problem, read up the appropriate chapter in Part 2, as well as relevant bits of the chapters on investigation and treatment. Aim to read the whole of the first two parts in the first week of your time in the department of psychiatry.

Parts 3 and 4 can safely be left until the earlier parts have been absorbed, although all parts are equally important.

Preparing for the OSCE

The OSCE (objective structured clinical examination) is now used in most medical schools around the world to ensure reliability and objectivity in the assessment of clinical competencies.

The student may be subjected to an OSCE in which a patient presents with a particular set of problems and the student is set a particular task. Usually the student is presented with a patient, or an actor playing a patient, and the task is often to establish a brief assessment based on history, mental state examination and sometimes a brief physical examination focused on one or two systems (e.g. central nervous system, cardiovascular system) or anatomical sites (e.g. thyroid gland). The information required for such a brief assessment has been placed into boxes at the end of each chapter; these boxes are titled brief history and/or mental state examination. For instance in Chapter 15 on severe mood disorder, Box 15.1 summarizes the findings of a 10-minute history and mental state examination for a severe depressive episode. However, the information in the box should be read with the rest of the relevant chapter and Chapter 1 so that the necessary skills are developed to carry out a brief history and mental state examination, and the findings in Box 15.1 are placed in the correct context (otherwise the wrong inferences may be drawn from symptoms such as fatigue, sleep disturbance and social withdrawal, and mental state findings such as self neglect and psychomotor retardation).

We also think that these short summaries will help you to think about how to carry out brief focused assessments in any general medical setting.

Problem based short-answer questions

The second format widely used to test problem based learning is problem based oral examinations, or problem based short-answer questions. The typical scenario is that some basic information is given about a patient and the student is asked to generate possible diagnostic categories or methods of further assessment to reach a diagnosis. Further information on the same patient is then provided and the student is asked to refine their assessment based on the new information, or to suggest management options. Some examples of problem based short-answer questions are given at the end of the book. The answers to each question require only the factual information contained in this book, but the student will need to practise this format of question to apply the information about each disorder contained in the book in the context of the incomplete patient information usually provided in these scenarios.

THE CARD

We have included a card with this book, which you may wish to carry about with you until you have got used to carrying out clinical assessments. On one side we have shown you, in note form, the main headings to be used in taking a *history* and carrying out a *mental state examination* with special attention to assessments for organic damage. You will most often need this side of the card in the department of psychiatry, although you will find it useful on the general wards as well from time to time. We also give you the abbreviated mental test for the assessment of *cerebral impairment* in elderly patients.

On the other side we have reminded you of some of the common manifestations of *mood disorders* that accompany physical illnesses in the rest of the hospital. We also remind you of the useful screening questions for the detection of alcoholism in patients with medical problems. A further section reminds you of the questions that need to be answered when you make an assessment of *suicidal risk* in the accident room. Get into the habit of using all these questions in your routine clinical work. You will not be sorry.

In case you lose the card, we have reproduced its content at the end of the book.

PART 1

THE CLINICAL APPROACH TO THE PATIENT

2 INTERVIEW TECHNIQUES AND HISTORY-TAKING

A medical interview should allow you to obtain the most accurate possible account of the patient's illness, and the events in the patient's life that are relevant to it, within a reasonably short time. If time is not to be wasted, you must create conditions from the outset so that the patient finds it easy to talk to you. To start with, you must look like a member of the medical staff. On the general wards this is quite easy since you will be wearing a white coat, but in settings like the department of psychiatry or in general practice it is important that you dress in such a way that patients who may be much older than you nevertheless see you as someone from whom help may be sought.

First we will look at how to take a 'long' psychiatric history, which is required for a full and comprehensive assessment. However there are occasions when you will need to know how to carry out a briefer 'focused' history, and this will be covered later in the chapter. For both of these types of assessment you need good interviewing skills, so we will cover not only 'what' to ask but 'how' to approach the interview.

Start by saying who you are, and explaining the purpose of the interview. Show consideration by asking whether it is a convenient time for the patient: it usually will be, but people like to feel that they have been consulted. Let us suppose that you have been asked to see a 29-year-old woman called Angela Cooper who has been referred to the out-patient clinic by her GP because she has been feeling depressed and has had thoughts of harming herself.

> *Good morning, Miss Cooper. My name is Stephen Davies . . . (shake hands) . . . I am a student doctor and I am working with Dr Phillips. He has asked me to see you to ask you about the problems that have brought you up to the clinic. After we have spent some time together, I will be talking to Dr Phillips about what you have told me, then we will both see you again together. Is that all right with you?*

In places where interview rooms are available, you should now lead the way to the room, resisting the temptation to start the interview until you are both seated and the patient is comfortable.

In the medical wards you should establish some privacy by drawing the curtains so that others in the ward will not be able to eavesdrop on what the patient tells you. If you can do anything to make the patient more comfortable – for example, helping an orthopnoeic patient to sit up on his pillows – this also shows consideration, and you will be rewarded by a better history.

You should be aware that communication between yourself and the patient will be affected by the distance between you, and your relative positions. For example, a doctor who stands at the foot of a patient's bed while taking a history is making three mistakes at once: he is too far away, he is face to face, and he is looking down on the patient. You should be sitting about a metre from the patient, on the same level, and sitting in such a way that you can always look at the patient, but he can look away from you without difficulty. In out-patient work this is usually achieved by having the patient sit beside the doctor's desk, while on the wards one draws up a chair beside the bed.

Would you prefer me to call you Miss Cooper or Angela?

*Angela? That's fine. Angela . . . I'm going to have to ask you quite a lot of questions about yourself, but I'd like to **start** by asking you to tell me about the problems that have brought you up to the clinic. I'll need to jot down a few notes while you are talking, but the notes I make are confidential, and will be kept with your other medical notes. Is that okay with you?*

In fact, don't dream of writing down anything yet. Look at your patient and, as you listen to the first few sentences, notice as much as you can about the sick person who is seeking help. There is a great deal to take in, and eventually it will become as automatic as the complex series of actions taken by a driver as he starts a car and drives off into a busy city street. However, at first you will have to break it down into its component parts. We will concentrate on those aspects of the patient's non-verbal behaviour that should alert you to the possibility that he or she is psychologically unwell. These are called **non-verbal cues**.

The **posture** may be dejected, with the patient slumped in his chair; or it may indicate anxiety, with the patient being so tense that either the back of his chair does not take the weight of his body, or as he lies in bed the weight of his head is unsupported by his pillow. Valuable cues are also in the handshake: the warm dry feeling of health contrasting with the cold, clammy feeling of anxious over-arousal. The **voice** also contains valuable information quite apart from what is being said: the monotonous, uninflected sound of depression; the strained, distressed sound of pain and anxiety; the altered pitch of anger; and the whining note of someone who feels he is always left with the dirty end of the stick. The patient may **avoid eye-contact** with you, sometimes because he is distressed and perhaps ambivalent about confiding emotional problems, but sometimes just because he is feeling ill. There may be motor activities that suggest inner tension: either tremor or **restlessness**.

In addition to these non-verbal cues, the patient may mention things that suggest that they have been worried or depressed, or have had unusual experiences: these are of course **verbal cues.**

THE HISTORY OF THE PRESENT CONDITION

This is a clear account of the development of the patient's symptoms starting from the time the patient last felt well until before the time of your assessment (which might, for example, be on admission to hospital, or attendance at an out-patient clinic or GP's surgery). It is up to you to leave out things that are clearly irrelevant, and to arrange symptoms and events into chronological order. All times are given relative to the date of admission to hospital: thus, *'Angela Cooper started to feel depressed about 6 months ago following the break-up of the relationship with her boyfriend'*, rather than *'. . . on 3rd January'* or *'. . . on the day of the World Cup Final'*.

The topics that you should try to cover to obtain a full picture of the history of the present condition are shown in *Box 2.1*. However, you also need to pay attention not only to *what* you ask, but also to the *way* in which you ask about these topics.

Box 2.1 Topics to cover in the history of the present condition

Nature of the problem
Time of onset
Development of problems or symptoms over time
Precipitating factors or possible links with life events
Key events since onset
Alleviating or exacerbating factors
What help has been given or offered
What is the patient's view of what is wrong and what help has been offered so far?
What help would the patient like?

'Probe' questions like 'And what happened after that?' help to emphasize to the patient your interest in a sequential account of her problems.

It encourages the patient to speak in the early minutes of the interview if you utter **facilitations** – these may take the form of noises like *'uh-huh'*, words like *'yes, I see'*, or by repeating what the patient has just said with a different inflection *'you fell down the stairs?'* Sometimes patients start by telling us the most dramatic events, and only gradually tell us about what actually happened to them first. If you think that this is happening, say something like:

> *I need to know the order in which these things happened to you. What was the first thing you noticed that was wrong?*

It becomes apparent that the onset of Angela's emotional distress was probably earlier than she first indicated.

It was actually after my grandmother died. I couldn't stop thinking about her, I felt I'd let her down . . .

After each incident is described, remind her of the same need by saying:

And what happened after that?

Sometimes patients start by pouring out an account of their current social problems without really mentioning medical symptoms at all. If this happens you will need to interrupt quite soon, saying something like:

How did that affect you? or

I'd like to come back to that in a minute. Could you start by telling me about your health (or about how you have been feeling in yourself)?

During the course of giving the history patients will often mention key symptoms about which you will need to know many details. **Pain** is the most obvious example: you will need to know its site, quality, intensity, radiation, things that make it worse, and things that ease it. Sleep disorders, symptoms of anxiety and depression, suicidal thoughts, alcohol and drug use, and unusual or strange experiences such as 'hearing voices' are other examples where there are many questions that need to be answered before you can pass on to the next topic. In your anxiety to leave nothing out, you have perhaps already got into the habit of asking patients many probe questions about each of these areas, but this is not the right way of going about things. It takes too long, and patients who are suggestible often agree to things that they have not actually experienced. Get into the habit of asking **directive questions** about such important topic areas:

You say you developed a pain in your chest. Could you describe it to me?

How have you been sleeping?

The student has indicated to the patient that this is an important area, but phrases his question in such a way that the patient must use her own words to convey her experience, rather than having words put into her mouth. It is often necessary to ask several directive questions.

Patients often use vague phrases to describe their symptoms – such as 'these heads of mine', or 'my dizzy turns' – and when this happens you must try to find out exactly what the patient is experiencing:

Please describe your dizzy turns to me exactly.

and follow this up with any probe questions that are necessary, like 'do they come on at any particular time?', 'how do they start?', can you do anything to influence them?', and so on. This technique is called **clarification**, and you must get into the habit of doing it carefully. Occasionally you will ask **closed questions** that the patient can answer with a simple *'yes'* or *'no'*, but generally only when the patient has told you what he can, but has left out some detail that is potentially important. Specific 'checklist' questions that you need to ask about certain topics, such as symptoms of depression or anxiety, can be introduced using **transition statements** – think of them as a form of professional good manners – the signpost to the patient of a change in the direction of the interview

Angela, you've told me about feeling very low in your spirits – there are a few things that often go along with feeling low, I wonder if I could just ask you a few questions about them . . . how have you been sleeping?

Sometimes you will notice that the patient looks emotionally unwell as she describes her physical symptoms, a **non-verbal cue** suggesting psychological illness. The thing you notice could be any of the cues already mentioned, but in Angela's case, she avoids eye contact, then when she does look up you see that her eyes are red and swollen.

As she mentions the break-up of her relationship, she dabs her eyes with her handkerchief. Instead of politely ignoring this, the student deals with it by drawing attention to it. This in effect gives the patient permission to talk about her feelings:

Angela, I can see you're very upset. Have you found yourself crying a lot?

This procedure is called a **reflection** of the patient's feeling, and it can be used for other feelings as well, such as anger or tension.

Sometimes patients mention their feelings at the same time as they give you important information about a physical symptom. An insensitive interviewer simply picks up the physical symptom and asks further questions about that, never returning to the abnormal mood. Remember to prick up your ears when you hear these **verbal cues** relating to psychological illness. You may well want to finish hearing about the pain first, but remember to come back to the abnormal mood, and ask a **directive question** about it:

You mentioned a moment ago that you've been feeling hopeless and you don't see any point in going on. Could you tell me more about that?

It has been known for some time that some doctors are very good at detecting psychological disorders, while others miss most of these illnesses. The way that you interview the patient will affect the number of both verbal and non-verbal cues that they show you: doctors who hurry the patient, or tend to interrupt the patient, who ask many questions derived from theory, or who ask many 'closed questions', will inhibit the release of these cues; while those who ask questions that follow on from what the patient has just said, who make sympathetic comments when they are appropriate, and who make a habit of asking directive questions, will find that patients are prepared to allow their distress to show.

Your questioning therefore proceeds in a systematic way moving gradually forward in time, so that eventually you arrive at the day of your assessment. This should remind you to carry out a brief **systems review**. In psychiatry some parts of this are particularly important, so be sure you remember to ask for:

1. Changes in **appetite**.
2. Changes in **weight**.
3. Changes in **sleep**.
4. Changes in **sexual feelings**.
5. Changes in **bladder and bowel habit**.
6. Decreased ability to **enjoy oneself**, including **loss of usual interests**.

Sometimes students feel embarrassed asking older people about their sexual feelings. You need not be. The patients aren't embarrassed if you aren't. Everyone knows what sexual feelings are, whether or not they are currently having a sexual relationship with someone. If the patient isn't consulting for a sexual problem, it is usually sufficient just to ask whether there has been any *change* in their sexual feelings recently, in the same part of the interview as you are asking about other functions such as appetite and sleep.

Anyway, when you have completed the 'systems review' questions you should be thoroughly up to date. This should remind you to **recapitulate** the history to the patient. This only takes a few moments, and it is an excellent habit to get into. Patients frequently correct things that (often through no fault of your own) you have got wrong, and they are often reminded to put in something important that they forgot to tell you the first time:

> *Well, Angela, you seem to have been feeling quite well in yourself until the death of your grandmother about 18 months ago. After that you were understandably very upset indeed and in the few months after this the relationship with your boyfriend started to deteriorate. Then, 6 months ago you discovered that he was having an affair and confronted him with this, and he told you that he wanted to finish the relationship, which you did not want. You have been very distressed and upset since then. You blame yourself for the break-up and feel that you should not have got jealous and angry with him for spending time with his own friends occasionally. You had been feeling depressed at times before the break-up but things got much worse afterwards and you have felt low on most days, with difficulty getting to sleep, poor appetite, no interest in your friends or family and loss of half a stone in weight. There have been times when you have felt that life has not been worth living and you recently took an overdose of medication and you were admitted to the general hospital overnight. You still have thoughts of harming yourself but are able to resist them. You have also been drinking a couple of glasses of wine each evening to help you to go to sleep.*

THE FAMILY HISTORY

Now that you have heard the nature of the present illness, you are in a far better position to know how much detail to take about the family history. Not everything is equally important. In Angela's case, for example, we want to know about her early relationship with her own family as this might help us to understand her difficulties in her adult relationships. We want to know if her family are a source of support, or of stress. We also particularly want to find out if there is a history of depression or other mental health problem in the family – particularly substance misuse. These are questions in our minds, but we do not ask them right away. However, they will influence us in the amount of detail that we collect. The family history is a voyage of discovery.

However, before we embark we need to use a transition statement again to let the patient know that we have finished one area, and are about to go on to another:

> *Now that I've heard about your present problems I'd like to go on to ask you a few questions about your family. Could we start with your father? Is he still alive?*

We are aiming to get answers to the following questions about each parent: Age, or age at death and year of death (so that you can work out how old the patient was at the time); occupation; health; whether parent suffered with 'nerves' (if so, details: were they seen by a psychiatrist; did they have any treatment?); what the parent was like; how the patient got on with them.

Go on to siblings. List them in order, showing where the patient comes in the family. If the patient uses first names, use these both in your notes and in questioning the patient, otherwise use the patient's terminology: *'so your older sister was always your mother's favourite, and you found that you never really could please her?'* You are interested in the health of all first-degree relatives, but not of relatives by marriage. The family history should tell us whether any of Angela's first-degree relatives have had mental illnesses, as well as giving us some idea of the sort of family she comes from. Do not ask about the patient's spouse, or partner, or children yet: they come later. It can be helpful to draw a small family tree in your notes at this point (see p. 81).

We started our family history with some hunches about the patient: we should by now have begun to confirm or refute them, and often we now have some new insights: the voyage of discovery can continue . . .

THE PERSONAL HISTORY

At first you will take very full and detailed personal histories, because you won't really know what is relevant and what is not. Don't worry about that, you need the practice, and you will discover some very interesting things about your patients in the process. However, once more, not everything is equally relevant. How a girl received her sex education will have great relevance if the patient is asking for help because she has not been able to consummate her marriage, but it will probably matter very little in a spinster of 75 who is complaining of loss of memory.

Childhood

It is helpful to take the personal history in chronological order, starting from childhood. A patient's mother may be able to tell you what her health was like in the pregnancy that produced your patient, and to give you details of the delivery and age on reaching

17

'milestones': however, information on the same points from the patient is likely to be unreliable. Students often begin their account of the personal histories of their patients with an air of spurious accuracy: *'Angela Cooper was born in Manchester as a full-term, normal delivery. Her milestones were normal, and there were no neurotic traits in childhood . . .'*

Don't do this unless you can obtain information that seems to be reliable. It doesn't matter whether she was born in Manchester or Salford, and she probably doesn't really know whether her delivery was normal or not. Nor does she have much idea whether her motor milestones were normal, and it doesn't matter in the least whether or not an adult patient reports 'neurotic traits' in childhood! Although birth injury and delayed motor milestones are of great medical interest, it is better to say that you have no information than to say that things were normal when they in fact were not. However, if the patient has been told that her birth or early years were abnormal this is certainly worth recording; otherwise confine yourself to facts the patient can actually remember, and that are of interest in understanding disorders in adult life.

So, start the personal history with a transition statement:

> *Now you've told me a bit about your family I'd like to ask a few questions about your early life. Were you ever told anything about your birth?*

Go on to ask:

> *Do you remember your childhood as happy or unhappy?*

Happy childhoods can be passed over quickly, but get details about unhappiness. What was wrong, and how did it affect her? Was she separated from her parents? (If so, for how long, and how did they manage?) In patients with mixtures of physical and psychological symptoms, ask about physical health in childhood, and the attitudes of care-givers to them when physically ill. It is helpful to ask routinely whether or not there were serious physical illnesses in childhood.

School

If you are taking a detailed history start with primary school – how did they get on? What were they good at? Did they make friends? (If not, were they teased; what about?) How did they get on with teachers? Then, pass on to secondary school. The briefest school history will record age of entering and leaving full-time education, and the highest level of education achieved. Make a note of any public examination passed, since this information is especially important in the assessment of possible organic cerebral damage.

Sexual history

Move on to the sexual history by asking female patients about their age at the menarche, and go on to a menstrual history. Ask whether their mother prepared them for their menarche, and whether sexual matters could be discussed at home. Go on from there to ask about boyfriends. You are interested in their capacity to form loving relationships, as well as obtaining a detailed account of any problems encountered in the physical side of sexual relationships.

Ask male patients at what age they learned the facts of life, whether sexual matters could be freely discussed at home, and so on through a similar sequence of questions. Once more, do not confine yourself to an account of the purely physical problems that the patient may describe, but try to assess the patient's capacity to form loving relationships.

Do not ask about homosexual activities unless the patient volunteers information, or unless there is some reason to suspect it and it is relevant to the patient's present problems. If you need to discuss such problems, do so without embarrassment. If anal intercourse has occurred, has the patient been worried about the possibility of AIDS?

If the patient presents with a sexual problem you will of course need to get fuller details than this brief outline suggests: these are given in Chapter 21.

Marital and relationship history

The marital history follows naturally on: once more, happy marriages can be recorded briefly. If the patient has been married more than once obtain a description of the first marriage and how that marriage ended. At what age did they meet their spouse, and get married? What is the age, health and occupation of the spouse? Can they confide in their spouse? Have there been problems? (An example of a problem would be separations, or threatened separations.) If there have been no problems, record this briefly; otherwise obtain a description of the problems. Long-term relationships and partnerships may of course also be established without marriage.

Is the sexual side satisfactory? Ask about children, recording separate notes about each child: age, health, any problems?

Occupational history

The occupational history gives valuable information about the patient's personality, as well as the range of his abilities. What is the patient's current occupation: if none, how long has the unemployment lasted? How many jobs have there been, and how long did the longest one last? Why do changes occur? Promotions and changes forced by circumstance require no explanation, but get someone who is constantly changing jobs to tell you what goes wrong. A list giving exact names of employers and dates is of little value: but this part of the history and the marital history give you some idea of the patient's capacity to form enduring relationships and stick at things, as well as allowing you to judge his strengths.

Present social circumstances

Finish this part of the history by trying to assess the patient's present living circumstances. Who is there at home? How do they get on? What sort of accommodation do they live in?

Forensic history

Whether or not you take such a history depends largely on the patient's presenting problem. They should routinely be taken in patients with drug or alcohol problems.

Start with truancy and problems at school, both with teachers and with other students. Go on to ask if they have ever been in trouble with the police. If they have, be sure to start with the first time, not the most recent! Have they appeared before a court, either juvenile or adult? If so, what was the charge, were they convicted, and what was the sentence?

Previous medical history

If there are important medical, surgical or psychiatric illnesses in the **past history** these should be recorded in the usual way.

Life charts

If there appear to be relationships between life events, physical illnesses and psychiatric illnesses it is very helpful if these are brought together as a **life chart**. An example of Angela Cooper's life chart is shown as *Box 2.2*.

THE PRE-MORBID PERSONALITY

Some personality types are at greater risk than others of developing psychiatric illnesses: for example, people with cyclothymic traits are more likely to develop bipolar disorder, or those with obsessional traits are more likely to experience obsessional symptoms when depressed. This is discussed more fully in Chapter 18 (pp. 276–284).

However, there are two major problems in relying on information from the patient. Unless you're very careful, patients tell you what they are like now, rather than what they used to be like. Also, people cannot tell you things that they don't know themselves, and if they are depressed they will tend to see themselves in a bad light. Always see a relative if you want accurate information. Nonetheless, there are some things that the patient can tell you about himself, and you should start, as usual, with a transition statement:

> *Angela, I want to ask you some questions now about the sort of person that you were before you became ill. Could you remember how you were a year or so ago? Could you start by telling me about your interests?*

Aim to collect information under headings: interests, mood, friendships, habits – including alcohol and drugs.

Age	Year	Life events	Physical illness	Mental illness
		Box 2.2 Example of a life chart for Angela Cooper		
	1978	Born 10.9.78		
1	9			
2	1980			
3	1			
4	2	Started school		
5	3			
6	4			
7	5			
8	6			
9	7			
10	8	Family problems – violence	Appendicectomy	
11	9	Parents divorced		Saw child psychiatrist,
12	1990			nightmares, anxiety
13	1			
14	2			
15	3	Left school – clerical work		
16	4			
17	5	First serious boyfriend		
18	6			
19	7	Relationship ended		
20	8			
21	9			
22	2000	Met future fiancé		
23	1			
24	2			
25	3			
26	4			
27	5	Death of grandmother		
28	6			
29	7	Broke off engagement		Onset of depression
				Started drinking heavily
				Overdose

INTERVIEWS WITH SPECIAL GROUPS

Children and old people

Special points that should be borne in mind with patients at either end of the life cycle are discussed in Part 3: interviews with children on pp. 297–300 and interviews with old people on p. 349.

21

Deaf people

Don't shout at them. Make sure that they can see your mouth, and speak slowly and clearly. Ask them to let you know if they cannot hear any of your questions, as you will be pleased to repeat them. If a particular question is really important, and you are unsure whether the patient really understood it, write it down.

People who do not speak English very well

Often you can manage just by speaking slowly and clearly, and *avoiding long words*. If this does not work, you will need an interpreter: these are usually available, so make proper enquiries. When the interpreter appears and you have introduced yourself, put the patient in the usual chair and address your questions to him or her, *not to the interpreter*. Watch the patient's face as they reply to each question: even if you do not understand a word of their language, you will learn a great deal. Ask the interpreter to tell you exactly what the person has replied to you, and not to summarize this or add their own assessments. It is never good practice to ask a family member to interpret for you.

INTERVIEWING A RELATIVE

Use the same headings when you see a relative, but be sure to include your impression of your informant. Include any anecdotes that are mentioned. You should learn about the patient's capacity to form friendships, as well as patterns of relationship within the family. Look now at the following example:

Ms Angela Cooper
Cleveland Community Mental Health Centre
25 July 2005

Informant: Mother
Mrs Sharon Cooper
s/a as patient

Impression of informant

Mrs Cooper works as a practice nurse in Salford. She seems very concerned about the problems that her daughter has been having, and was in tears at one point during our conversation. She feels guilty, she says, about Angela's problems because of the disrupted childhood that she experienced. She said that their relationship has always been 'up and down' but at the moment they are getting on better and Angela has moved back home, however she has been particularly concerned with how much Angela has been drinking, she thinks it is about half a bottle of wine per night and sometimes more.

Present illness

Little to add to patient's account except that she thought that Angela had really been very depressed since the death of her grandmother and this might have contributed to the problems that she was having in her relationship with her boyfriend. Mrs Cooper described her mother as a 'rather cold person'. Angela had spent a considerable amount of time with her grandmother in childhood because of problems at home and still visited her every day up to her death.

Early life

Angela's father was violent towards her mother and also hit Angela sometimes too, although not causing serious injury. Mrs Cooper divorced him when Angela was 11 and her sister was 13. Angela has always accused her of favouring her sister and protecting her from her father, but she insists this was not the case. Her father used to pick on Angela because she 'answered him back'.

Marital and relationship history

Angela had been with her boyfriend for 5 years. Mrs Cooper says that she liked him very much and that Angela was unreasonable with him at times, preventing him from spending time with his friends. They had been engaged and were living together when they broke up. Angela had one previous serious boyfriend whom Mrs Cooper didn't like because he was 'unreliable'. She couldn't remember exactly how long Angela had been with him for, possibly a couple of years, but they did not move in together. He ended the relationship.

Previous psychiatric history

Angela saw a child psychiatrist at the time of her parent's marital problems. She had nightmares, lost weight and couldn't sleep.

Pre-morbid personality

Always a bit anxious. Worries a lot about problems and does tend to brood on things. Doesn't make friends easily. Enjoys reading, watching TV and going to the cinema. Good at her job as a personal secretary, and proud of her ability to cope with quite a lot of pressure at work.

Stephen Davies
Medical Student

THE BRIEF 'FOCUSED' ASSESSMENT

In many medical settings outside the psychiatric setting, such as in general practice or in the emergency department, you will have much less time to take a history. You therefore also need to practise how to take a briefer, more focused history that covers the essential points and provides you with the necessary information, often to decide whether you need to obtain a fuller assessment (see *Box 2.3*).

Box 2.3 The brief 'focused' history

History of the present condition
Specific key questions (focused history)
Relevant past history
Family history of relevant illness
Current social circumstances
Drugs/alcohol screen

For example, you might have been asked to see Angela in the emergency department on the occasion that she took the overdose of tablets. At this time you would have approached the history of the present condition in a similar way as described above – except that you would be particularly concerned with the *details of the events just prior to her coming to hospital*. You would focus in more detail on getting a clear picture of the episode and her suicidal thoughts and actions – what she has taken, when and why – as well as finding out about her depression and alcohol history, as these are important cues that you would want to clarify further. You would not need (or indeed have time) to take a full family and social history, but you would want to know about relevant past history, and in particular about her current social circumstances: Where is she living? Who with? Is there anyone at home? Even if the question of alcohol and drugs is not raised, you should always consider asking about these as they frequently complicate the presenting condition.

We will specifically address the key questions to ask when you focus on certain topics in psychiatry in the relevant chapters of this book.

3 EXAMINATION OF THE MENTAL STATE

The examination of the mental state is an orderly and systematic procedure like that of the physical examination. It is carried out routinely for each new patient and is repeated, either in whole or in part, on every subsequent occasion that the patient is seen. A summary of the main aspects of the mental state follows this introduction. Each of these aspects is then considered in turn, with a description of the observations that are to be made and the tests that will be carried out, the interpretation of these observations, and their relevance to diagnosis. The division of the mental state into these parts is convenient, but to some extent arbitrary, because they tend to overlap.

The emphasis in this chapter is on the accurate evaluation of the most important symptoms and signs of mental illness. The student is advised to start by learning how to carry out well the tests presented here and how to evaluate the significance of the results. Many other symptoms, particularly those seen in schizophrenia, are described in the chapters on those disorders.

As in other branches of medicine the history of the disorder should suggest the diagnosis, and the examination should help to confirm it. Although an experienced clinician will be able to concentrate on certain aspects of the mental state, the inexperienced student will only learn to carry out the mental state examination rapidly and effectively by keeping to the routine described for each patient examined. The novice can expect to take as long as an hour to carry out the examination in some cases, but by the end of a few weeks should be able to carry out at least an initial examination in about 20 minutes.

A full and accurate account of the mental state should always be recorded in the medical notes, for both clinical and medico-legal purposes. As with all medical records each note must be dated and signed. Observations must be noted separately from opinions. For example:

> *The patient insists that Dr Smith is his father, refers to him as 'Dad' and describes his real father as an imposter when he comes to visit. He cannot be argued out of this belief*

should be recorded, and separately the opinion:

> *(This belief appears to be a delusion)*

The latter might not be the only interpretation of the finding. It might be an overvalued idea, or intentional play-acting. Records that contain only opinions, for example 'The patient is suffering from delusions', are of little value. Another doctor, seeing the patient a few days later, may find no evidence of delusions and will probably decide that the recorded opinion is wrong and based on inexperience if he does not also have available the data on which the opinion was based.

Negative findings are as important as positive findings and should be recorded. For example, the note of orientation in time should specify the patient's replies to questions on the time, day of the week and date, together with the correct answers, rather than the opinion 'Well orientated in time'. Similarly 'Mood normal' is not an acceptable alternative for 'Describes his mood as "contented" and shows appropriate modulation of mood throughout the interview'.

Verbatim accounts by the patient should be recorded if they are particularly illuminating or provide an example of some morbid phenomenon, and should be indicated by using inverted commas. It is especially important to record examples of speech that you consider to be abnormal: once more, a note that reads 'patient's speech grossly thought disordered' is valueless – you must record an actual example. You should also record the context in which the statement is made, or whether it is in response to a question.

Some of the words to be found in this chapter are also used in colloquial English, when they often have a less precise meaning. For example, 'obsession' is a term used generally only to mean a preoccupation, whereas in psychiatry it has a more specific meaning, which is precisely defined, and should only be used in this way. Throughout the following account we shall use technical terms, some of which may be unfamiliar to you. Rather than break up the text each time this occurs, we have gathered these together at the back of the book in a **Glossary**, and have used asterisks to indicate that a Glossary definition is available. Thus, if you come across the word **'akathisia** (*p. 369)' this means that a full account of that term is to be found on page 369.

APPEARANCE AND BEHAVIOUR

General description

The mental state examination should start with a brief description of what the patient looks like, so that another person hearing the account might recognize the patient in a crowded room. Include the physique, clothes, cleanliness, hair, make-up and whether these seem appropriate to the age, sex, cultural group and social class of the patient.

Signs of self-neglect (poor hygiene, stubbly beard, body odour, stained clothes, or loose clothes because of weight loss) occur in many mental illnesses, particularly depressive disorders, dementia and schizophrenia, as well as being a result of poverty.

Always note any evidence of disorders of the **level of consciousness**. Is the patient fully awake and alert, responding normally to stimuli, drowsy or unrousable? Apart from normal tiredness, an impaired state of consciousness is strongly suggestive of an organic cerebral disorder, particularly delirium, but inattention also commonly occurs in affective disorders. Tests of orientation (see p. 37) may help to differentiate these.

Reaction to interviewer

The manner of the patient towards the interviewer should be described next. Is he friendly, cooperative, complaining, suspicious, or critical? Students tend to assume either that they themselves are at fault when occasionally a patient refuses to cooperate, or alternatively that the patient is being 'difficult'. However, this is an important part of the patient's mental state and provides some indication of how the patient relates to others at the present time. One must then consider whether such behaviour is the patient's reaction to an unfamiliar and stressful experience, is a symptom of illness, or is an indication of personality problems.

Motor activity

This is sometimes referred to as 'psychomotor activity'. Included here are the facial expression, posture and gait. Note particularly the speed of movement, the quantity and the presence of abnormal movements. Is there any evidence of repetitive, apparently purposeless or involuntary movements?

There may be *too little* movement. Distinguish between **akinesis** (*p. 369), in which there are reduced voluntary movements especially affecting the face, and **retardation** (*p. 373), in which all movements are slowed. Loss of **volition** is where the patient generally doesn't have much 'go' in him, and **stupor** (*p. 373) is when the patient does not move at all, although fully conscious.

There may be *too much* movement. Distinguish between a generally increased level called **over-activity** (*p. 372), or an anguished, driven restlessness that leads to **agitation** (*p. 369). **Akathisia** (*p. 369) is a state of restlessness and over-activity produced by neuroleptic drugs. Ask yourself whether any increased level of activity is associated with **disinhibition**.

There may be **involuntary movements**. Some of these are of special interest to psychiatrists. You are probably already familiar with **tics** (*p. 374), and will have seen **choreic** movements on the neurological wards. The movements of **acute dystonia** (*p. 369) are painful spasms, and **tardive dyskinesia** (*p. 373) refers to a wide variety of repetitive and distressing movements, both brought on by neuroleptic drugs.

DISORDERS OF TALKING AND THINKING

Knowledge of another person's thoughts is only available through speech or some other form of communication, such as writing or gesture. Talking and thinking are closely related, in that thought usually precedes speech; however, thoughts may remain unspoken. We therefore consider talking and thinking together.

Students often have some difficulty in understanding the essential difference between the form and the content of talk. Briefly the **form** is how we talk, while the **content** is what we say. For example, we may talk quickly in a disjointed manner (the form), but this gives no indication of whether we are talking about the weather or our next meal (the content).

The speed of talk

The speed of talk varies greatly from one person to another, so that a moderately fast or slow rate of talk cannot be assumed to be morbid. Extremes of speed may be associated with changes in volume and also in the quantity of speech.

RETARDATION OF SPEECH

Retardation of speech (*p. 373) refers to a delay in starting to speak as well as to the rate of speech.

MUTISM

Mutism (*p. 371) is total absence of speech. **Elective mutism** (see p. 309) is characterized by mutism that occurs in some settings but not in others.

Changes in the amount of speech occur in depression and mania. A reduction in talk may sometimes be seen in dementia, where patients may say very little; alternatively, they may talk a great deal but communicate little.

PRESSURE OF SPEECH

Pressure of speech (*p. 372) describes a rapid outpouring of ideas that is often difficult to interrupt.

Continuity of talk

Note whether talk is hesitant, with longer than usual interruptions for thought, and whether it is coherent and relevant to the current conversation. Remember that this should be judged more by what is relevant to the patient, who may be preoccupied with a crisis in his life, than by what is relevant to you the interviewer. Hesitancy in speech is a common feature in those who are anxious or depressed, indecisive, or preoccupied with worries. Deafness, often unsuspected, is also a common impediment to the free flow of conversation.

Does the patient use words of his own making (**neologisms**: for example, 'my mind is *spired*') or strange grammatical constructions?

Does talk **follow a sequence** in which consecutive ideas follow logically, working towards an identifiable goal, or is it circumstantial, tangential or over-inclusive? If any disorder is possibly present, record verbatim samples of speech to illustrate this, together with the question that you asked beforehand:

How long have you been in hospital?

I came in last Wednesday: that was a fine day for mushrooms. Do you like omelettes?

The patient may talk circumstantially, or he may wander from one subject to another, apparently with little purpose other than social contact. This must be differentiated from a breakdown of normal associations of ideas, in which talk apparently attempts, but fails, to follow a logical sequence.

Schizophrenic thought disorder

In **schizophrenic thought disorder** the logical sequence of ideas may break down so that consecutive sentences are unconnected; a single sentence may contain two unrelated elements:

> I want to go home because this hospital is nearer to the shops than the last one.

Here there is an apparent attempt to provide an explanation in the second half of the sentence for the wish expressed in the first half, yet there is no real explanation, and the two ideas appear to be disconnected. Always ask the patient to explain the association between ideas if you are unable to discern a meaningful connection. This may result in an even greater breakdown in logical thinking or a logical explanation that was not initially evident. Asked to explain the previous statement, the patient may say:

> Shops frighten me and if I stay here I may be expected to go to the shops. I wouldn't mind going to the other hospital.

This now begins to make sense. Alternatively, he may say:

> I mean I want to go home because it's near the shops and the shops are near the hospital.

This makes even less sense than previously. In extreme disorder there may be a jumble of unrelated words (**word salad**).

Flight of ideas

Flight of ideas describes the way in which the speech of manic patients may move rapidly from one subject to another, usually with some discernible association, which may be rather flimsy. For example:

> I don't like this place. It's really rather boring. The patients keep snoring. It's just a great yawn: I'd rather have soft porn. Are you a softie, doc?

Here the ideas are associated and there is a return at the end to the initial theme. Such 'flight' is usually associated with pressure of speech, unlike schizophrenic thought disorder. However, the form of the disorders of thinking and speech in schizophrenia and mania may be so similar in practice as to defy differentiation.

If the patient suddenly seems to go blank during your examination the most likely explanation is just that he is anxious, but consider the possibility of **thought block** (*p. 373) and ask him what was happening during the pause. Another possibility is **epileptic absence attacks** (see pp. 152–153)

Perseveration

Perseveration is the repetition of a response when it is no longer appropriate. For example:

> *What day is it today?*
> *Monday. (Correct)*
> *Which day did you come into hospital?*
> *Monday.*
> *What is the name of the ward?*
> *Monday*

Verbal perseveration is often associated with motor perseveration: 'Hold up your left hand.' The patient does so. 'Hold up your right hand.' The patient again raises his left hand. Perseveration is usually an indication of organic brain disease.

DISORDERS OF MOOD

The examination of mood has four main components: subjective mood, objective observation, autonomic activity and thought content. The last of these is considered further in the next section.

Subjective mood

Always ask first about the patient's subjective mood state with an open-ended question:

> *How have you been feeling recently?* or

> *How have you been in your spirits?*

If the response is non-committal, follow up with:

> *Have you been feeling mainly happy or sad?*

If the reply indicates sadness, ask:

> *How sad? Can you snap out of it?*

30

If the patient describes depressed mood, always remember to ask:

What do you find yourself thinking about when you feel like that?
How do you feel about the future?
Do you ever feel completely hopeless?
(If 'yes' to previous question:)
As though life isn't worth living?
(If 'yes', continue with questions about suicide, see pp. 49–53)

Objective observation of mood

Moods of sadness, anxiety or happiness are conveyed through facial expression, posture and motility. 'Normal' mood modulates frequently, depending on the thoughts and experiences of the individual.

There are two separate points to note:

1. What is the predominant mood during the course of the interview?
2. To what extent does the mood fluctuate, are fluctuations appropriate, and in what direction are these fluctuations?

Occasionally patients deny unpleasant mood states, such as depression, perplexity or suspicion, although there may be ample alternative evidence to show this is present. In particular there may be a deliberate attempt to conceal depression by refusing to answer questions, and this should alert the interviewer to the risk of suicide.

Sadness is a feature of depressed mood, but it is not of course in itself indicative of mental illness. **Weeping** is commonly associated with sadness, although it may merely be a way of releasing pent-up tension.

In less severe depressive states the mood may improve when the patient is distracted by amusing incidents, that is to say the mood reacts to the circumstances (this is the proper meaning of '**reactive depression**'). In more severe depressive states weeping is less common, and there tends to be a more constant melancholic mood, lacking normal modulation, which may easily be mistaken for **affective blunting** (see below). The patient may describe the experience of an inability to have feelings or to care about others, such as family members or friends.

Smiles and laughter are associated with cheerfulness and **euphoria**, in which case they usually have an 'infectious' quality. However, they can also be produced in the unhappy as an indication of irony or of social expectation, when they fail to convey real enjoyment. The manic patient is not always cheerful: he will often display irritability and impatience if frustrated by those trying to limit his activities. **Irritability** is commonly seen in all affective illnesses.

The patient may display **labile mood** (*p. 371), in that he has little control of emotion. Less commonly, you may notice examples of inappropriate or **incongruous affect** (*p. 371), or he may display **blunting of affect** (*p. 370), in that the capacity to experience emotion seems to have been lost.

Autonomic activity

Affective changes are accompanied by fluctuations in autonomic activity. You may have noticed a cold, sweaty palm as you shook hands with the patient.

Increased arousal is characterized by sweating, palpitation, dry mouth, hyperventilation, frequency of micturition which may be evident during mental state examination, while raised diastolic and systolic blood pressure, tachycardia and increased gastrointestinal motility may be found on physical examination. High arousal commonly occurs in all psychiatric disorders associated with anxiety, including anxiety states, depressive illness and both acute and chronic schizophrenia.

THOUGHT CONTENT

The content of thinking is evident primarily through the patient's talk, but also through aspects of behaviour. In this respect 'actions speak louder than words'. For example, the patient may deny that he is suspicious of others, but opens the office door to see if anyone is listening outside.

Preoccupations

Themes that are predominant in a patient's thought content are likely to be revealed in his spontaneous speech. Note any topics to which he may return repeatedly during the course of the interview and the difficulty that you encounter in trying to steer him from these subjects back to other aspects of the history and mental state examination. If preoccupations are not evident, ask:

What are your main worries? or

Do you have some thoughts that you just don't seem to be able to get out of your head?

Many people have preoccupations, but these are appropriate to the circumstances. For example, it is appropriate for a patient about to undergo major surgery to be preoccupied with the possible hazards, the likely outcome, the provision for dependants, and so on, even though there may be encouragement from others to keep these thoughts to himself. However, some preoccupations are morbid, and their content may be important in understanding the diagnosis of the disorder:

Ruminations are repetitive ideas and themes, usually having an unpleasant content, on which the patient may brood for prolonged periods. They commonly occur in anxiety states and depressive illnesses, when their content reflects the **affective state**: for example, they may include ideas of guilt, low self-esteem or hypochondriasis. These should be differentiated from delusions (see below) in which the content may be the same but the form is different. Ruminations also occur in **obsessional states** (p. 271, *p. 371), in which case they reflect the state of indecision.

Suicidal ideas are of special importance, because of the risk to the patient's life. A patient who has said that life is not worth living should be asked:

Have you ever thought of ending your life?
Have you planned what you will do?
Do you intend to carry it through?

Perhaps surprisingly most patients answer such questions honestly, but be particularly wary of the patient who avoids answering. Although commonest in depressive illness, suicidal ideas are by no means limited to that disorder.

Abnormal beliefs

Ideas that are shared by many people within a particular cultural or ethnic group may seem strange to others; for example, particular religious beliefs and practices. Individuals too may have ideas that seem idiosyncratic or eccentric, but are not necessarily symptomatic of mental illness.

Overvalued ideas are beliefs that are strongly held about matters that are of special importance and preoccupy the subject. They are not delusions, because they lack the quality of unshakeable conviction. For example, a patient with anorexia nervosa may develop the characteristic belief that they are fat although they know that they are grossly underweight; indeed, they would regard others of the same weight as dangerously thin. Overvalued ideas are not necessarily indicative of illness.

Delusions are mistaken beliefs that are held with conviction, that are not shared by others of the same cultural or social background and intellect, and that persist despite all the evidence to the contrary. For example, a patient insists that there are men plotting to kill him, hidden in the hospital grounds behind the shrubs and trees. The doctor takes him round the grounds and they look carefully in potential hiding places. Eventually they return to the ward, and the doctor points out that there was no one there.

'Of course not,' says the patient, 'they knew we were going to look for them and they left, but I know that they're back in the grounds now.'

Primary delusions are not secondary to other morbid processes such as abnormal moods or hallucinations. However, they may be prompted by non-morbid processes. For example, a patient may see three clouds in the sky (a normal perception) and realizes that these are a personal message to him from God telling him that he is a member of the Holy Trinity. Primary delusions are generally associated with schizophrenia provided that they occur only in a setting of clear consciousness. There are several kinds of primary delusion, but of particular importance is the **delusional perception**, of which an example is presented above. Here the perception is normal, but it is given delusional significance.

Secondary delusions are secondary to some other morbid process. For example, a patient wrongly believes he is being persecuted by his neighbours. This belief may be secondary to an abnormal mood state of depression in which he believes he is guilty and worthy of punishment; or secondary to voices that he identifies as belonging to the neighbours, saying 'Kill him'. Secondary delusions occur in many different disorders, but their content may be related to the diagnosis. For example, delusions about having disease or dying are usually associated with depressed mood, while grandiose delusions are more likely to occur in mania.

The possible presence of delusions usually becomes evident whilst taking the history. For example, the patient with delusions of persecution may tell you about the way others are acting against him, and his efforts to stop them by complaining to the police or consulting solicitors, or he may appear suspicious in the course of an interview.

Do not ask about delusions routinely; only when other aspects of the history or mental state indicate that they might be present. Then ask:

> *Do you think that others are trying to harm you?*
> *Do you ever feel guilty, or to blame?*
> *Do you think that your body has changed in any way?*
> *Do you think that you have been specially chosen, or have special powers?*

If the patient agrees to any of this, detailed questioning will be necessary to discover whether such ideas, if present, satisfy the criteria of delusions. Is there evidence supporting the patient's views? Do others share his views and encourage him in them? Are his beliefs shakeable?

Delusions occur in many different mental illnesses, in fact all those commonly labelled as **psychoses**, where there are alterations in the patient's perception of reality. Persecutory and hypochondriacal delusions occur in many disorders and are of little help with diagnosis.

PERCEPTION

Most of the time we are aware of our own thoughts, our bodies and the world around us only to a limited degree, but we can focus our attention on each of these, and they have qualities and order that we recognize and take for granted. This sense of familiarity may be morbidly disrupted. Disturbances may occur in each of the modalities of our perception of ourselves and the outside world.

It is not necessary to ask every patient detailed questions about disorders of perception but it is useful to ask most patients a few 'screening' questions and to pursue these more vigorously if indicated by the history or mental state examination.

> *Have you noticed any changes in yourself or your surroundings that you can't account for?*
> *Have you heard voices of people that you couldn't see?*

The patient may have an unpleasant feeling that although his environment is the same, he or his body has changed – this is suggestive of **depersonalization** (*p. 370) Alternatively he may feel that although he is the same, the surrounding environment has altered in some way – this suggests **derealization**.

Depersonalization and derealization do not necessarily indicate morbidity, but occur commonly in states of fatigue and high arousal, particularly in association with anxiety and depression; and less often in schizophrenia, epilepsy and drug-induced states.

Illusions

Illusions are misinterpretations of external stimuli. They may affect each of the sensory modalities. Commonest are auditory illusions, in which the patient misinterprets what is heard, and visual illusions, in which there is a misinterpretation of visual stimuli. Illusions are not necessarily morbid, and most people are familiar with 'optical illusions' or with the tendency to 'hear' footsteps following them when walking alone in the dark. Emotional states, such as anxiety, often result in such misinterpretation.

Probably the commonest pathological cause of illusions is sensory deficit, as in partial blindness or deafness, and a similar effect may result from diminished sensory input, such as the effect of darkness. Lowering of the state of consciousness has similar effects, and illusions are particularly liable to occur in delirium. In this state it is common for the movement of shadows to be misinterpreted as, for example, the movement of dangerous animals, or the movement of bedclothes against the skin may be misinterpreted as the movement of insects. Not surprisingly, patients experiencing such illusions often appear terrified.

Hallucinations

Hallucinations are perceptions that are not based on external stimuli. For example, a voice is heard talking, but no one is there speaking, and others present hear nothing. Like illusions, hallucinations can occur in any modality of perception, but auditory hallucinations are by far the commonest.

AUDITORY HALLUCINATIONS

Ask:

Do you ever hear voices when there is no one there, or no one is talking?

If 'yes':

Are these real voices, coming from outside your head, or your own thoughts inside your head?
Do you ever hear your own thoughts, spoken aloud, outside your head?

Also ask about the content of the voices:

What do the voices say?
Give me an example of what you heard today, or yesterday.

Always record verbatim accounts of the patient's experiences, including the content of the hallucinations.

Auditory hallucinations can occur in many disorders, including schizophrenia, organic brain syndromes and serious mood disorders and their content tends to be related to the nature of the disorder. For example in manic states they may be grandiose, such as a voice telling the patient that he has special powers; whereas in depressive disorders they are likely to be abusive and consistent with the state of low self-esteem. Features suggestive of schizophrenia are described on pages 186–188.

VISUAL HALLUCINATIONS

Visual hallucinations are uncommon and most likely to occur in acute organic states (e.g. intoxication with drugs such as amphetamines, or other delirious states), although they occur occasionally in schizophrenia and in affective disorders. Disorganized visual hallucinations (lacking normal form) may result from occipital lobe disease.

OTHER HALLUCINATIONS

Olfactory and gustatory hallucinations may occur as symptoms of temporal lobe disease, for example in complex partial seizures. **Tactile and somatic hallucinations**, that is, perceptions arising from the body surface or internally, are described, but are difficult to differentiate from illusions. All of these occasionally occur in schizophrenia.

Hallucinations occur commonly during dreams, and also in the twilight state between waking and sleeping (**hypnagogic hallucinations**), in which case they have no morbid significance. Simple hallucinations – that is to say, bangs or flashes of light – may occur in conditions of extreme fatigue. You should therefore always ask about the circumstances in which hallucinations are experienced:

Was it during the day or at night?
Were you in bed with the lights out?
Were you awake or dozing?

It is sometimes difficult to differentiate between an illusion and a hallucination. If, for example, a patient says he heard a voice saying 'You have been specially chosen', ask:

Where did the voice come from?
Was anyone else present at the time?
Were they speaking?

Pseudohallucinations lack the qualities of vividness and reality that are possessed by normal perceptions and by hallucinations: they have an 'as if' quality, and they are experienced in inner subjective space. Thus a voice is heard inside one's head, or a vision is seen as if by an 'inner eye'. Ask:

Did it sound just the same as a real voice, like listening to my voice now?

Pseudohallucinations, like illusions, have little diagnostic specificity. They may occur in any mental illness, and also in those who are not mentally ill, particularly those who are highly imaginative or of dull intellect. Failure to discriminate between pseudohallucinations and hallucinations sometimes results in a patient being wrongly regarded as psychotic.

INTELLECTUAL FUNCTIONS

These tests should be used for most patients seen in the department of psychiatry and in particular should be carried out whenever there is a possibility that a patient is suffering from an organic brain syndrome. The tests described must be presented accurately if the results are to have any value. You should start by explaining what you are going to do, and why.

Now I am going to ask you some other questions to find out how well you are keeping up with things. It's important that you try to do your best even if you find them very easy or very difficult.

Record correct and incorrect answers. Also note the patient's attitude to the tests. Is he really trying? Is he *unable to cooperate* because he is very anxious, or very depressed? Does he lose patience or refuse to attempt them, for example on the grounds that they are too trivial? When interpreting the results remember that to some extent they are affected by both intelligence and education, and the history of education and occupation should, therefore, be taken into account when trying to decide the significance of difficulties that are encountered.

Orientation

Orientation in time and place should be examined first. Ask:

What day of the week is it today?
Without looking at your watch, about what time is it now?
Can you tell me the date and the year?
What is the name of this place?

If these are inaccurate ask more detailed questions:

What sort of place is it?
What town are we in?
How would you get here from your home?
What is your name?
Who am I?

If the patient is unable to do any of these, ask:

>*Is it daytime or night time?*
>*Is it nearer to 9.00 a.m. or midday?*
>*Would you say it's Monday or Tuesday today?*
>*The beginning or end of the month?*

All patients should be able to answer the questions about identity correctly. They should also know they are in hospital and its name. They should have an accurate knowledge of the day of the week and of the time of day to within about one hour. Record verbatim replies to your questions together with the correct answers (in brackets).

Note any other observations suggesting disorientation. For example, the patient may have difficulty finding his way about a hospital ward several days after arrival, or he may get into the wrong bed.

Disorientation is the cardinal sign of clouding of consciousness, which is a feature of delirium. This may be accompanied by a diminished awareness and grasp of the surroundings, and attention is also likely to be impaired. Delirious patients may be unaware of the time of day, the nature of the place, or of the function of people around them. However, inaccurate replies to questions about orientation may also be a result of poor memory (in dementia), or of a narrowed range of interest in the affective disorders.

Attention and concentration

Defects in attention and concentration will usually be evident while the history is being taken. It may be difficult to attract the patient's attention, or once attracted it may be poorly sustained. The patient may be distracted by events in the environment that would usually be ignored during a medical consultation, such as birds singing in the garden or a book on the table, and attention may flit rapidly from one object to the next. Attention may be diverted by experiences not shared by the interviewer, such as voices to which the patient listens. Specific tests of attention are based on the ability to keep track of sequences of material that is familiar to the patient and does not, therefore, require new learning.

Allow the patient as much time as he needs to complete each test, but note unobtrusively how long the patient takes and record this:

>*Tell me the days of the week backwards, starting with Saturday.*
>*Tell me the months of the year backwards, starting with December.*

As usual, record the patient's replies verbatim and the length of time taken for each task. Unimpaired subjects should be able to complete these rapidly, without mistakes:

>*Starting with one hundred, subtract seven and then continue to subtract sevens as far as you can.*

If the patient does not understand the task, ask:

What's seven from one hundred?
And seven from ninety-three?

Carry on like this until he's got the idea. If the patient still does not understand, or says it is too difficult, ask him to subtract threes from twenty.

Performance here is more dependent on educational and intellectual attainment than in the previous tests, and results must, therefore, be interpreted in the light of the history of schooling and employment. Disorders of attention are common and can occur in almost any psychiatric disorder, particularly organic states and affective disorders.

(Patients who show definite evidence of impaired attention on these tests will usually be unable to attend to the following tests of memory, in which case they will not provide any additional information and need not be carried out.)

Registration and short-term memory

The patient can be asked what tests the examiner has carried out, or to say what they have been talking about in the interview so far.

DIGIT SPAN

This is a test of registration and immediate recall. Start by explaining:

I am going to give you some numbers to remember. When I stop I want you to repeat them to me. For example, if I say '2 4 7', you would repeat '2 4 7'.

Give a series of three digits, at an even speed of about one per second, and avoid laying emphasis on some more than others. Ask the patient to repeat them immediately.

If he is correct, give four digits, using a new sequence, then five, and so on, until the patient makes a mistake, say at seven digits.

Finally note the maximum number of digits that can be correctly repeated in sequence. Most unimpaired adults of average intelligence can manage seven digits forwards. Five or less is strongly suggestive of impairment.

STANFORD-BINET SENTENCE

This is a test of registration and immediate recall, which makes allowance for intelligence. Explain:

I am going to ask you to remember a sentence. Listen carefully and then repeat the sentence as accurately as possible.

One of the following sentences should then be read out slowly. Select the one best suited to the patient's probable intellect. Then immediately ask him to repeat it. If he makes a mistake, try an easier sentence. If his repetition is accurate, try a more difficult sentence. Only read out a sentence once, slowly and clearly. Then record the response verbatim.

Sentence to be given to adults of dull intellect (completed successfully by 50 per cent of 11-year-olds):

Yesterday we went for a ride in our car along the road that crosses the bridge.

For dull average adults (50 per cent of 13-year olds):

The aeroplane made a careful landing in the space that had been prepared for it.

For adults of average intellect:

The red-headed woodpeckers made a terrible fuss as they tried to drive the young away from the nest.

For adults of superior intelligence:

At the end of the week the newspapers published a complete account of the experiences of the great explorer.

NAME, ADDRESS AND FLOWER

This tests registration, immediate recall, and short-term memory. Explain:

I am going to give you the name and address of an imaginary person, and the name of a flower that he likes. It is a routine test of your memory which we give everyone. I want you to try to remember it and repeat it back to me as soon as I have finished. The name is:
Mr William Thompson
118 Hamilton Terrace
Chorlton
Manchester 13
The flower is a daffodil
Now please repeat that back to me.

Record both the name and address that you give the patient and his immediate response. Note that there are nine items to be remembered, apart from 'Mr'. In selecting a name and address avoid very common names, such as John Smith, or local addresses that are familiar to the patient. If the patient makes a mistake, read back the same name and address as before and ask him to repeat it. Continue until he is entirely accurate, noting the number of trials required. When the patient is entirely correct, say:

I want you to try to remember that name and address and I will ask you again later on.

Then continue with other tests, for example remote memory. After 2 minutes ask the patient to repeat the name and address. This time do not correct any mistakes. After a further 3 minutes again ask for a repetition. Record the responses each time. Was there evidence of poor registration? Once the material has been correctly registered, is there accurate recall? If mistakes are made, are they the same on each occasion, or is performance worse after 5 minutes than after 2?

If the same test is used on subsequent occasions, use different names and addresses each time, of similar length and complexity to the example provided. Most people are able to repeat the name and address without mistakes immediately and after 5 minutes. Three mistakes or more at 5 minutes are strongly suggestive of a clinically significant deficit.

Longer term memory

Recent memory can be tested by asking about personal experiences in the last few days: if possible ask questions to which the correct answers can be verified. For example, ask:

How long have you been in hospital?
Who brought you here?
Can you tell me which tests we have been doing since I came in to see you?

Test remote memory by asking about personal experiences, for example:

Can you tell me the name of your last school?
And the name of the headteacher?
What was the date when you got married?

Past general events, for example the dates of the Second World War or the names of the last five prime ministers, are concerned with general knowledge rather than long-term memory, and answers depend on intelligence and education as well as memory. Thus, poor performance can be a result of poor education as well as dull intellect or organic brain disease:

Can you tell me the names of five cities in England?
And five sorts of fruit?

What is the name of the prime minister?
And the one before that?

Evidence of difficulty with longer term memory often comes to light during the process of taking the history. For example the patient may show major contradictions in his age, the year of his retirement, or when his wife died.

Defects in short-term memory alone, as revealed by the above tests, are actually defects of new learning. Memory of events prior to the onset of brain disease remains intact, but there is a disorder in the registration and retention of new experiences.

Defects in longer term memory may involve **retrograde amnesia**, that is, the loss of memories of events experienced before the onset of brain disease.

Patients with dementia often have difficulty with short-term memory, but appear to have remarkably good memory for the details of early life. However, beware of **confabulation** – the invention of replies to questions to hide poor memory. As dementia progresses, eventually even long-term memory deteriorates.

INTELLIGENCE

An impression of the patient's level of intelligence will be gained during the course of history-taking, from the extent of the vocabulary used, the complexity of the concepts expressed and from the Stanford-Binet sentence remembered correctly. If these appear to be consistent with the patient's known history of education and employment, and if there is no evidence of impairment in tests of memory, then tests of intelligence are unlikely to be helpful.

Possible **mental retardation** may be assessed by simple tests of comprehension, such as:

> *What is three times nine?*
> *Sixteen divided by four?*
> *What is the difference between a fence and a wall?*
> *If a flag is being blown towards the west, from which direction is the wind coming?*

Illiteracy may be a serious handicap, which patients often fail to mention and may not be suspected. If in doubt, ask:

> *Did you learn to read and write at school?*
> *Would you mind reading to me from this newspaper?*

Abstraction

Tests of abstraction can be helpful in eliciting thought disorder, and should be given only if this is suspected. Ask the patient to explain the meaning of one or two **proverbs**. Start by giving an example:

> *Proverbs are sayings which have general meanings. For example, 'Too many cooks spoil the broth' means 'If too many people do the same job it is likely to go wrong'. Have you heard people say 'Make hay while the sun shines'?*
> *(If yes) Could you tell me what it means?*

Record the reply and if it is satisfactory ask a more difficult proverb:

Now tell me the meaning of 'People who live in glass houses shouldn't throw stones'.

Consider the extent to which the patient's answer shows thought disorder (which may indicate schizophrenia) on the one hand, or concrete thinking (suggestive of organic damage or dull intellect) on the other.

INSIGHT AND JUDGEMENT

An understanding of the presence and nature of mental illness and of its causes is never complete and is rarely totally absent, therefore avoid generalizations, such as 'good insight' or 'bad insight'. The patient's insight may be indicated at different stages through the history and examination. The following are all quite common:

There's nothing wrong with me. I'm not ill. It's my doctor who wanted me to see you.
My wife's the one who needs to see you.
I just need some stronger sleeping pills.

Sometimes a patient's statements about insight appear to contradict his non-verbal behaviour. For example, he may insist that he is not mentally ill, but agrees voluntarily to admission to a psychiatric unit and to take medication for mental illness. So, ask:

Do you think you are ill?
What sort of illness do you think you have?
Do you think it might be a nervous or mental illness?

To what extent does he correctly identify the relevance of his symptoms? For example, does he recognize that feelings of guilt and suicidal thoughts are a result of depressive illness from which he may recover? Does he regard his auditory hallucinations as abnormal experiences, indicative of mental illness and requiring treatment; or as a normal experience, shared by others and not requiring medical attention?

Further questions may be needed to find out the patient's views about the cause of his illness and the appropriate treatment:

What do you think might have caused this illness?
Has anything happened to upset you?
What sort of help do you think you need now?

How realistic are the patient's views?

The assessment of insight has important implications for management. A patient who does not recognize that his suicidal thoughts are symptomatic of a treatable illness with good prognosis is more likely to act on such thoughts and, therefore, will require closer observation, possibly as an in-patient. The patient with persecutory delusions who is unaware that his fears are a result of illness is more likely to defend himself by attacking others. A patient who shares the doctor's opinion of appropriate management is more likely to be compliant, for example either by taking medication or involving himself in psychotherapy. Insight has, therefore, an important bearing on prognosis (see Chapter 9).

INTERVIEWER'S REACTION TO PATIENT

What is your own subjective response to the patient? Did you enjoy meeting the patient, or did he make you feel sad, frustrated or angry? Was it easy or difficult to control the interview in order to obtain necessary information? Ask yourself what happened in the interview that caused you to feel this way. Your responses indicate something about you, as well as about the patient, and your relationship with each other. Is the patient a passive, dependent person, who induces in you frustration as much as sympathy; an aggressive, bombastic or egocentric person, who took over the interview, prevented you from obtaining essential information and left you feeling inadequate and angry; or one who makes frequent statements about how others, particularly doctors, have let him down and, therefore, induces feelings of guilt?

If you found some difficulty in developing a working relationship with the patient, consider to what extent this is determined by the patient's behaviour and whether this is symptomatic of his present illness. Alternatively, have you elicited evidence of life-long difficulties the patient has had in his relationships with family, workmates or others? It is likely that your own reaction to the patient is similar to the reactions of others and may tell you much about the patient's personality.

EXAMPLE OF A MENTAL STATE EXAMINATION

Appearance and behaviour

Angela Cooper is a rather thin young woman dressed in jeans and a stained T-shirt. She has a tattoo on her right upper arm. On introduction she refused to shake hands and at first avoided eye contact but later in the interview her eye contact improved and we were able to establish a rapport. She maintained the same tense upright posture throughout the interview and on occasions rocked slightly backwards and forwards in her chair. She became very tearful at times during the interview particularly when talking about the end of the relationship with her boyfriend and the death of her grandmother.

Speech

Talk is slow with slight delay before replying to questions and there is little spontaneous speech except about her physical health. However her answers are coherent and to the point, and there is no evidence of formal thought disorder.

Mood

She describes her mood as 'very down'. Appears sad but also very tense through most of the interview, weeps when talking about her ex-boyfriend. Describes frequent thoughts that life is not worth living but no specific plans. 'I don't know what I would do it didn't work last time, I can't even do that properly.' At the moment feels able to resist these thoughts.

Thought content

Very preoccupied with how the relationship with her boyfriend ended. Blames herself for being very jealous of him spending time with his friends. 'I drove him away – it's all my fault, I'm just a stupid useless bitch.' Worried about the impact that all her problems are having on her mother and feels very guilty too about that. 'I'm no use to anyone.'

Perception

Angela admits on direct questioning that she has heard a voice telling her to harm herself. 'Just go on and do it, get it over with.' She has heard this two or three times. Most recently the night before coming up to the hospital. It was very frightening. She thought it sounded like the voice of her father. (These seem to have been auditory hallucinations.) There are no other disorders of perception.

Orientation

'Thursday, about ten o'clock, November 2006; I'm not sure, is it the 26th?'
(All correct except 28th November)
'In the Meadowbrook Unit, Hope Hospital Salford.' (correct)

Attention and concentration

Generally attentive during the interview except when preoccupied with recent events.

'Saturday, Friday, Thursday, Wednesday, Tuesday, Monday, Sunday.'
(Slow and hesitant in 25 seconds)

'December, November, October, September . . . September, August, July March . . . no, where was I? I'm sorry.'
(40 seconds)

'100, 93, 86, 80, 73, 65, 60, did you say seven from a hundred? 60, 50, no 53, 45, no, I'm sorry.'
(4 mistakes; 2 minutes 10 seconds)

'20, 17, 14, 11, 9, 7, 5 . . . no, that's not right is it?'
(25 seconds)

Registration and short-term memory

Not tested in view of obvious problems with attention

Long-term memory

Gives detailed and consistent account of early life.
Cities: Manchester, London, Birmingham, Liverpool, Chester, Southampton.
Knows the name of the prime minister and the president of the USA but cannot remember their predecessors.
Dates of world wars 1915–1919, 1939–1945.

Intelligence

Probably average in view of school to age of 16 and semi-skilled work; consistent with present use of vocabulary.

Insight

'I suppose there's something wrong with me. I don't know what it is. The doctor says its depression, but I don't agree with that. This is just the way I am. I don't want tablets.'

Box 3.1 gives a summary of the mental state examination.

FURTHER READING

Casey, P. and Kelly, B. (2007) *Fish's Clinical Psychopathology: Signs and Symptoms in Psychiatry*, 3rd edition. London: Gaskell.
Sims, A. (2002) *Symptoms in the Mind: An Introduction to Descriptive Psychopathology*, 3rd edition. London: W.B. Saunders.

Box 3.1 Summary of the mental state examination

1. **Appearance and behaviour**
   Description; reaction to interviewer; motor activity
2. **Speech**
   Speed; quantity; continuity; relevance
3. **Mood**
   Subjective account; observed mood; autonomic reactivity
4. **Thought content**
   Preoccupations; morbid thoughts; abnormal beliefs
5. **Perception**
   Illusions; hallucinations; depersonalization
6. **Intellectual function**
   6.1 Orientation
       Time and place
   6.2 Attention and concentration
       Days of week and months of year backwards
       Serial sevens or threes
   6.3 Registration and short-term memory
       Recent news; your name; consultant's name
       Digit Span; Stanford-Binet Sentence
       Name, address and flower
   6.4 Long-term memory
       Early life; six cities
       World leaders; world wars
   6.5 Intelligence
       Assessed from personal history
7. **Insight**
   Nature of illness; causes of illness; appropriate treatment

4   RISK ASSESSMENTS

There are risks to the person with mental disorder through suicide, self-neglect and incitement of aggression from others. Risks to other people arise from the person with mental disorder through verbal and physical aggression, recklessness and impaired judgement, and neglect as a carer for others (children, frail elderly, people with learning or physical disability, other people with severe mental illness). Accurate assessment and management of the mental disorder is necessary but not sufficient. Specific assessment and management of the risk of harm to the self or others has also to be employed to manage mental disorder safely. For instance a doctor may correctly recognize that a person has depression and requires antidepressants. However, such a person contemplating suicide might decide to take an overdose of antidepressants as part of a suicide attempt. Therefore the suicide risk needs to be correctly identified. The patient should be followed up within the following week and prescribed only 1 week's supply of an antidepressant.

In most countries, there are steps in law that can be employed when a patient with a mental disorder or a suspected mental disorder is at high risk of harm to themselves or other people, especially if they lack the mental capacity to accept treatment, or refuse to accept treatment. In these circumstances people can be compelled against their will to accept treatment. However, there are ethical issues concerning the circumstances in which such compulsion should be employed.

THE RISK OF SELF-HARM

Suicide and self-harm

The characteristics of those who successfully commit suicide and those who harm themselves without apparent intent to kill themselves may seem separate. The elderly man who takes himself to a lonely place with a lethal dose of paracetamol represents a different phenomenon from the young girl who impulsively takes a handful of tablets in front of her boyfriend in the context of a row. However there is an area of overlap between these extremes.

This section will examine the overlapping phenomena of suicide and self-harm and then consider two types of risk assessment – detailed assessment of suicide risk as part

48

of a mental state assessment in a person who is presenting in a crisis, and assessment of a person who has self-harmed.

SUICIDE

There are about 5000 deaths from suicide in England and Wales every year. In the last 20 years there has been a rise in the suicide rate in young males, and in males under the age of 35 suicide is now the commonest cause of death. The elderly are still at greatest risk, although the rate is falling in this age group. In all groups, men are at greater risk than women.

Methods used vary according to access and availability but also to sex. Men are more likely to use violent methods such as hanging and shooting; women tend to use either prescribed medication (the older antidepressants are particularly lethal) or over-the-counter medications such as paracetamol. Before the change in the domestic gas supply from coal gas to natural gas in the 1970s, carbon monoxide self-poisoning usually took place in the home. More recently, car exhaust fumes have been used. In the 1970s, the majority of people who killed themselves had seen their GP within the previous month. This is still true for those over the age of 35 but not for those under 35, the group in which the rate of increase is greatest.

Based on 'psychological autopsy' research, in which all available information is collected after a person's suicide and key informants are interviewed, there is evidence that over 90 per cent of people who kill themselves are mentally ill (see *Box 4.1*). The most common psychiatric disorders are affective disorders and substance misuse. Factors known to be associated with suicide are shown in *Box 4.2*.

SELF-HARM

A person who 'attempts suicide' is not always intent on ending his or her life. The term 'attempted suicide' has been superseded by 'parasuicide', 'self-poisoning', 'deliberate self-harm', and now 'self-harm' and 'self-injury', which includes cutting, burning and other self-mutilatory acts. There was a massive increase in the rate of self-harm in the 1960s and 1970s; the current incidence is between 300 and 400 per 100,000 per year, and self-harm is the commonest reason for acute medical admission in women and the second commonest in men. This may help to explain some of the negative attitudes often encountered among doctors and nurses to people who harm themselves. There has been a steady decrease in the female:male ratio; whereas previously twice as many women as men harmed themselves, currently the numbers are almost equal. Peak ages are 15–24 years for women and 25–34 years for men. There are some suggestions of an increased incidence in certain ethnic groups; for example, in the UK young women of South Asian origin are 2.5 times more likely to harm themselves than white women. Factors associated with non-fatal self-harm are shown in *Box 4.3*.

The most common diagnosis associated with self-harm and self-injury is affective disorder (70 per cent). Eating disorders (bulimia nervosa) and personality disorders (anti-social or borderline) are also associated with self-harm, and drug and alcohol

Box 4.1 Mental disorders in people who kill themselves (range of findings from psychological autopsy studies)

Disorder	Percentage
Depressive disorders	36–90
Alcohol dependence or abuse	43–54
Drug dependence or abuse	4–45
Schizophrenia	3–10
Organic mental disorders	2–7
Personality disorders	5–44

Box 4.2 Factors associated with suicide

- Male sex
- Depression
- Alcohol- or drug-related problems
- Separated, widowed or divorced
- Social isolation
- Recent discharge from psychiatric care
- Serious physical illness
- Impending or recent job loss
- Current involvement with police
- Prison
- Certain occupations, e.g. farmer, doctor, dentist, lawyer

Box 4.3 Factors associated with non-fatal self-harm

- Female sex
- Divorced
- Under 25 years old
- Social class V, i.e. unskilled workers
- Unsuitable, overcrowded accommodation
- Unemployment
- Debt
- At present address for less than 1 year

misuse is common. Fifty per cent of men and 25 per cent of women take alcohol within a few hours of harming themselves. In most cases, individuals report that the episode was precipitated by interpersonal or social problems. One view is that episodes of self-harm are a maladaptive form of communication with significant others in response to relationship problems and other life stresses.

Repetition of self-harm: The 1-year repetition rate for self-harm is in the region of 15 per cent, and repetition tends to occur quickly: 25 per cent of patients repeat within 3 weeks. Those who are more likely to repeat the behaviour tend to be people who:

- have done it before
- have a personality disorder
- have been in psychiatric treatment
- are unemployed
- are in social class V (i.e. unskilled workers)
- misuse alcohol and/or drugs
- have a criminal record or history of violence
- are aged between 24 and 35 years
- are single, divorced or separated.

Suicide following self-harm: Follow-up studies have shown rates of suicide to be 1 per cent in the year after an episode of deliberate self-harm (100 times the general population rate), 3 per cent at 5 years and around 7 per cent for periods longer than 10 years. Those who do kill themselves tend to be:

- older
- male
- have a mental illness
- have poor physical health.

They might have made repeated attempts and there is also an association with long-term use of hypnotics (sleeping pills). Approximately half of successful suicides have previously deliberately harmed themselves.

Assessment of suicide risk in a person who is in crisis

Suicide risk should be assessed as part of any mental state examination. **Talking about suicide will not result in a person being more likely to harm themselves**. It is usually a relief to people who feel suicidal to be able to talk about these thoughts with a person who is prepared to listen (see *Box 4.4*).

ASSESSMENT AFTER AN EPISODE OF SELF-HARM

Patients seen in casualty or admitted to the general wards who have taken an overdose or deliberately injured themselves may present acute problems of management (see *Box 4.5*).

Box 4.4 Assessment of suicide risk in a person who is in crisis

- **Clarify current problems** – what has been going on in the person's life?

Specific questioning about **suicide intent**:

- Explore **hopelessness** *How do you see the future?*
- **Wishes to be dead** *Fleeting or persistent?*
- **Specific plans for suicide**
  Have you ever felt that you would prefer to get away from it all?
  Have you ever felt that life isn't worth living?
  Have you ever thought that you would do something to harm yourself?
  How recently have you thought that?
  What exactly would you do? Do you have plans?
  What has stopped you from carrying that out so far?
- Ask about any measures that were taken to **prevent detection**
- Evidence of recent/current **psychiatric illness**, notably symptoms of depressive or psychotic illness, drug or alcohol problems
- **Past history** of self-harm, family history of mental illness and/or self-harm
- **Current social circumstances and support**

Box 4.5 Assessment of suicide risk after an episode of self-harm

- Exactly **what was taken**, where and when, and was anyone else present? Were any precautions taken to avoid discovery?
- Was there a **suicide note?** (If so, could you see it, please? – the content may indicate increased or decreased risk) Was there any other act in anticipation of death?
- Was action taken to **alert potential helpers** after taking the overdose?
- What was the patient's **stated intent**?
- What was the patient's **estimate of lethality** of the substances taken? (Even though you consider 10 diazepam tablets relatively harmless the patient may have thought that dose would kill her: it is what the patient thinks that is important – not the actual lethality of the substance).
- Evidence of recent/current **psychiatric illness**, notably symptoms of depressive or psychotic illness.
- Is there a **past history** of psychiatric illness or previous episodes of self-harm?
- Is there any evidence of **alcohol or drug abuse**?
- Recent **precipitating life event**, such as bereavement, redundancy, break-up of a close relationship. Are there job problems or unemployment, marital, family or other interpersonal conflicts? Are there financial or other social difficulties?
- Is there a **family history** of mental illness or self-poisoning? Does the patient **live alone**, if so can he or she go and stay with someone for a while if necessary?

The **history from a relative** or other informant is especially important. If the patient is drowsy or in a coma, do this right away; otherwise do it after you have seen and examined the patient. This covers the same areas as the interview with the patient.

When **interviewing the patient** you need a quiet private place for the interview and to allocate a sensible amount of time for it. *Do not attempt to interview a patient who is drowsy after an overdose and expect to get a clear history.*

The patient may be reluctant to talk. She may be preoccupied with guilt about the episode of self-poisoning, still be angry after a row (this anger can be displaced onto you), or depressed and retarded. These will exercise your interview skills and may appear as apparent refusal to cooperate with you, or refusal to see the psychiatrist. However an assessment must be made and it is usually best to make this clear to the patient: be polite, but firm.

The **history** is taken in the usual way but the points in *Box 4.5* are most directly related to assessment of suicidal risk. The **mental state examination** is performed in the usual way but evidence of depressed mood and **continuing suicidal ideation** (see *Box 4.5*) is sought. Is the patient relieved or sorry to find himself still alive? The presence of psychotic phenomena and a brief assessment of cognitive functioning are also important.

Now record your opinion about the whole episode. Why did the episode occur? What was the seriousness of suicidal intent? Who may continue to care for the patient?

> **Opinion**: *Overdose of 10 paracetamol tablets taken from mother's handbag following a row with boyfriend. Episode seems to have been demonstrative, and without real suicidal intent: told mother what she'd done an hour later when she came home as expected; has been treated with parvolex. No suicidal ideation now. Discharge to care of mother.*

Does the patient need to be seen by a psychiatrist? Some hospitals have a policy that all people who harm themselves are seen by a psychiatrist, but this is gradually changing. Compare the above patient with this one:

> **Opinion**: *Overdose with 50 aspirin, having hidden herself in garden shed. Increasing depression since death of husband last year, and pain from rheumatoid arthritis. Left note saying she could take no more, and disposing of her property. Discovered by son on chance visit to the house. Seems severely depressed with nihilistic ideas. She lives alone.*

It is necessary to make your assessment sufficiently detailed for a decision regarding discharge to be made on the assumption that there is no continuing suicidal risk. Clearly, the last note should end with the words: 'Will psychiatrist please advise on further management?'

If in doubt, or if there is continued suicide risk, psychiatric illness, or the possibility that the patient may have to be compulsorily detained, it is essential to request advice from a more senior doctor on your own unit, or from a psychiatrist.

The patient who tries to leave before your assessment is complete

If, as a general hospital doctor, you have grounds for supposing that the patient may be a risk to him/herself it may be necessary for him or her to be detained under the Mental Health Act (see p. 364).

Long-term management

The patient may be discharged to the care of the GP and local social services or other agency, in which case it is essential that you inform that person of the episode and the patient's discharge. This is best done by a phone call in addition to a letter. The patient may be discharged with an appointment for the medical clinic. If this is to review social or psychological factors it is best done quickly (1 or 2 weeks) or the patient may not attend.

Responsibility for the patient may be transferred to the psychiatrist. If this is by means of transfer to a psychiatric ward it is usually straightforward. But if the patient is being discharged, ensure that the appointment and any instructions regarding prescription are understood by the patient, psychiatrist and GP before the patient leaves. Do not prescribe any potentially lethal drugs for the patient to take away with them.

THE RISK OF HARM TO OTHERS

Aggression and mental health

Verbal and physical aggression are features of human behaviour in general. They can also be symptoms of mental disorder. Alternatively a person who is often prone to aggression can develop a mental disorder. Despite newspaper reports, aggression, and in particular homicide, by people with mental disorder is not rising over time compared to aggression in the general population; figures have risen and fallen in line with trends for aggression and homicide in the general population. In England and Wales, there are around 500 homicides per year. However, there are many more assaults, with 40 per cent of medical and nursing staff reporting being assaulted on at least one occasion during their work. Ten per cent of homicides are committed by people with symptoms of mental illness at the time of the offence. Most of these were not in regular contact with mental health services at the time of the homicide. Alcohol and drug misuse play a major role in the homicide in about 7 per cent of cases. A third of all homicides are committed by people with a history of mental illness. One sixth have a history of both mental illness and drug or alcohol misuse or dependence.

ASSESSMENT OF RISK OF AGGRESSION

Verbal aggression is a feature of irritability, a mood state that is associated with a range of mental disorders such as depressive episodes, mania and anxiety disorders. However, irritability is also a feature of normal or severe stress in everyday life, such as being late

54

or problems at work. Verbal aggression may have the intent to harm or intimidate others. It is not usually a feature of mental disorder except as a coping response to ward off an interpersonal threat in a person who has paranoid ideation or marked anxiety, or as a feature of an anti-social or explosive personality disorder. The risk factors for physical violent behaviour are shown in *Box 4.6*.

Box 4.6 Risk factors for physical violent behaviour

Personal history
History of disturbed or violent behaviour, especially in a similar situation
History of alcohol or drug misuse
Previous expression of intent to harm others
Previous use of weapons or martial arts
Previous dangerous impulsive or reckless acts
Rootlessness and inability to stay long in any one place or form lasting relationships
Threats of violence
Recent severe stress
One or more of the above in combination with: cruelty to animals, reckless driving, history of bed-wetting in adolescence, loss of a parent before the age of 8 years

Clinical variables
Current alcohol or drug misuse
Drug effects (akathisia, disinhibition)
Morbid jealousy
Delusions or hallucinations focused on a particular person
Command hallucinations
Preoccupation with violent fantasy
Delusions of control by other people or things
Agitation, excitement, overt hostility or suspiciousness
Poor collaboration with suggested treatment
Anti-social, explosive, paranoid or impulsive personality traits
Delirium, Capgras phenomenon (misidentification syndrome where familiar person is thought to have been replaced by an imposter), disinhibition resulting from organic brain disease

Situational variables
Availability and quality of social support
Hostility, threat and criticism perceived by potential perpetrator of violence
Access to a potential weapon
Difficulties in relationship with a potential victim
Access to potential victim

As with suicide, sometimes the risk of violence is unmistakable. On other occasions however, it may be much less so. While apparently obvious, it needs to be emphasized that recognition that the risk exists is the essential first step in the assessment of the likelihood of self-harm and violence to others.

Assessment of risk is in three steps. First, define the risk and estimate the **seriousness** of the potential harm. Central to this is a thorough review of the 24-hour period leading to any past aggressive incident. In addition, the severity of the aggression, its imminence and the resources available to prevent or contain it must be taken into account. Then, make an estimate of the **probability** the risk will become reality. Finally, estimate the **imminence** that the risk will become reality. *The assessment of risk of serious harm to others is always difficult, and the beginner would be well advised to ask for help from a more experienced clinician.*

MANAGEMENT OF IMMINENT AGGRESSION

Health professionals need to be aware that attitudinal, situational, organizational and environmental factors could provoke disturbed or violent behaviour. An attitude conveying irritation, hostility or lack of concern for the person's views or predicament in the face of the signs shown in *Box 4.7* is likely to increase the likelihood and severity of aggression. A situation that conveys threat and does not allow a non-violent course of action without the person losing dignity is likely to escalate the risk of aggression. Similarly an organization that seems insensitive to the person's needs, or is muddled or confrontational, can escalate aggression. Also an environment that is enclosed, noisy, allows poor vision of potential threats and has weapons readily to hand such as chairs,

---

Box 4.7 Warning signs of imminent physical aggression

- Tense and angry facial expression
- Increased or prolonged restlessness, body tension, pacing
- Signs of over-arousal (increased rate of breathing, dilated pupils, sweating, flushing of face, muscle twitching)
- Increased volume of speech
- Prolonged or staring eye contact
- Irritability, discontentment, increased suspicion, fear, refusal to communicate, withdrawal
- Verbal threats or gestures
- Reporting anger or violent feelings
- Blocking escape routes or intimidating forward movement towards health professional
- Replicating behaviour similar to behaviour exhibited just before a previous violent incident
- Unclear thought processes, poor concentration
- Delusions or hallucinations with violent content

---

knives, bottles, breakable glass, may provoke or increase physical aggression. The health professional needs to de-escalate the risk of physical aggression as a clinical priority before carrying on with other aspects of assessment or management of the condition.

The person's anger needs to be managed by the doctor using an appropriate, measured and reasonable response. The need is for the doctor to remain calm, monitoring their own verbal and non-verbal behaviour first and foremost. The doctor must also observe the person at risk and others in the vicinity at the same time. The person who is becoming angry needs to have their dignity preserved. They must not feel under threat and if possible they should feel listened to and supported. The doctor needs to remove other people who are at risk of aggression, or who might provoke the situation, such as other patients in the same physical space. If necessary move everybody who needs to be in the situation to a safer environment (without weapons, less enclosed, quieter and with better lighting). The doctor should have enough people in the same physical space or close by and in direct communication to manage the situation safely in case the person becomes physically aggressive. However, these people must not be in such close proximity that they appear threatening, otherwise safety would be compromised. The person who is angry, and other people in the situation, need to be given clear, brief, assertive instructions explaining exactly what the doctor intends to do before and at the same time as he or she is doing it.

The doctor should ask the person who is angry for the facts about the problem, try to encourage reasoning, and try to get the person to use anxiety management techniques to control over-arousal (look for signs of over-breathing, flushing, tensing of the body, dilation of the pupils, restlessness). The doctor should attempt to establish a rapport, ask open questions, ask about the reasons for the person's anger, listen carefully, and show concern and assertiveness. The doctor should take care not to patronize or seem dismissive of concerns even if they appear trivial, irrelevant or illogical. The doctor must avoid issuing threats. Realistic options are negotiated but not options that would put the person or other people at increased danger, or lead to a worsening of the underlying mental health problem. If the person has a serious mental health condition that requires immediate treatment to prevent further deterioration in the mental state, then treatment for the underlying mental health problem should be negotiated.

MEDICATION FOR THE MANAGEMENT OF VIOLENT BEHAVIOUR

Oral sedative medication such as lorazepam, which is quick-acting and reversible if necessary with flumazenil, for patients without psychosis, or a single neuroleptic drug with or without lorazepam if the person is psychotic (acute symptoms of schizophrenia, mania, delusions or hallucinations) may be given if the risk of further aggression is thought likely to recur. Rapid tranquillization with lorazepam and/or a neuroleptic drug (in those with psychosis) must only be attempted in people who are medically fit for such an intervention and using drugs prescribed within British National Formulary (or other similar national formulary) limits. Oral medication using liquids or dispersible under-the-tongue tablets is preferable rather than rectal or intramuscular medication. Intravenous medication should only be used exceptionally. Rapid tranquillization should not be attempted in people who are already compromised in terms of respiratory or cardiac function, those who have consumed large quantities of alcohol, or who are dehydrated or physically ill. No more than one drug from the same drug group should be given at any one time and drugs should not be mixed in a syringe if they are given parenterally.

PHYSICAL RESTRAINT

Physical intervention such as restraint, seclusion or rapid tranquillization medication may have to be employed when reasoning and negotiation of oral medication have failed to control the situation. It is helpful to have sufficient staff to control each limb using sufficient force to prevent injury but not inflict pain. Often the angry person will cooperate with restraint if the team is assertive but preserves the dignity of the individual as much as possible. Physical interventions should not be attempted unless they can be managed safely without injury or pain to anyone and with the dignity of the person preserved as much as possible. Restraint should never be attempted without someone in charge of the restraining procedure taking care of the head and neck so that the airway and circulation are preserved.

Seclusion in a locked room must only be attempted when there is clear unimpeded observation of the person in seclusion, and this must be done at regular intervals no longer than 15 minutes apart. It should be continued until the risk of aggression can be managed by other means. Restraint should be avoided in the frail or those who are easily injured, such as those with brittle bones or problems with blood clotting.

After every incident of aggression, there should be a period of observation until the risk of aggression is clearly reduced, and a review of the incident. Observation may be unobtrusive with the person's whereabouts and behaviour monitored at regular intervals. Sometimes one or more members of staff will need to be assigned to the aggressive patient. Such close observation is only really practical on an in-patient ward and requires considerable tact if the dignity of the patient is to be preserved and the situation is not to escalate further.

A review of the incident is used to understand triggers to the aggression and warning signs of further aggression, and to learn the best way of preventing, containing or managing it in the future. It should also be used to understand if there are improvements to be made in terms of the organization of the service, the procedures used in the service, attitudes and knowledge of the staff, and the physical environment where the aggression occurred.

5 SYNDROMES AND DIAGNOSIS

THE PURPOSE AND LIMITATIONS OF DIAGNOSIS

The purpose of a diagnosis is to bring together illnesses that have the same characteristics. Ideally, a diagnosis should identify disorders having the same underlying pathology, the same causes, and the same likely response to treatment. However, such an ideal is rarely achieved. Thus a diagnosis of **Huntington's chorea** identifies a necessary cause (an autosomal dominant gene), a pathology (cortical and extra-pyramidal degeneration), a clinical presentation (dementia and choreiform movements with onset usually between ages 30 and 50) and a course (progressive deterioration resulting in death). Ideally the diagnosis should also indicate an expected response to treatment, which in this example is at present limited to genetic counselling and symptomatic care. Although this diagnosis identifies a disease process, there are some limitations in its value, because not all those who suffer the disease will conform to this typical pattern. For example, some will show choreiform movements with little or no evidence of dementia. The age of onset will vary, and occasionally presentation may occur in childhood or old age. This illustrates the fact that all disease processes are subject to considerable variability.

Pulmonary tuberculosis is a diagnosis that deviates further from the ideal. All patients will have a similar basic pathology in the same organ, but the clinical presentation will vary from a chance radiological finding with no clinical features to an acute fulminating disorder. The course of these will differ widely, as will the management. All cases will have a similar necessary cause (the tubercle bacillus), but this is not a sufficient cause, and many other different factors will play a part in the aetiology of different cases (for example, the state of nutrition, accommodation, and socio-economic status).

Other 'diagnoses' tell us even less and are mainly a means of identifying clinical syndromes. A common example is **congestive cardiac failure**, which identifies a set of symptoms and signs, but provides only limited information about the underlying aetiology or pathology, and little about the course or response to particular treatments. However, even such a limited clinical label may alert us to a range of possible causes.

Most psychiatric diagnoses are syndrome diagnoses. Like the example of congestive cardiac failure, they tell us the symptoms and signs that characterize the disorder, but only a little about the aetiology, which must be considered separately. A diagnosis of **delirium** (see pp. 159–162) will convey the clinical presentation, but does not tell us

59

which of the many different causes of this syndrome is relevant to a particular case, and therefore does not tell us which specific treatment will be appropriate.

However, it does direct our attention to known causes of delirium, just as the diagnosis of depression directs our attention to known causes of depressive illness. Cause and treatment should usually therefore be considered separately.

A further complication arises because not only may a syndrome have a different cause in different cases, but often there are multiple interacting factors all contributing to the aetiology of a single case. In the example of pulmonary tuberculosis, contact with a case of pulmonary tuberculosis exposes an individual to the risk of developing the disorder, but he will not necessarily become infected unless other factors are also involved. Similarly a woman's susceptibility to the development of a **depressive illness** will be increased by the death of her mother before the age of 11, having no close supportive relationship and having three children or more below the age of 14. However, not all women with these experiences will develop depressive illness. Just as malnutrition may predispose an individual to many different physical illnesses, the same aetiological factors may increase susceptibility to several psychiatric syndromes.

THE TRADITIONAL ORGANIZATION OF DIAGNOSTIC CATEGORIES

It has been traditional to differentiate between categories of psychiatric disorder in two ways. The first divides them according to clinical presentation, into **psychoses, neuroses (now called internalizing disorders)**, and **personality disorders**. The second has regard to aetiology, and divides them into '**organic**' disorders that are secondary to known brain disease, and '**functional**' disorders whose physical basis is unknown.

Both the psychoses and the neuroses share a widely accepted criterion of illness, that is, a deterioration from a presumed previous state of health and the development of symptoms. By contrast **personality disorders** do not involve change. They are identified by the presence of personality characteristics (traits) that are relatively constant throughout life and cause the subject and/or society to suffer.

The differentiation between the psychoses and neuroses is essentially arbitrary, and based mainly on historical beliefs and practices. The **psychoses** include those disorders traditionally regarded as madness, in which strange beliefs and perceptions, often accompanied by violent and destructive behaviour, at one time resulted in incarceration in mental asylums. It has long been recognized that some of these illnesses are secondary to structural disease of the brain and these are therefore called **organic psychoses**, while others occur in brains that appear normal on CAT scans, and are therefore called '**functional' psychoses**.

However, recent research shows that demonstrable structural or neurochemical changes also occur in the functional psychoses, so that the distinction between them and organic psychoses no longer has much substance.

The term **neurosis** was first used in 1769 by William Cullen to describe what were believed to be organic diseases of nerve tissue. Patients with these disorders presented to physicians with complaints generally thought to indicate physical illness, such as lassitude, dizziness, weakness and poor appetite. They were considered to be suffering literally from 'weak nerves', and the terminology survives, even though there is usually no corresponding underlying physical disease of nerve tissue. During the nineteenth century there was increasing awareness that these physical complaints could have their foundation in mental rather than physical mechanisms. The development of psycho-analysis from the 1890s, and behavioural psychology from the 1920s, led to increasing awareness of the way in which mental mechanisms might operate to produce these symptoms.

By the beginning of the twentieth century psychiatrists saw those who presented with physical symptoms that were without known organic cause (hysterical neuroses and hypochondriasis), and also began to see patients with wholly psychological disorders such as anxiety state, obsessional neurosis and phobic neurosis.

In the United Kingdom psychiatrists only began to be appointed to the staff of general hospitals in any numbers in the 1930s, and departments of 'psychological medicine' arose, to which patients with somatic symptoms unaccompanied by physical disease – the 'neurotics' of the previous century – were referred. However, most psychiatrists continued to work in mental hospitals, where their clinical work was mainly concerned with 'psychotic' illnesses. Thus patients with neuroses and psychoses were seen and treated in different hospital settings and often by different groups of psychiatrists. Although these barriers have almost disappeared, the separation between neuroses and psychoses lingers on as a vestigial remnant.

By the middle of the twentieth century psychiatrists were working more closely with colleagues in general hospital settings, were seeing patients referred by general prac-titioners, and were beginning to be asked to see increasing numbers of patients with **externalizing disorders** that cannot be fitted into the categories of either psychosis or neurosis. These include disorders such as alcohol dependence, anorexia nervosa, bulimia nervosa, and drug dependency; self-damaging behaviours such as self-poisoning and self-mutilation; and certain sexual disorders.

We will now consider the distinction between each of the various categories we have discussed so far.

Organic versus 'functional' psychosis

The disorders at present referred to as 'organic' should more accurately be thought of as those where we have a clear idea of an aetiology, and that aetiology is a physical disease. They include conditions where the structure of the brain is abnormal such as Alzheimer's disease or psychoses secondary to cerebro-vascular disease, and conditions where the brain is structurally normal – such as delirium associated with typhoid fever, pneumo-coccal pneumonia or alcohol withdrawal ('delirium tremens'). It could be argued that the latter group are in a sense 'functional', and that as knowledge of neurochemistry advances we can expect to gain a greater understanding of many – if not all – of those psychoses at present referred to as 'functional', such as schizophrenia and bipolar disorder. For the present, there are clear advantages in making a distinction between those conditions where the aetiology is either coarse brain disease or physical disease

61

elsewhere in the body, and those where the disorder arises from disordered functioning of the brain itself.

Neurosis versus psychosis

Previous claims that psychoses differ from neuroses because they are more 'severe' are not valid, because many neurotic patients also suffer from chronic severely disabling illnesses. Although psychotic patients are said to be less in touch with reality (or to show 'defects in reality testing') and to have less insight into their illness, it will be remembered from Chapter 3 that insight is never completely present or absent. Psychotic patients rarely have no insight at all, and neurotic patients seldom have perfect insight. It is a matter of degree, so insight cannot be a basis on which two categories of disease can be separated.

The only criterion by which these groups of disorders can be separated reliably involves an arbitrary operational definition. Psychotic illnesses are characterized by the presence of 'psychotic symptoms', specifically delusions and hallucinations. Such symptoms occur only in the psychoses, whereas 'neurotic symptoms' occur in both the neuroses and the psychoses. Thus if delusions or hallucinations are found in a particular mental illness, by definition it is a psychosis; if absent, it is a neurosis. The reason for making the distinction at all is that patients experiencing psychotic phenomena are more likely to have grossly deranged neurochemistry, and are therefore more likely to respond to physical treatments such as psychotropic drugs and ECT. They are also more likely to have severely disturbed behaviour requiring in-patient treatment.

However, the word 'neurosis' applies to a kind of illness that can come and go, while the word 'neurotic' refers to long-standing attributes in a person. There are many individuals who have episodes of allegedly 'neurotic' illness, such as depressive illness, who are not especially 'neurotic' people. The term 'neurosis' should really be abandoned, but it will probably obstinately live on, if only because it is a pithy way of saying 'non-psychotic'. However, we shall not be using it in the remainder of this book, and prefer to speak of **internalizing disorders**, where the patient tends to introspect about problems, and experience inner distress and dysphoria.

Non-psychotic illnesses therefore form a large residual category of disorders. Within this category the mood disorders – those related to depression and anxiety – are most like medical syndromes such as migraine, but there are also other disorders where the abnormality is seen only in external behaviour, such as drug and alcohol problems, eating disorders, anti-social behaviour in adults and conduct disorders in children. These are termed '**externalizing disorders**'. However, it is important to note that in clinical practice people with externalizing disorders may on occasion experience considerable inner distress, dysphoria and sometimes serious suicide intent.

THE HIERARCHICAL MODEL OF DIAGNOSIS

We have seen that the various syndromes of psychiatric disorder can be arranged in a rough hierarchy, where the top level (*'level one'*) represents those conditions that have a known 'organic' aetiology; the second ('*level two*') those psychotic conditions where there are likely to be severe neurochemical derangements in cerebral functioning, and then there is a rather heterogeneous residual group. It is reasonable to make a distinction between disorders where concepts of treatment and recovery are appropriate ('*level three*'): affective disorders, externalizing disorders, and abnormal illness behaviours; and those that represent stable attributes of human functioning ('*level four*'): personality disorders and disorders of gender identity and sexual orientation.

The latter should not be thought of as illnesses, but they are often relevant to understanding the aetiology of illness, they may complicate treatment plans, and they are associated with suffering – either for the patient, or for those with whom he lives. The scheme is shown in *Table 5.1*.

From the student's point of view, the main advantage of such a hierarchy is to remind you that certain symptoms have more specificity than others in leading to a syndrome diagnosis.

Thus symptoms in the 'intellectual function' section of the mental state examination indicate that serious consideration must be given to the possibility that the patient can be recruited to the top of the hierarchy. If we decide to do this, we will give less attention to other symptoms from lower in the hierarchy that might be present. For example, if we decide a patient has delirium, we will pay little diagnostic attention to anxious mood since we will be preoccupied with finding (and treating) the cause of the delirium. However, once the diagnosis is made, the presence of anxiety may still be important in relation to the management of the patient, for example indicating the need for nursing staff to explain to the patient with delirium what is going on and to reassure them that they are being looked after.

Within the psychotic stratum, it is now usual to put clear manic symptoms 'above' schizophrenic symptoms, and to put these in turn 'above' depressive symptoms (see below). This is because many studies have shown schizophrenia-like symptoms in manic patients who have recovered completely from such illnesses and gone on to develop clear manic-depressive (or 'bipolar') illnesses. However, providing manic symptoms are absent, 'disintegrative delusions' (thought reading, thought withdrawal or ideas of passivity) are suggestive of schizophrenia, *providing that features indicating an organic disorder are absent*. This is because certain organic illnesses can cause schizophrenia-like symptoms (see p. 191), and if these illnesses are present it is usual to diagnose them rather than schizophrenia.

In this way 'schizophrenia' becomes a name attached to disorders that have certain typical symptoms, but for which no organic aetiology has been identified and that are not clearly manic: and it is in this sense that organic illnesses and mania are 'above' schizophrenia in the hierarchy. On the other hand, mood disorders such as depression and anxiety occur commonly in the setting of schizophrenia, but do not alter the diagnosis of schizophrenia since they are said to be 'below' schizophrenia. Thus, a depressive illness would only be diagnosed if signs of schizophrenia and of an organic state were absent.

The third level of the hierarchy contains all possible symptoms except those pathognomonic of organic disorders or strongly suggestive of psychotic illness. These

Table 5.1 *The hierarchical model of diagnosis*

Level one: ORGANIC DISORDERS	**Delirium** ('Acute brain syndrome') **Dementia** ('Chronic brain syndrome') **Korsakow's syndrome**
Level two: 'FUNCTIONAL' PSYCHOSES	**Schizophrenia** **Bipolar illness** Mania Psychotic depression
Level three: NON-PSYCHOTIC DISORDERS	**Internalizing disorders** **'Anxious misery' disorders** Depressive illness Anxiety state **Fear disorders** Specific phobias Agoraphobia Panic disorder Post-traumatic stress disorder **Abnormal illness behaviour** Somatization disorder Persistent somatoform pain disorder Hypochondriacal disorder Factitious illness Malingering Dissociative disorders **Externalizing disorders** Alcoholism Drug dependence Anorexia nervosa and bulimia Obesity Obsessive compulsive disorder
Level four: PERSONALITY DISORDERS	**Paranoid** personality **Schizoid** personality **Dissocial** personality **Emotionally unstable** personality **Histrionic** personality **Obsessional** personality **Dependent** personality

symptoms are non-specific in the sense that they can also occur at the higher levels, but if they do they will not alter the diagnosis. They only attract syndromal labels when they occur on their own. You will notice that the concept of 'depression' appears in both levels 2 and 3. This is because in its severe form depression can be accompanied by psychotic symptoms, whereas the commoner forms of depression have symptoms that are more readily understandable. This alerts you to the fact that the distinction between 'functional psychoses' and less severe forms of mental disorder is but a convenient fiction.

ONE DIAGNOSIS OR TWO?

In the case of externalizing disorders it will often be useful to diagnose these *in addition* to a diagnosis based on experienced symptoms.

For example, if a patient with schizophrenia (*a level 2 diagnosis*) also has symptoms of alcohol dependence (an externalizing disorder) we should diagnose both conditions, since the second diagnosis gives important information not contained in the first. There is no underlying assumption about their relationship: they might be coincidental, or either might be a factor contributing to the aetiology of the other. It is usual to ask ourselves whether there might be a relationship whenever we make more than one diagnosis: in this example the patient may have developed a typical form of auditory hallucinosis after many years of heavy drinking (in which case we speak of **alcoholic hallucinosis**), or he may only drink because the voices tell him to (primary diagnosis therefore **schizophrenia**), or there may be no obvious relationship, in which case we simply make two diagnoses, putting the one highest on the hierarchy first.

Further examples of related diagnoses, where the second label gives information not implicit in the first, would be:

1. *Agoraphobia*
2. *Alcohol dependence*, or

1. *Anorexia nervosa*
2. *Depressive illness.*

The second diagnosis is necessary since by no means all agoraphobics develop alcohol dependence, and not all anorexics are depressed. In each case, the presence of the second diagnosis is likely to influence the treatment plan proposed for the patient. Note that the externalizing disorder has been put first in the latter example, implying that it may be causally implicated in the depression.

Diagnosis of a personality disorder may also be complementary to other diagnoses, and either help us to understand the aetiology, or influence our management of the problem; for example:

1. *Paranoid psychosis,*
2. *Paranoid personality*, or

1. *Self-harm*
2. *Emotionally unstable personality.*

65

Having said this, it should be emphasized that two diagnoses should only be made if one will not do, so one tries first to find a single diagnosis that will accommodate all the symptoms and signs. Only if this is not possible consider a second diagnosis.

Differential diagnosis is a quite separate process, which is concerned with alternative rather than complementary diagnoses, and is discussed in the chapter on formulation.

CLASSIFICATORY SYSTEMS

The terminology used to label the different syndromes is embodied in various systems of classification. The tenth revision of the International Classification of Disease (ICD-10) includes a classification of mental disorders in its fifth chapter. There are 458 categories of mental disorders listed in this chapter, and they are combined into 10 major groups. Most of these are rare disorders, or are sub-varieties of some of the larger groupings described in this book. The 51 disorders described in this book are shown in *Table 5.2*, grouped according to their official codes in the ICD-10. This is the system that has been most widely used, both in the United Kingdom and abroad. It has been shown that different psychiatrists working in different hospitals, and in different countries, reach a high level of agreement in making diagnoses for the same patients when applying this classification. The World Health Organization has produced a much simpler version of this classification for use in primary care and general medical settings, called the ICD-10 PHC: each of the 24 conditions included in this classification is accompanied by clear advice on the management of the disorder. The British version of ICD10-PHC can be accessed on-line at http://www.mentalneurologicalprimarycare.org

The *Diagnostic and Statistical Manual* of the American Psychiatric Association (now in its fifth revision, thus DSM-V) provides another classification that has recently aroused much interest. It differs from the *International Classification of Disease* in some important respects, notably in that it tends to give more emphasis to clear operational rules in making diagnoses.

FURTHER READING

American Psychiatric Association (1993) *Diagnostic and Statistical Manual of Mental Disorders. DSM-IV*. Washington, DC.

Kendell, R. E. (1975) *The Role of Diagnosis in Psychiatry*. Oxford: Blackwell Scientific.

World Health Organization (1992) *The ICD-10 Classification of Mental and Behavioural Disorders: Clinical Descriptions and Diagnostic Guidelines*. Geneva: World Health Organization.

Table 5.2 *Ten major groups of Chapter V of ICD-10, and their relationship to the 42 disorders described in this book*

F0   Organic, including symptomatic, mental disorders

F00	Alzheimer's disease
F01	Vascular dementia
F02	Other dementias
F05	Delirium

F1   Mental and behaviour disorders due to psychoactive substance use

F10	Disorders due to alcohol
F10.2	Alcohol dependence
F10.5	Korsakow's psychosis
F11–19	Disorders due to other substances

F2   Schizophrenia and delusional disorders

F20	Schizophrenia
F22	Persistent delusional disorder ('paranoid psychosis')
F25	Schizoaffective psychosis

F3   Mood (affective) disorders

F30	Manic episode
F31	Bipolar affective disorder
F32	Depressive episode
F32.3	Depressive episode with psychotic symptoms

F4   Neurotic, stress-related and somatoform disorders

F40	Agoraphobia
F40.2	Specific phobias
F41.0	Panic disorder
F41.1	Generalized anxiety state
F42	Obsessive compulsive disorder
F43.1	Post traumatic stress disorder
F43.2	Adjustment disorders
F44	Dissociative (conversion) disorders
F45	Somatoform disorders
F45.2	Hypochondriacal disorder

F5   Physiological dysfunction associated with mental factors

F50	Anorexia nervosa
F50.2	Bulimia nervosa
F51.0	Non-organic insomnia
F52.0	Lack of sexual desire
F52.11	Lack of sexual enjoyment
F52.2	Failure of genital response (includes male impotence; female lack of arousal)
F52.3	Orgasmic dysfunction
F52.4	Premature ejaculation
F52.5	Vaginismus
F52.6	Dyspareunia
F53	Puerperal mental disorder

continues overleaf

Table 5.2 *(continued)*

F6	**Abnormalities of adult personality and behaviour**	
	F60.0	Paranoid ('sensitive') personality
	F60.1	Schizoid personality
	F60.2	Dissocial ('anti-social') personality
	F60.3	Emotionally unstable personality
	F60.4	Histrionic personality
	F60.5	Obsessional ('anankastic') personality
	F60.7	Dependent personality
	F64	Gender identity disorder
F7	**Mental retardation**	
	F70–73	Mild; moderate; severe; profound
F8	**Developmental disorders**	
	F84.0	Autism
F9	**Behavioural and emotional disorders of childhood or adolescence**	
	F90	Hyperkinetic disorders
	F91	Conduct disorders
	F93	Emotional disorders

6   AETIOLOGY

In this chapter we will look at the general principles that underlie the causes of mental disorders, and the way in which these can be used to form hypotheses about the aetiology of an individual patient's illness. An accurate assessment of aetiology is important but should be based on well-observed data rather than wild speculation. It then serves as a logical basis for the plan of management (Chapter 8). The particular causes of each syndrome will be considered in Part 2.

AETIOLOGICAL FACTORS

When we look for the aetiological factors of a patient's illness we are in effect trying to answer the following questions:

Why this disorder?
Why this particular time?

In more chronic disorders we must also ask:

Why no recovery?

Aetiological factors can contribute at different stages: first by predisposing to illness, then as precipitants and finally as maintaining factors. The first of these questions deals with predisposition, the second with precipitation and the third with maintaining factors.

Predisposing factors

Predisposing factors are those that increase an individual's vulnerability to develop an illness at any time in the future. They address the *'Why this disorder?'* question. **Genes** may operate in a highly specific way (e.g. a genetic predisposition to Huntington's chorea) to increase the risk of one particular disorder, or they may increase the risk of both psychotic disorders and common mental disorders. A careful family history is therefore an essential first step. The predisposition may also operate in a general way (e.g. **personality traits** of anxiety, which are partly under genetic control, but also exacerbated by adverse early experiences). Some kinds of **abnormal personality** are at higher risk of particular illnesses, probably because personality traits modify the type and number of stressful life events experienced during adult life. Abuse and neglect during childhood will also increase the risk of later disorder.

Precipitating factors

Precipitating factors determine when the illness starts (*'Why at this particular time?'*). Some people are vulnerable to mental illness but may go for many years without becoming ill, so we have to determine the factors that bring about this change from health to illness. Usually precipitating factors act in a non-specific way, that is they determine when the illness starts but not the type of illness: for example, **life events** (see page 74) that involve loss or threat can help to precipitate almost any disorder to which the patient has a predetermined vulnerability.

Maintaining factors

In addition we have to consider whether there may be additional maintaining factors that prolong a disorder, if it continues for longer than would usually be expected (*'Why no recovery?'*). For example, the majority of affective disorders lead to recovery within weeks or months so, if the condition persists for longer, is there any evidence of causes that continue to affect the patient and prevent recovery?

A systematic approach

We should use the available data to answer these questions for each patient that we assess. *Table 6.1* provides a guide to a systematic approach and each stage needs to be considered in turn. At each stage the aetiological factors may be divided into biological, social, and psychological. Consider whether you have discovered anything about your patient that might fit into these categories in turn, but you are only likely to use a few of these for each patient.

Aim to write a systematic account of the possible aetiological factors that you have discovered after you have taken the history and completed the examination of the mental state. This will form part of the formulation (see Chapter 10).This initial hypothesis will have to be tested, and perhaps modified, when you attempt to support it by investigations (see Chapter 7).

In the past there was some controversy about whether the origins of mental illnesses are mainly genetic or acquired: nowadays it is more appropriate to consider the extent to which each makes a contribution.

THE GENETIC CONTRIBUTION

Evidence for the inheritance of a mental illness is based on the following:

Table 6.1 *Examples of aetiological factors*

1. *Predisposing*

A biological: genetic; intra-uterine disadvantage; birth trauma; or disorders of later onset resulting in cerebral disease or physical handicap. Some forms of personality disorder

B social: physical or emotional deprivation during childhood due to family discord, bereavement or separation. Chronic difficulties in work, marriage, housing, or finance, lack of supportive relationships

C psychological: inappropriate parental models, e.g. agoraphobic mother or violent father: constitutional predisposition to neurotic traits (may be partly biological), low self-esteem. Some forms of personality disorder. Habitual use of particular defence mechanisms

2. *Precipitating*

A biological: recent physical disease, e.g. infections, injury resulting in disability, malignant disease with threat of disfiguring surgery or death

B social: recent life events, particularly those involving threat and loss, such as redundancy, child leaving home, separation, or divorce, loss of a supportive relationship

C psychological: subject's responses to biological or social factors, e.g. following bereavement or mutilating surgery; feelings of loss of self-esteem; helplessness; hopelessness

3. *Maintaining*

A biological: physical handicaps; pain from physical disease; failure to take medication or unwanted effects of medication

B social: adverse social circumstances; no intimate relationships; negative interactions at home; no support from key relative; inappropriate medical management

C psychological: hopelessness (no expectation of recovery); marked adverse personality traits, e.g. low self-esteem, excessive dependency or anxiety traits

---

1. *Higher prevalence rates in first-degree relatives than the risk for the general population.* There is considerable variation in the extent to which different diagnostic categories have a genetic contribution. For example, the concordance rates for first-degree relatives of schizophrenics is between 5 per cent and 15 per cent, compared with a life-time prevalence of about 1 per cent in the general population. The concordance rates for monozygotic twins is between 40 and 60 per cent and this remains almost as high in twins that are raised separately by adoptive parents. The picture for bipolar affective disorder follows a similar pattern.

   From these figures there can be no doubt that there is an important genetic contribution to the aetiology of these illnesses. However, the nature of this contribution is in doubt. It cannot be determined by either a simple dominant or recessive gene because concordance rates are too low. It has therefore been suggested that inheritance is likely to be the result of either polygenic interactions (i.e. a number of different minor genes acting to complement or modify each other) or of a single gene with incomplete penetrance.

2. *Higher prevalence rates in children whose biological parents were mentally ill, despite being adopted by healthy parents.*

3. *Higher concordance rates in monozygotic than dizygotic twins.* The relative contributions of genetic and environmental factors for a particular disorder are determined by measuring the degree of similarity between a set of identical (monozygotic, or MZ)

twins, and comparing this with similar figures for a set of non-identical (dizygotic, or DZ) twins. The analysis proceeds by assuming that the genes are indeed identical in the MZ twins, and that they therefore have perfect correlation for variance because of genetics, but since they only share half their genes in the case of the DZ twins, it is assumed to be 0.5. Variance as a result of common family environment is also assumed to be perfect for both MZ and DZ twins, and anything left over is attributed to a residual term covering unique (or non-shared) environment. The similarity between the MZ twins is now considered to be the result of the sum of the effects of genetic factors and shared environment, while the similarity between the DZ twins is the result of half the genetic factor, plus the shared environment. Comparisons of the within-pair correlations for the two sets of twins will thus result in rough estimates of the variance resulting from genes (a), shared environment (c) and unique environment (e).

4. *The persistence of this increased concordance, even when monozygotic twins have been separated in infancy and reared apart.*

Gene/environment interactions

However, there are considerable interactions between genes and the social environment, so that some illnesses require the combination of an abnormal gene and a particular life situation to manifest themselves. These effects are called 'gene/environment inter-actions', and they are contained within the 'a' term. We will mention three examples:

1. People with an abnormal 5HT transporter gene are much more likely to become depressed under stress, while those with the gene normal are relatively resilient in the presence of stress.
2. The gene monoamine oxidase A (the 'MAO-A gene') is related to anti-social beha-viour. An abnormality of this gene results in an individual with high levels of all the transmitters metabolised by this enzyme – noradrenaline, dopamine and serotonin. However, the manifestation of the gene in later life depends on the environment. Children who are maltreated but have normal MAO-A activity are only slightly more likely to develop anti-social behaviour than those who have not been mal-treated – but if the gene is abnormal, then the risk of anti-social behaviour increases greatly with increasing degrees of maltreatment. This relationship holds true for all later measures of anti-social behaviour: anti-social personality disorder, conviction for violent offences, childhood conduct disorder and an index of 'disposition towards violence'.
3. Those with a positive family history of schizophrenia – who are more likely to be carrying the recessive gene or genes that predispose them, are very much more likely to develop schizophrenia if they take cannabis than those without such a history.

The fact that the concordance rates in monozygotic twins are considerably less than 100 per cent demonstrates the importance of the contribution from environmental factors.

There are few mental disorders in which the genetic contribution is substantially greater than this and these are the result of single gene transmission following the recognized Mendelian patterns. Examples are:

Huntington's chorea (autosomal dominant inheritance)

and some of the uncommon causes of severe mental handicap such as:

tuberose sclerosis (autosomal dominant) and
phenylketonuria (autosomal recessive).

ENVIRONMENTAL FACTORS

Secure attachment to the care-giver (usually the mother) in the first few months is of critical importance in modifying the excitability of the hypothalamo-pituitary axis (HPA), and thus the vulnerability to later life stress. Attachment theory proposes that infants develop 'internal working models' of relationships that serve as a psychological blueprint for interpersonal functions with others in childhood and later life. Insecure attachment produces a baby with poor social development and more anti-social behaviour, which in the presence of negative experiences leads on to anxious traits. Thus, maternal attachment is the first life experience that can modify – in either direction – the excitability of the HPA axis. Maternal separation increases HPA sensitivity, as does maternal depression. Severe chronic privations, such as being brought up in an orphanage since birth, are also associated with changes in the sensitivity of the HPA axis – with cortisol hypersecretion frequently reported.

It has become increasingly apparent that maltreatment of children (physical and sexual abuse) has significant biological consequences for neural systems and chemical codes for behaviour. Child maltreatment is associated with cortisol hypersecretion in some studies, but also with hyposecretion in others. Girls are at greater risk than boys for sexual abuse.

Abused and neglected children are more likely to develop anti-social behaviour, but many do not do so. Children with anti-social behaviour are more likely to have soft CNS signs, under-controlled temperaments and hyperactivity, and poor performance on intelligence test. These disorders are substantially more common among boys. The experience of parental divorce increases the rates for conduct disorder and anti-social behaviour. Children subjected to physical or sexual abuse display a wide range of common mental disorders in adolescence – not only much higher rates of depression, but self-harm behaviours and eating disorders, as well as problems in obtaining satisfactory sexual relationships.

In contrast to the effects of poor attachment, the effects of poor parenting practices are less dramatic: poor parenting – whether over-involved or depriving – carries increased risks of common mental disorders later, but each can occur without the other. Marital discord – often associated with separations and violence – exerts an effect on common mental disorders in the children independent of the effects of parenting. Children who have experienced parental divorce and parental death also have higher rates of common mental disorders in adult life. Concepts of self-worth, peer popularity and social competence develop during childhood and have important later consequences for common mental disorders. Of these, the development of friends is the most important non-family activity. Those who do not develop friendships may have difficulties handling negative life events in later life.

During middle childhood children begin to adjust their self-perceptions as a result of failure at key tasks, with the first emergence of feelings of shame, helplessness and hopelessness. It is at this stage that the germs of later depressive illness become manifest as early cognitive changes occur, especially in those who have a tendency to persistently ruminate and perseverate about real or supposed shortcomings.

LIFE EVENTS

Life events refer to discrete changes in a person's environment that may cause some form of threat or stress to the individual. Research into life events prior to the onset of depressive disorders shows a five-fold excess only of undesirable events, and these may occur throughout at least the 6-month period preceding the onset of illness. 'Loss events' such as bereavement, divorce, severe illness in a close relative, or redundancy have been shown to be particularly important.

Events that can precipitate an episode of schizophrenia are any that involve change and include such 'desirable' events as promotion, getting a new job, and moving house, in addition to undesirable events. In the 3 weeks prior to an episode of schizophrenia there is a three-fold increase in life events of all types compared with controls. The brevity of this increased period of risk indicates that the event is merely concerned with the exact *timing* of an episode of illness – we must look elsewhere for predisposing factors.

This means that the contribution of life events to the precipitation of a particular episode of depression is relatively greater than in schizophrenia. Of course most people experience such events without developing schizophrenia, depressive disorders or any other mental illness, and this demonstrates that many people are relatively resilient to life stress. This resilience is likely to be partly a result of genetic causes such as the 5HT transporter gene, and partly from favourable post-natal events. Resilience and vulnerability are two sides of the same coin.

Normal personality variations and the experience of life events

There is a substantial genetic component to the experience of stressful life events, but this is entirely mediated by personality variables, notably neuroticism (harm avoidance) and a personality dimension called 'openness to experience'. About half the variation in normal personality is genetically determined.

In a similar manner those who score highly on a dimension called 'novelty seeking', or another called 'reward dependence', or who score low on a related dimension called 'constraint', may be expected to experience more dangerous and threatening events. Such events include taking recreational drugs, and participating in dangerous sports.

These findings remind us that people create their own environments, and provide us with an entirely separate genetic pathway for the influence of genes on the later development of adult illness.

PSYCHOLOGICAL DEFENCE MECHANISMS

Psychological defence mechanisms stems from the psychoanalytic work of Sigmund Freud (1856 to 1939). These are *unconscious* processes (the subject is not aware of them) used to *protect the individual from anxiety* arising from inner impulses or environmental threat. The subject is consciously unaware of painful experiences and of the unpleasant feelings attached to them. Individuals tend to have particular mechanisms that they acquire in childhood and use habitually, although sometimes these may emerge for the first time in the face of an unusual crisis. However, if a particular mechanism is used habitually it sometimes helps us to answer the *'Why this disorder?'* question, since different mechanisms tend to be used in different illnesses.

Repression and denial

Defence mechanisms are a part of the healthy repertoire of all people, since we all need to ward off anxiety. **Repression**, for example, refers to the exclusion from our awareness of impulses or emotions that would otherwise cause us distress. It would be difficult to remain healthy if we were unable to suppress unpleasant material, but it is easy to see that the process could go too far. Sometimes the defence against anxiety may prevent the subject from being aware that there are problems in his life that require constructive action. At other times the defence mechanism used may lead the subject to act in inappropriate ways that are maladaptive.

Thus defence mechanisms play another part in the aetiology of mental illness: sometimes helping to protect against them, at other times contributing to their predisposition or precipitation. We shall be concerned only with those mechanisms that are of particular importance to an understanding of illness.

Denial is a mechanism by which experiences or feelings that might cause anxiety are denied, or are prevented from entering conscious awareness:

> *A widow may keep all her late husband's personal possessions intact, cook meals for him, and anxiously await his return: she is said to be denying his death.*

Patients who have been told by their doctors that they have malignant disease may afterwards not remember that they have been told and behave as though they are certain of recovery: they have *denied* the information.

Projection

Projection is a process by which your own feelings or impulses are attributed to others:

For example, Angela Cooper who was experiencing self-doubt, depression and guilt caused by grieving for her grandmother, was unable to accept her boyfriend's assurance of his affection for her and instead accused him of infidelity.

Projection is an important mechanism in paranoid psychoses, which are illnesses in which the patient is convinced that others are persecuting him: his own self-critical feelings are being attributed to others.

Introjection

Introjection is the reverse process, by which aspects of another person may be incorporated into the subject's perception of himself:

A patient may constantly criticize himself for being a failure in life, even though objectively he has done well. His criticism of himself stems from his father's critical attitude towards him which he has now introjected: it has become part of his perception of himself.

Idealization

Idealization is a means by which ambivalent feelings towards another person may be split, so that the bad feelings are denied, or sometimes introjected, and the other person is then regarded as perfect. It is thus a feature of being in love. However, it is also a common feature of morbid grief:

For example, Angela Cooper had a close but extremely ambivalent relationship with her maternal grandmother, being very dependent on her but never able to please her. Following her grandmother's death Angela responded by unconsciously using idealization so that she remembered only her grandmother's good qualities and her own feelings of affection towards her grandmother. Her more negative feelings of anger and resentment were introjected and took the form of ideas of guilt and self-blame: it was no longer her grandmother whom she regarded as at fault, but herself.

Somatization and conversion

The term 'somatization' can be used in a descriptive sense to indicate a psychological disorder presenting primarily with physical symptoms (see p. 234) but can also be used to describe a defence mechanism by which the focus on physical complaints serves to divert the subject from awareness of anxiety-provoking conflicts. Closely associated with this is the concept of conversion. This refers to the process by which the affect caused by a conflict is replaced by (or 'converted' into) a physical symptom. Idealization is also commonly associated with conversion: in extreme cases the patient claims that he has no problem of any kind in his life other than physical illness and if this is cured his life will be perfect in all respects (a truly remarkable state):

An example was a man who had been severely disabled due to headache for 3 years. He insisted that he could not remember any distressing event that occurred in the year prior to the onset of his symptoms. The history from his wife revealed that during that year he had experienced the bereavement of his father, a brother and his closest friend, and had been so distressed that he could not attend the funerals.

Dissociation

Dissociation is a defence mechanism that involves the splitting of two (or more) mental processes that would otherwise be integrated, one part then becoming unconscious. The splitting of conscious awareness is thought to result in such phenomena as **hysterical amnesia** or **fugue states** in which highly organized behaviours are carried out despite gross disturbance of memory or grasp of the environment. These symptoms are typical of what are now termed **dissociative** and **conversion disorders** (see p. 240), and were previously called 'hysterical neuroses'.

Example of aetiology

Now let's return to Angela Cooper for an example of how to write an account of aetiological factors:

Angela Cooper appears to be predisposed to the development of emotional problems that include depression, self-harm and alcohol misuse, due to a family history of depressive disorder in her mother, and to her own childhood experiences of physical abuse and emotional turmoil within the family. She developed an over-dependent relationship with her grandmother who was nevertheless emotionally withholding, and this made her particularly vulnerable to her loss. The present illness appears to have been precipitated by the death of her grandmother 18 months ago and exacerbated by the end of her relationship 6 months ago.

Notice that these factors are not independent. Angela's early experiences of physical abuse and insecure emotional attachment in childhood predisposed her to having difficulty in making satisfactory relationships in her adult life. The relationship with her grandmother makes her particularly vulnerable to her loss, and her reaction to this loss probably contributed to the deterioration in her relationship with her boyfriend. She projected her feeling of insecurity into the relationship and accused him of infidelity. Subsequently he did indeed have an affair and then ended their engagement, which precipitated a further worsening of her condition.

This example demonstrates another feature in the aetiology of mental illness: the interaction of **nature** and **nurture**. To some extent Angela's predisposition to depressive disorder may be genetically determined (suggested by the family history – her mother has also suffered from depression), although social and psychological factors have also played their part.

7   INVESTIGATIONS

After dealing with biological investigations, this chapter includes an important section on how to deal with suicide, self-harm and aggression.

HOW TO PLAN INVESTIGATIONS

It is best to plan the investigations methodically. First consider whether it is necessary to get further information about the history and then remember the familiar categories of **biological**, **psychological** and **social** factors. *Table 7.1* shows some examples of the commoner investigations that are needed together with some of their indications. As usual, this is only a guide: it is not intended to provide an exhaustive list of all possible investigations. Now let's find out how to apply this procedure: back to Angela Cooper.

*First consider the **history**. We already have an independent account from Angela's mother – but as her mother has emphasized the importance of the death of Angela's grandmother more than Angela herself in her account and indicated Angela's alcohol consumption might be more than two glasses of wine each night it would be helpful to talk to a close friend with Angela's permission. It would also be helpful to obtain Angela's previous records from her contact with child psychiatric services and her mother's previous psychiatric records.*

*Next we have to sort out the **differential diagnosis**. The likely diagnosis is depressive illness, but there is also a question of associated alcohol misuse and an episode of recent self-harm. **Biological** investigation will certainly have to include physical examination, liver function tests and full blood count. As we examine Angela we find small scars in her upper arms, indicating where she may have injured herself.*

*At this stage **social investigations** do not seem to be indicated.*

***Psychological investigations** might include serial observations of her mood and other aspects of the mental state, and if she is an in-patient we will want to ask the nurses to observe the daily pattern of her mood, sleep and appetite and to keep a weight chart. This will help to confirm the presence of depressive illness as the preferred diagnosis. Later on these will also provide a base line for assessment of change in response to treatment. Further*

Table 7.1 *Examples of investigations*

1. *History*

Always at least one additional **informant**, but sometimes others.
Include employers or teachers if likely to be useful (*with patient's consent*).
Patient's past **general medical and psychiatric records**, and information from general practitioner.
Relative's medical records, if there is positive family history of mental illness.

2. *Biological*

Includes any necessary assessment of physical disease (whether or not related to the mental state) including:
   Physical examination (if not yet done).
   Haematology: e.g. ESR or plasma viscosity, white cell count in infections.
   Biochemistry: liver function tests – alcoholism; thyroid function tests – hyperthyroidism; electrolytes – delirium or anorexia nervosa.
   Bacteriology, virology, serology: for urinary tract infection, herpes zoster, neurosyphilis.
   Electroencephalogram: epilepsy, delirium, dementia.
   Radiology: CT scan – dementia or space-occupying lesion, MRI scan if suspected demyelinating or vascular lesion.

3. *Social*

Assessment of family members: by interview (alone or with patient) to see what they are like and how they relate to each other.
Home assessment: (if necessary) by psychiatric social worker or others to determine adequacy of accommodation and services and home atmosphere.
Financial assessment: (if appropriate) balance of family income from all sources, expenses and debts.
Occupational: by occupational therapist, to determine nature and severity of disablement, in self care or employment.

4. *Psychological*

Exploratory psychotherapy (see p. 213)
Standardized psychometric tests: organic psychosyndromes, mood disorders.
Behavioural assessment: to identify maladaptive behaviours and their environmental reinforcers, e.g. in agoraphobia or obsessive compulsive disorder.

interviews with Angela in order to explore her early family relationships and in particular her relationship with her grandmother and her reaction to the grandmother's death may help to confirm their central importance as **aetiological factors** *(and may also be therapeutic).*

So far we have seen in the earlier chapters that the data collected from the history and mental state examination are used to formulate hypotheses about the differential diagnosis and aetiology. The next logical step is to start to test these hypotheses by planning the investigations. These provide additional data that will either support or fail to support our initial hypotheses.

The **purpose** of investigations can be summarized as follows:

1. To support the preferred **diagnosis** if possible and rule out the alternatives.
2. To confirm the identified **aetiological factors** if possible or, if this is obscure, collect new data that will lead to new hypotheses about aetiology.

3. To assess **change**, e.g. to monitor progress in response to treatment.
4. To assess likely response to treatment.

The investigations are therefore planned for each patient according to their particular needs. There are no 'routine' investigations. In this chapter we will consider how to plan investigations and then go on to describe a few special procedures that the young doctor should know about. Investigations that are particularly relevant to individual diagnostic categories are noted in Part 2.

Although in many branches of medicine it is customary to think of investigations mainly as those sources of data derived from laboratory or radiological procedures, in psychiatry we also include all additional sources of information that are required after the initial history and mental state examination. For example, these will include interviews with other informants, examination of past medical records, in-patient observations of mood, sleep pattern and weight chart, or a home assessment.

You will already be familiar with most of the physical investigations that may be needed but a number of procedures mentioned above will almost certainly be new. However, the following procedures require further explanation.

THE FAMILY TREE

When there is a possibility that a patient is suffering from a familial disorder (genetic or otherwise), it is often helpful to draw up a family tree. The data is gathered from interviews with the patient and relatives. It can be supplemented, if thought necessary, from hospital and general practice health records and from death certificates. It should include all consanguinous relatives for whom accurate data is available.

Figure 7.1 is an example for a patient, Jane Smith, aged 43, who has been referred on account of memory difficulties and involuntary movements. It illustrates the spread of a disorder through a family in a manner consistent with autosomal dominant inheritance. The following conventions are used:

- The **patient**, Jane Smith is indicated with an arrow.
- **Marriages** are joined by horizontal lines, e.g. Simon Smith and Ellen.
- A **marriage ended by death** can be indicated by a double sloping line, e.g. John Smith and Mary.
- A **marriage ended by divorce** can be indicated by a double cross, e.g. William and Elizabeth Morris
- **Children** are shown joined to parents by vertical lines and siblings to each other (in chronological order) by horizontal lines.
- **Abortions and still births** are included, as shown for Mary Smith's first two pregnancies.
- **Twins** are indicated by a vertical line that branches at an acute angle, e.g. Keith and Lawrence Morris.
- For each person the year of birth (and death) is shown.

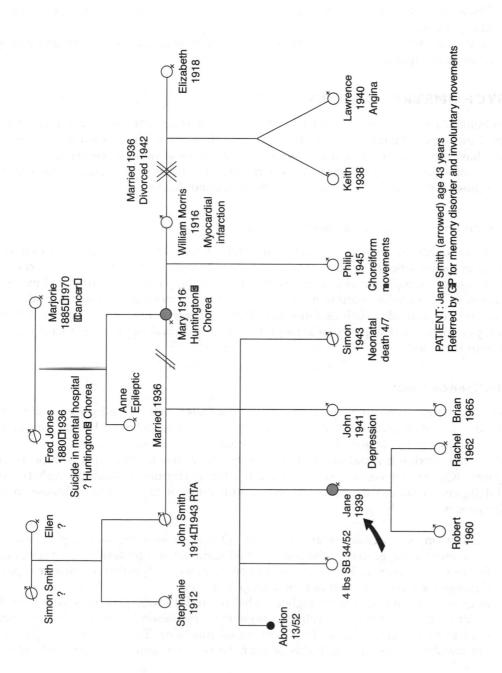

Figure 7.1 *Example of a family tree*

- **Death** is also indicated by a sloping line through the idiogram, e.g. Simon Smith, Fred Jones, and the cause of death is given.
- Important illnesses are also shown for living relatives.
- Those with illnesses (possibly) related to that of the patient are shown by a shaded idiogram, e.g. Fred Jones, Mary, Jane and Phillip.
- Any other information that might be useful can be added such as place and date of birth or occupation.

PSYCHOMETRIC TESTING

Psychologists have devised standardized tests to measure virtually every conceivable aspect of human thought and behaviour. Although many of these, such as personality tests, have no place in clinical psychiatry, others make a valuable contribution to the process of assessment; particularly in differentiating patients with organic brain disease from those with affective disorders or without mental illness.

Assessment of cerebral organic disease

Many standardized tests are available to detect deterioration in brain functions that occurs in the presence of organic disorders. Some of these are designed to assess specific functions, for example the visual–spatial functions of the parietal lobe or visual memory function of the non-dominant temporal lobe. Others are more general and include tests of a range of aptitudes such as those found in intelligence tests. While you are doing your psychiatry clerkship, try to arrange to watch a clinical psychologist carrying out some of these tests.

Intelligence tests

The most widely used intelligence test is the **Wechsler Adult Intelligence Scale**. This provides an intelligence quotient (IQ), in which the scores obtained by the subject are expressed as a percentage of the mean scores obtained by the samples on which the tests are standardized. It is usual to sub-divide the test score results and express these as two separate IQs, one for verbal tests and the other for 'performance' (i.e. non-verbal) tests.

Intelligence tests can contribute to the identification of organic brain disease in the following ways:

1. Testing on one occasion may reveal an IQ that is well below the past level of attainment as suggested by the history of educational and professional achievement. For example, an overall IQ of 100 would be definitely suggestive of possible organic damage for a physicist but not for a shop assistant.
2. A gross disparity between a higher verbal IQ and a lower performance IQ (in the order of 20 or more) is suggestive of organic deterioration because verbal functions tend to be preserved longer than non-verbal functions. The reverse discrepancy is not usually of significance in this respect. Tests of vocabulary are particularly well

preserved in early organic damage, and are therefore sometimes used to estimate premorbid ability.

3. Repetition of intelligence tests over a period of months or years may show a deterioration that usually provides a much better guide to the effects of organic cerebral disease than tests on a single occasion.

Mood assessments

Mood assessments are based on standardized self-rating questionnaires such as the **Beck Depression Inventory (BDI)** or the **State-Trait Anxiety Inventory (STAI)**, which can be easily administered and scored. However they are not diagnostic instruments: for example the BDI can provide a measure of the severity of depressive symptoms, but cannot differentiate between the affective symptoms that may occur in the setting of a depressive illness, dementia or schizophrenia. It does not take into account objective signs of illness but is based on the patient's subjective experience. It does not differentiate between mood 'state' and 'trait', although the STAI does attempt to do this. Despite these limitations they provide a useful measure, particularly if administered repeatedly in order to assess change, for example to monitor the response to treatment. In primary settings the **Personal Health Questionnaire (PHQ-9)** is now widely used for this purpose (see 'Further reading' for how to obtain), and in general hospital settings the **Hospital Anxiety and Depression Scale (HAD)** or the **General Health Questionnaire (GHQ-12)** is often used. Mood scales are also available for both depression and mania based on observations by the nurses looking after the patient.

THE ELECTROENCEPHALOGRAM (EEG)

This is essentially a voltmeter that measures changes in potential transmitted from the brain to the scalp. Electrodes (usually 8 or 16) are placed bilaterally on the scalp in standard positions, and simultaneous tracings are made on a polygraph. The healthy adult, relaxed, awake and with eyes closed, shows a characteristic **alpha rhythm** of about 10 cycles per second and low frequency. On opening the eyes, or with increased mental activity, the tracing flattens. The records of young children normally show **delta waves**, which are much slower (less than 4 cycles per second) and of greater amplitude. During adolescence these are replaced by **theta waves** (4 to 7 cycles per second). These slow waves are not usually present in the adult except during sleep.

The most valuable contribution of the EEG is in the diagnosis of **epilepsy**. 'Spikes' (brief high amplitude discharges) or 'sharp waves' (more prolonged but also high amplitude) are characteristic. Alternating spikes and delta waves at 3 cycles per second are a classic feature of generalized absence attacks.

The EEG may be a valuable adjunct in identifying the presence of organic brain disease. In delirium there is usually an irregular slow wave pattern. In dementia the most useful findings are the loss of normal alpha activity and the emergence of delta activity in the waking state. These changes also tend to occur gradually in the normally ageing brain, so they have to be interpreted with care. Negative findings do not exclude the possibility of organic disease, but a grossly abnormal record is very highly suggestive. It can therefore be valuable in helping to differentiate between dementia and depressive pseudo-dementia, particularly as it is relatively cheap, non-invasive and painless. The EEG can also be useful in helping to localize a lesion because the abnormal findings may then be limited to tracings from a few leads rather than appearing as a generalized abnormality. A major limitation is the non-specific nature of the abnormal findings, which tend to be similar regardless of the underlying pathology.

BRAIN IMAGING

Brain imaging can be divided into **structural**, where brain structure is shown, and **functional**, where regional brain activity is seen. There are two forms of structural brain imaging in common clinical use. **Computed tomography (CT)** gives a picture of the head in terms of its X-ray density. This means that it is good for showing bony and calcified structures, but less good for showing soft tissue structure of the brain itself. The main structures that can be seen are the interfaces between fluid and brain tissue in terms of the brain ventricles and the cerebrospinal fluid over the surface of the brain. Both these are enlarged in progressive dementias. A straightforward CT scan of the head takes about 15 minutes but involves exposure to ionizing radiation. **Magnetic resonance imaging (MRI)** gives a picture based on the proton density of tissues. This equates to water content, and so soft tissue structures can be differentiated much better than with CT, which can show demyelinating lesions, congenital deformities and ischemic damage. It gives a high resolution picture of white matter, grey matter and the ventricular system. MRI involves no ionizing radiation and is safe. However, it involves being enclosed in a smaller space than for a CT scan and can be unnerving. Usually, neither procedure involves an injection. In psychiatry CT or MRI scanning is indicated in new cases of dementia, new cases of psychosis, and atypical presentations of severe depression or cognitive deficits in adult life.

Functional brain imaging usually involves the visualization of regional blood flow, which increases significantly a few seconds after a particular area of the brain becomes active. A version of MRI, called functional MRI, can do this. Alternatively, there are techniques such as single photon (computed) emission tomography (SPECT or SPET) and positron emission tomography (PET), which use radioactive isotopes to look at brain blood flow, or to image metabolism or receptor activity. These functional techniques are important research tools but have no widespread clinical application in psychiatry at present.

THE CONTRIBUTION OF OTHER PARAMEDICAL WORKERS

Social workers (SWs)

SWs have special training in the management of the mentally ill and their families. They contribute to the social aspects of assessment and treatment with regard to material welfare such as financial status and living conditions; the impact of the mentally ill and their families on each other; and the patient's social interactions, sources of support, and satisfaction. In addition some social workers have **approved social worker** status, which carries particular responsibilities with regard to the Mental Health Act (1983) (see p. 364).

SWs may contribute to assessment, for example by interviewing family members to collect additional histories or to assess the attitudes of the relatives to the patient; or by carrying out a home assessment to determine the adequacy of material resources and to observe the nature of family relationships within the home environment.

Psychiatric nurses

Psychiatric nurses have received special training in mental nursing and play a major part in the care of severely ill patients. It is unwise to judge patients entirely on what you observe at interview: the nurses observe the patient closely for long periods of time in a variety of settings, and regularly provide invaluable additional information about patients. They are responsible for administering medications and they participate in group therapy on the ward as well as providing intensive care for individual patients. **Community psychiatric nurses** are trained to provide nursing care in people's homes.

Occupational therapists

OTs have special skills in the management of disability in the mentally ill. They help those with acute illnesses to regain their self-confidence and to interact with others. They discover a patient's assets and exploit them, as well as helping patients to cope with disabilities. They may be involved in the assessment of 'activities of daily living', which include the essentials of self-care such as washing, dressing, cooking and the use of public services; in the assessment of work, leisure, and recreational activities; and in the assessment of psychological problems through the use of 'projective techniques' such as art and drama. The contribution of OTs is particularly valuable in the rehabilitation of those with chronic disorders, and much useful work can be done by 'community OTs' developing rehabilitation programmes in their patients' homes.

FURTHER READING

The Personal Health Questionnaire (PHQ-9) can be downloaded and *used free of charge* from http://www.depression-primarycare.org/clinicians/toolkits/materials/forms/phq9/

8   TREATMENT

Treatment in psychiatry should always be considered under the headings **physical**, **psychological** and **social**. This may seem different to treatments in general medicine but the example of epilepsy will serve to illustrate the model.

- **Physical**: anticonvulsants, and folic acid if necessary.
- **Psychological**: supportive psychotherapy and reassurance about the diagnosis and its implications; advice about avoiding stressful situations and alcohol if these precipitate fits; appropriate treatment for depression or anxiety if these occur.
- **Social**: counselling the patient about employment, driving, marriage and having children, helping the family coping with the epileptic fits. The person may require being registered as disabled.

Doctors vary in their inclination to regard the psychological and social aspects of treatment as important. For example, anxiety, depression and sexual problems frequently follow mastectomy and can respond to appropriate treatment. However, some surgeons are more likely than others to detect and treat these symptoms among patients who have undergone the operation. We give separate accounts of physical treatments and psychological treatments.

Negotiating the management plan

The ideal management plan is one that reflects current best evidence on treatment, is tailored to the situation and preferences of the patient, and addresses emotional and social issues. Both patient and doctor should be involved in developing the plan, although one or the other may have the greater input depending on the nature of the problem and the inclinations of the patient (see *Box 8.1*).

PHYSICAL TREATMENTS: DRUGS

History

The use of medications to treat mental illness and behavioural disturbance is described from the beginning of history, for example in the famous Ebers papyrus (1550 BC), and

86

Box 8.1 Negotiating a management plan

Ascertain expectations
- What does patient know?
- What does patient want? – Investigation? Management? A particular outcome?

Advise on options
- Elicit patient's preferences

Develop a plan
- Involve patient
- Tailor preferred option to patient's needs and situation

Check understanding
- Ensure that patient is clear about plan
- Consider a written summary

Advise on contingency management
- What should patient do if things do not go according to plan?
- Agree arrangements for follow-up and review

---

occurs in all cultures. Various plant products have sedative effects that would have been useful in the past in calming disturbance in the short-term, but curative treatments are relatively recent – the first antipsychotics and antidepressants were discovered by chance about 50 years ago. In fact the main classes emerged in part from observing the effect of changing the structure of antihistamine drugs. Indeed, it has taken several decades to design out the sedative antihistamine effect of some drugs used in psychiatry.

Classification

There are five main groups of drugs used in the treatment of mental illness and they are defined by their effectiveness in four broad categories of mental illness:

1. **Antipsychotics** are effective in the treatment of schizophrenia and mania.
2. **Antidepressants** are effective in the treatment of depression, but they are also effective in the treatment of anxiety states, somatization disorder and obsessional compulsive disorder (the neuroses in old terminology).
3. **Mood stabilizers** for preventing relapse in bipolar affective disorder.
4. **Anxiolytics** for treating anxiety.
5. **Cognitive enhancers** for the treatment of dementia. In addition, drugs active at the benzodiazepine binding site of the GABA-A receptor have useful short-term sedative (calming), hypnotic (sleep-promoting) and anxiolytic effects. They are also anticonvulsants.

Golden rules of good prescribing

CHOOSE ON THE BASIS OF THE EVIDENCE

Drug companies have to satisfy stringent government regulatory requirements in demonstrating that a drug works in its indicated condition better than a matching placebo (dummy) treatment under double-blind multi-centre conditions over the short term (usually 6–8 weeks) and in the long term, typically 6–12 months. However, trials of treatments known to be effective sometimes fail to show it – for reasons that are not always known. This has two implications. One is that it is wise to include an effective treatment (positive control) in a new clinical trial so that if the new drug fails, researchers can know whether this is because of a genuine lack of effect or a failure of the trial itself. The second implication is that it is important to consider the results of all clinical trials in evaluating efficacy, and statistically this can be done with a formal procedure called meta-analysis.

In the UK the government has set up the National Institute for Clinical Excellence (NICE), which issues regular guidelines about optimal treatment of all medical disorders in all modalities including drugs. The judgements are based on meta-analysis of available clinical trials. Good medical practice requires that doctors read the guidelines. They are not legally binding but there should be positive and recorded reasons for deviation from them.

Clinical trials cannot cover all contingencies, especially concerning the effectiveness of combining treatments, and here we rely on less certain assessments of effectiveness, where elements of the ideal trial are missing such as a placebo group, random allocation, blind raters or large-sized treatment groups. Case-reports of a small number of patients treated are the weakest component of the evidence-base. Choosing solely on the basis of personal experience of one or two successes has no rational basis because the placebo response rate is very great even in severe psychiatric illness.

ADEQUATE DOSE AND ADEQUATE DURATION

Antipsychotics and antidepressants take weeks to exert their full effects, and it is important to ensure that the treatment has been given in a full therapeutic dose for a sufficient time before concluding that there is lack of efficacy requiring a change in treatment. Often in reviewing patients who seem resistant to treatment, it turns out that basic treatments have not been tried at a therapeutic dose, or that it has not been sustained for long enough. Where an acute effect is required, it is important to know how rapidly drugs are absorbed by different routes of administration, and how rapidly they are eliminated, so that doses are not administered so rapidly that the delayed cumulative dose dangerously overshoots safe levels.

MONOTHERAPY AND RATIONAL POLYPHARMACY

Where a treatment has reached recommended limits and there has been no recovery, there is sometimes a temptation to add a different drug that works in the same way as the current treatment. This can be dangerous because excessive action at a receptor can have toxic effects – for example two antipsychotics each at a sub-therapeutic dose could cause severe Parkinsonian rigidity because of excessive dopamine receptor blockade. Furthermore, the risk of causing pharmaco-kinetic interaction is obviously increased by polypharmacy. Nevertheless, it may be necessary to treat some patients with more than one drug and there are established combinations with a clear pharmacological rationale and demonstrated efficacy. For example, the addition of lithium to an antidepressant can sometimes complete a partial recovery.

BE AWARE OF DRUG INTERACTIONS

Drugs are often metabolized by the liver through the cytochrome P450 (CYP450) system. Different drugs are preferentially metabolized by one or more of the five main P450 isoenzymes. Some drugs inhibit the activity of particular isoenzymes, and so inhibit the metabolism of other drugs, which then accumulate to high concentrations producing toxicity even at therapeutic doses. In psychiatry the main P450 inhibitors are the serotonin-selective re-uptake inhibitor (SSRI) antidepressant drugs, notably fluoxetine and paroxetine. Co-prescribing them can inhibit the metabolism of some calcium channel blockers and of older antidepressant drugs, which may then cause toxicity. This is one of the main arguments for avoiding polypharmacy. It is difficult to remember such interactions, therefore interactions should always be checked, for example, in the back of the British National Formulary or an accessible website.

KNOW THE SIDE-EFFECTS AND REPORT NEW ONES

It is important to be aware of side-effects the patient may experience so that they can be warned. An unexpected minor and harmless side-effect can cause alarm that the drug is having a toxic effect and so the patient stops taking it (non-compliance or non-adherence). Some side-effects are rare and only emerge after the drug has been in use for some time. Any unexpected side-effect should be reported to the Medicines and Healthcare Products Regulatory Agency (www.mhra.gov.uk) using the 'Yellow Card' scheme. Patients can also complete a yellow card. This post-marketing surveillance has detected many unexpected adverse effects of drugs that have then been withdrawn.

INVOLVE THE PATIENT

It is important that drug treatment is discussed with patients and that they join in decision-making. They need to be aware of side-effects and what the target symptoms and expected benefits are. All too often, patients know nothing about their drug treatment and so cannot provide important information to the doctor when they require further or new medical treatment. Furthermore, the patient's experience of the benefits and side-effects of previous treatments can be an important guide for future episodes of their disorder. Patients will often check what is prescribed on the internet and this can be seriously misleading; involving the patient can counteract such misunderstandings.

RECORD THE TREATMENT AND MONITOR THE OUTCOME

When deciding what to prescribe, it is vital that the effectiveness and side-effects of previous treatments are assessed to ensure that previously ineffective, unpleasant or even dangerous treatments are not prescribed. A record should be made of recommended treatment in the same place as each mental state examination is recorded, together with an assessment of the response to previous treatment. In this way, a retrospective assessment of previous treatment response can be made at any time in the future in order to guide future treatment.

1. Antipsychotic drugs

CLASSIFICATION

Antipsychotics improve symptoms of psychosis – hallucinations, delusions and thought disorder in schizophrenia and bipolar disorder – and can help treat symptoms resulting from organic causes. Two obsolete synonyms for 'antipsychotic' are still occasionally used. The term 'neuroleptic' was coined by Delay and Deniker in 1952, who were struck by the then revolutionary ability of the drugs to cause calming and indifference without sedation. The term is outmoded because modern antipsychotics do not cause indifference. Antipsychotics are sometimes called 'major tranquillizers' but this belies their therapeutic actions in reversing psychotic symptoms rather than simply suppressing them.

A classification of antipsychotic drugs is shown in *Table 8.1*. Classification based on chemical structure has little utility because structure does not predict characteristic actions. They can be divided into older and newer drugs. Some older drugs are still in use because they have been safely and widely used for many years. Their main side-effects are acute dystonias and Parkinsonism (tremor, rigidity) known as extrapyramidal symptoms (EPS). Newer antipsychotics have been developed that lack EPS, and they have been termed 'atypical antipsychotic drugs' in distinction from the older, typical agents. Meta-analyses and recent naturalistic clinical trials suggest there is little to choose between antipsychotics in terms of their efficacy or their tolerability, despite the greater EPS tendency with typicals. One explanation is that the lack of EPS with atypicals is offset by greater side-effects of sedation and weight-gain associated with some of the atypicals.

The drug **clozapine** stands out from the others because it is the only one that has been shown to be effective where other antipsychotic drugs have been ineffective. Because it can cause fatal bone marrow depression, it can only be dispensed if the patient and the psychiatrist are first registered with the Central Patient Monitoring Service or equivalent organization. Each week's medication is dispensed only when a blood test has been received by the Monitoring Service. Treatment is stopped if white cells decline in three successive samples.

DOPAMINE RECEPTOR BLOCKADE

Antipsychotics of different classes have a common mode of action: they block post-synaptic dopamine receptors. Resperpine and tetrabenazine were occasionally used to

Table 8.1 *A classification of old and new antipsychotic drugs*

D2 receptor occupancy in basal ganglia at effective doses	Proper name	UK trade name	Comment
Older 'typical' antipsychotics			
High	Chlorpromazine	Largactil	Phenothiazine
	Trifluoperazine	Stelazine	
High	Haloperiodol	Haldol	Butyrophenone
High	Flupenthixol	Depixol	Thioxanthene
	Zuclopenthixol	Acuphase	
Newer 'atypical' antipsychotics			
Low	Clozapine	Clozaril	Dibenzodiazepine
Low	Quetiapine	Seroquel	
Medium	Olanzapine	Zyprexa	Sublingual preparation Available for rapid action
High	Sulpiride	Dolmatil	Substituted benzamides
	Amisulpride	Solian	
High	Risperidone	Risperdal	Depot preparation available
High	Aripiprazole	Abilify	Possible partial agonist

treat resistant psychosis but are of historical and pharmacological interest only – they block dopamine neurotransmission by depleting presynaptic dopamine nerve terminals. PET imaging studies consistently report that in living patients during psychosis there is more dopamine in dopamine synapses. Thus antipsychotics appear to work by blocking a disease-related pathological increase in dopamine neurotransmission.

The effects of antipsychotics are related to the four areas of the brain where dopaminergic synapses, and thus dopamine receptors, are located:

1. *Limbic system and neocortex*: Dopamine-containing neurones in the midbrain project to the limbic system ('mesolimbic pathway') and to some areas of the prefrontal cortex ('mesocortical pathway'). It is believed that the blockade of dopamine receptors at these sites is the basis of the antipsychotic effect for all antipsychotics, including the high potency second-generation antipsychotics. However, clozapine and quetiapine have a strikingly low affinity for the dopamine receptor and they are able to exert antipsychotic effects while occupying a much smaller proportion of dopamine receptors (< 50 per cent) than the 70 per cent occupancy necessary for older antipsychotic drugs to work. This property of the drugs is not understood.
2. *Striatum*: Dopamine-containing neurones in the pars compacta of the substantia nigra project to the striatum ('nigro-striatal pathway'). Blockade of striatal dopamine receptors is thought to be responsible for EPS. Atypical antipsychotic drugs are much less likely to cause EPS than the older drugs. This is not surprising in the case of clozapine and quetiapine because they are weak dopamine blockers. However, risperidone and aripiprazole occupy just as high a proportion of dopamine receptors

as older drugs, yet cause much less EPS. It may be that special 5HT antagonist actions of the drugs may offset their dopamine receptor blockade. Aripiprazole may cause weak activation of the dopamine receptors it occupies (partial agonism) that is just sufficient to prevent EPS while blocking the effect of high dopamine levels in psychosis. EPS do begin to appear at high doses of the second-generation antipsychotics, except for clozapine and quetiapine.

3. *Hypothalamus*: Dopamine-containing neurones in the arcuate nucleus of the hypothalamus release dopamine into the portal veins that drain to the anterior pituitary, where dopamine inhibits the release of prolactin. A common effect of new or old high-potency antipsychotics is therefore hyperprolactinaemia. This in turn causes amenorrhoea in female patients and troublesome gynaecomastia and lactation in both sexes. Aripiprazole causes prolactin levels to fall and this is one of the main reasons to think the drug may cause a slight stimulation of the dopamine receptors it occupies.

4. *Brain stem*: Dopamine receptors have been identified in an area of the lower brain stem that lies outside the blood–brain barrier in the chemoreceptor trigger zone. Neurones in this area project to the dorsal nucleus of the vagus, and their stimulation can result in vomiting. It is believed that the anti-emetic effect of antipsychotics is based on the blockade of dopamine receptors in the chemoreceptor trigger zone.

SIDE-EFFECTS

Dopaminergic effects

Anticholinergic drugs are effective in the treatment and prevention of acute dystonias and Parkinsonian side-effects. In addition to EPS, long-term use of typical antipsychotics is associated with a significant risk of tardive dyskinesia. This typically involves buccolingual masticatory movements, but may involve twitches and a wide variety of other involuntary bodily movements. Anticholinergics are ineffective but the symptoms can slowly resolve on clozapine and possibly other atypical antipsychotics. The **neuroleptic malignant syndrome** is a rare but serious side-effect that can occur at any stage of treatment, especially if there is rapid escalation of dosage. It is characterized by extreme muscle rigidity and hyperthermia. It requires intensive specialist treatment with a dopamine agonist such as oral bromocriptine or subcutaneous apomorphine if the patient is unable to swallow.

Non-dopaminergic side-effects

Older antipsychotic drugs had side-effects because of various pharmacological actions, including anticholinergic effects – dry mouth causing tooth-decay, aggravation of glaucoma, urinary retention, confusion; anti-noradrenaline effects – postural hypotension, impotence, sedation; antihistamine – sedation and weight gain; anti-5HT effects – weight gain. Clozapine shares many of these actions.

92

Some atypical antipsychotic drugs are potent 5HT and histamine receptor antagonists and this is thought to be responsible for the risk of very marked weight gain that can occur in some individuals on any antipsychotic but olanzapine.

Metabolic syndrome

The metabolic syndrome includes abdominal obesity, insulin resistance/glucose intolerance, hypertension, and dyslipidaemia. When found in combination, and with smoking, these factors increase the risk of cardiovascular disease by up to five times. They are common in schizophrenia, probably as part of the disorder, possibly a result of common genetic mechanisms but certainly considerably exacerbated by antipsychotic drugs. No antipsychotic should be regarded as free from this risk, but clozapine and olanzapine are associated with greatest risk. It is important that these parameters are actively monitored and that appropriate preventative steps are taken – patients with schizophrenia are much less likely than the general population to access healthcare or to have their physical symptoms recognized and treated.

INDICATIONS

Rapid calming of agitated patients

During acute psychotic episodes behaviour can be very agitated and disturbed because of the content of hallucinations and delusions. There may be ceaseless overactivity and violence to others and to the self. Rapid calming, commonly called rapid tranquillization, requires rapid sedation together with a rapid antipsychotic action. Rapid tranquillization algorithms often combine a benzodiazepine such as lorazepam and a rapidly absorbed antipsychotic drug. The antipsychotic may be administered orally, intramuscularly or intravenously. The sublingual preparation of olanzapine is also a convenient and rapid method that combines sedation and antipsychotic action. Zuclopenthixol comes in a depot form (Acuphase) that can be repeated daily for 3 days. The last dose lasts a week, at which time a longer acting depot can be given.

Treatment of acute psychotic states

In the first episode of schizophrenia, the NICE guidelines recommend oral medication with an atypical antipsychotic amisulpride, olanzapine, quetiapine, risperidone or zotepine because the risk of serious EPS is minimal. Marked dystonic reactions can occur with typical antipsychotic drugs, usually early in treatment, and this is an unpleasant introduction to drug therapy that can generate a long-term negative attitude to treatment that can drastically interfere with adherence.

If the response is unsatisfactory and the patient is taking the medication, it is probably wise to ensure he or she has tried an atypical with high-potency at the D2 receptor, such as risperidone or amisulpride. The NICE guidelines recommend the early introduction of clozapine after two failed trials with antipsychotics from two different families.

Table 8.2 *Side-effects of neuroleptics*

Central side-effects

extrapyramidal syndromes	Parkinsonism	Hypokinesia, rigidity, and tremor (alleviated by centrally acting anticholinergic drugs)
	Akathisia	'Inability to sit still', inner restlessness and compensatory foot-shuffling
	Acute dystonic reactions; coculogyric crises	Spastic contractions of the muscles of the neck and shoulders; relieved by an injection of procyclidine
	Tardive dyskinesia (late onset)	Orofacial dyskinesia Whole body chorea
	Neuroleptic malignant syndrome	Rigidity, hyperpyrexia, and coma (extreme dopamine receptor blockade: potentially lethal) treat with bromocriptine (dopamine receptor stimulant) and dantrolene (muscle relaxant)
lowering of the seizure threshold	fits	

Central autonomic side-effects

	Thermoregulatory failure	Body cools in cold temperature → dangerous hypothermia; in heat → heat stroke
	Orthostatic hypotension	Partly central origin (see below)
Endocrine complications	Hyperprolactinaemia	Galactorrhea, gynaecomastia, impotence and infertility
	Reduction in gonadotrophins, oestrogens and progesterone	Amenorrhoea and infertility
Psychiatric complications	Apathy, lassitude, lack of initiative	(Like chronic schizophrenia!)
	Disturbance of the sleep/wakefulness cycle	
	Depression	
	Acute brain syndrome ('atropine psychosis)	Esp. potent anticholinergic drugs (like thioridazine)

continues

Table 8.2 *(continued)*

Peripheral autonomic side-effects (phenothiazines > butyrophenones)		
	Blockade of muscarinic receptors	cycloplegia, dry mouth, constipation, urinary retention.
	Blockade of α_1 adrenoceptors	Miosis, orthostatic hypotension, nasal stuffiness, ejaculatory incompetence
Hypersensitivity reactions		
	Cholestatic jaundice	
	Blood dyscrasias	Agranulocytosis
	Allergic skin reactions	Urticaria, dermatitis
Skin reactions		
	Contact dermatitis	Affects nurses handling phenothiazine solutions
	Photosensitivity	Problem in sunny climates
	Patchy hyper-pigmentation (long-term medication)	
Drug interactions		
	Blockade of uptake of drug into peripheral noradrenergic neurones	Inhibition of the anti-hypertensive effect of guanethidine
		Potentiation of the effects of sedative drugs (including ethanol and opiates)

Maintenance treatment

Schizophrenia is a chronic and recurrent condition. However, the prognosis is generally good if there is good adherence to an agreed maintenance treatment. A psychotic relapse is very costly in terms of impaired social and occupational functioning. It is harmful to attempt slow withdrawal of an effective treatment or to have drug holidays because even with immediate treatment of the earliest signs of relapse, there is a very substantial risk of full-blown relapse. Of course the wishes of the patient must be respected, but sometimes maintenance treatment can be enforced where it is known that a patient is at serious risk of harm to self or others while psychotic. The side-effects and drug interactions of antipsychotics are shown in *Table 8.2*.

2. Antidepressant drugs

CLASSIFICATION AND MONOAMINE THEORY

All antidepressant drugs work by increasing the synaptic actions of the monoamine neurotransmitters 5HT (serotonin), noradrenaline and possibly dopamine. They accomplish this in three different ways and this is the basis of their classification. The synaptic actions of monoamines are terminated by a re-uptake or transporter mechanism that takes 90 per cent of monoamine molecules back into the presynaptic nerve terminal from which they were released. Within the terminal, monoamine oxidase removes the amine group and initiates the metabolism of monoamines. The primary actions of the two main antidepressant groups are to inhibit uptake and metabolism of monoamines, thus allowing monoamines to persist in the synaptic cleft. A small third group of drugs have primary actions on monoamine receptors. However, only mirtazepine has significant usage in the UK. Apart from this small group, no new effective ways of treating depression with medication have been devised since the development of uptake inhibitors and MAOIs 50 years ago. The only developments have been in designing more neurochemically selective drugs, safer in overdose, and with more tolerable side-effects.

MONOAMINE RE-UPTAKE INHIBITORS

Pharmacology

The primary pharmacological action is to inhibit the active re-uptake of monoamines back into presynaptic terminals. Re-uptake into nerve terminals is the normal mechanism for eliminating the actions of monoamines that have been released from the terminal into the synaptic cleft. When the re-uptake site is blocked then monoamines accumulate in the synapse. However, it is clear that this cannot be their sole mechanism of action because they are only fully effective after 4–6 weeks of treatment. Monoamine neurones are sensitive to the concentration of monoamines around the terminals and dendrites, which they detect with monoamine receptors on their surface called auto-receptors. Consequently, when extra-cellular concentrations begin to rise as a result of re-uptake blockade, terminal auto-receptors suppress further release of monoamine, and dendritic auto-receptors decrease the firing rate. This effectively neutralizes the increase in synaptic monoamine content. It is thought that auto-receptors may desensitize so that neurones come to tolerate higher concentrations of monoamine in the synapse and around the dendrites. This process of desensitization takes some time and may account for the delayed therapeutic effect of re-uptake inhibitors. In addition to monoamine re-uptake inhibition these drugs antagonize some post-synaptic monoamine receptors including α receptors and some 5HT receptor subtypes. This may be relevant to their therapeutic actions – by correcting imbalances between α and β noradrenergic neurotransmission or between different subtypes of 5HT receptors.

There are three major groups of re-uptake inhibitors: an older group that acts on both noradrenaline and serotonin; a group that predominantly act on noradrenaline; and one that specifically inhibits serotonin.

MIXED MONOAMINE RE-UPTAKE INHIBITORS (MARIs)

Imipramine was the prototype that established the effectiveness of MARIs, and clomipramine and amitriptyline followed soon after. They are still sometimes referred to

Table 8.3 *Pharmacology of side-effects of older antidepressants*

Antagonist action	Side-effects
Acetyl choline (muscarinic) receptor	Dry mouth (secondary tooth decay), urinary retention, constipation, aggravation of glaucoma
Noradrenaline receptor (alpha)	Postural (orthostatic) hypotension (secondary falls and fractures, myocardial infarction, stroke), sexual dysfunction, sedation
Serotonin (5HT) receptor	Weight gain
Histamine receptor	Sedation
Fast sodium channel	Cardiac arrhythmia
Serotonin re-uptake site	Nausea, anorgasmia

as tricyclics because of their three-ring structure. They have prominent anticholinergic, antihistaminic, and antiadrenergic effects (see *Table 8.3*). They can cause arrhythmias in patients with heart disease or in over-dosage. Venlafaxine and duloxetine are newer mixed uptake inhibitors that lack the side-effects and risks of the older drugs, but blood pressure needs to be monitored with venlafaxine treatment. It is clear that MARIs have broader effectiveness than selective uptake inhibitors and should be tried in treatment-resistant patients.

NORADRENALINE RE-UPTAKE INHIBITORS (NARIs)

These drugs were developed to select out the noradrenergic component of the MARIs and lose their side-effects. Prothiaden is an older NARI drug and has the tricyclic structure, side-effect profile and risk. Lofepramine is a newer agent, and the most recent and selective is reboxetine. Neither has appreciable affinity for other receptors but increased noradrenaline function can lead to disturbed sleep and micturition difficulty.

SEROTONIN SPECIFIC RE-UPTAKE INHIBITORS (SSRIs)

This is the youngest class of uptake inhibitors, but even so fluvoxamine was introduced over 20 years ago. The most commonly used are fluoxetine, paroxetine and citalopram together with its optically active isomer, escitalopram. They are almost devoid of other pharmacological actions and lack the side-effects listed in Table 8.3. There are three major side-effects, probably resulting from effects on 5HT function:

- Nausea is quite marked early on in treatment but tends to improve after the first week.
- Failure of orgasm in both males and females.
- In the first week of treatment there may be a transient exacerbation of anxiety and less commonly depression. Rarely, suicidal thinking has been provoked, but there is no evidence that they increase suicidal acts.

97

SSRIs have the important advantage that they alone among the antidepressant drugs do not cause weight gain. They are non-cardiotoxic and safe in over-dosage.

Indications

- NICE recommend **SSRIs** as the first line in treating major depression because of their superior safety and tolerability.
- **Venlafaxine** at full dose may work in depression if 6-8 weeks of an SSRI does not.
- Panic and generalized anxiety disorder are best treated with an **SSRI** initially.

Obsessive-compulsive disorder only responds to antidepressant drugs with a sero-tonergic action, NARIs are ineffective and should not be used.

MONOAMINE OXIDASE INHIBITORS (MAOIs)

Pharmacology

These drugs raise synaptic monoamine content by inhibiting their enzymic degradation by the two isoforms of MAO, MAO-A and B. Older MAO inhibitors (phenelzine, tranylcypromine and isocarboxazid) bind irreversibly to the enzyme. After stopping treatment, MAO remains inhibited because the drugs form a chemical bond with the enzyme. Return of normal activity requires synthesis of new enzyme and transport to the nerve terminal and this takes about 3 weeks. It is therefore dangerous to switch to an uptake inhibitor or to treat with any interacting drug until 3 weeks after cessation of an irreversible MAOI.

Moclobemide is the only competitive and therefore reversible antagonist of MAO. This means that MAO activity returns to normal as soon as the treatment stops and the drug is cleared from the circulation. This allows treatment to be changed to an uptake inhibitor within a day or two of stopping moclobemide. Moclobemide is selective for the MAO-A isoenzyme (older drugs block both MAO-A and B).

Side-effects

The irreversible MAOIs can produce troublesome side-effects, including excessive central stimulation (agitation, hypomania, convulsions); orthostatic hypotension (prob-ably because of sympathetic ganglion blockade); and hepatocellular jaundice (as a rare but severe hypersensitivity reaction).

Hypertensive crises and the cheese effect

Circulating and ingested amines are deaminated by very high levels of MAO in the liver and gut. Irreversible inhibition of both MAO-A and B therefore potentiates the circu-latory effects of drugs and substances that increase the release of monoamines in the periphery. The main risk is from eating tyramine-rich foods because tyramine is an indirectly acting sympathomimetic that releases monoamines from peripheral nerve endings. Furthermore tyramine is normally deaminated in the gut. Other sympathomimetic amines (e.g. phenylephrine) are taken as cold remedies. The potentiation of the effects of sympathomimetic amines can lead to a hypertensive crisis (as in the 'cheese reaction' following the ingestion of tyramine-containing foodstuffs, such as cream cheese, broad beans, pickled herrings, avocado pears, 'Marmite' and Chianti).

Moclobemide is much less likely to cause the cheese effect because it does not block MAO-B which deaminates tyramine. Furthermore, amines at high concentration can compete with the drug for the enzymic site of MAO-A and thus be inactivated.

Indications

- As a second line of treatment in the case of patients whose depression does not respond to treatment with other classes of antidepressant.
- They have been recommended for some atypical forms of depression characterized by features such as hypersomnia, weight gain and personality traits such as being sensitive to rejection by others.
- Phobic anxiety states. Relapse is common on withdrawal of the drug.

MONOAMINE RECEPTOR ACTIVE DRUGS

Pharmacology

Mirtazepine blocks presynaptic α_2 noradrenaline autoreceptors. These receptors sense the concentration of noradrenaline in the synapse to provide negative feedback inhibition of release. Blocking them thus 'fools' neurones into releasing more noradrenaline into the synapse. Increased noradrenaline is also thought to stimulate 5HT neurones, thus the drug may have twin noradrenaline and 5HT enhancing actions. Mirtazepine is also a 5HT2C antagonist and this is a property that seems to augment the antidepressant effect of 5HT release. It probably also contributes to the weight gain seen with the drug. Mirtazepine has sedative properties that can be useful.

Trazodone is a weak SSRI with 5HT2 antagonist properties.

Buspirone is a 5HT1A receptor agonist – it mimics the action of 5HT at the 5HT1A receptor. It was developed as an anxiolytic but it appears to have some antidepressant efficacy. There is weak evidence for its adjunctive use.

Indications

- Mirtazepine is a dual-acting antidepressant like venlafaxine. It is a reasonable first-line treatment when sedation is needed for insomnia or tension. It can be used alone or in conjunction with an uptake inhibitor in treatment-resistant cases.
- Trazodone is used in the elderly to promote sleep but its utility as an antidepressant is in doubt.

- Buspirone is occasionally used, mostly as an augmenting agent added to uptake inhibitors. There little evidence for efficacy.

TRYPTOPHAN

Tryptophan is the amino-acid precursor of 5-hydroxytryptamine. Administration of tryptophan results in increased 5-hydroxytryptamine synthesis in the brain, which in turn would lead to the replenishment of presynaptic stores. Tryptophan has only weak antidepressant properties, and is usually administered as an adjunct to enhance the effectiveness of uptake inhibitors or MAOIs in treatment-resistant depression. Several years ago, an outbreak of a dangerous eosinophilia-myalgia syndrome was attributed to tryptophan. Although the cause was probably a contaminant from a single manufacturer, the drug is only available on a named-patient basis.

MANAGING ANTIDEPRESSANT TREATMENT

The therapeutic effect appears gradually, usually after 1-3 weeks on the drug; therefore in severe retarded or psychotic depression a faster acting treatment, such as ECT, may be more appropriate. It is important to administer a therapeutically effective dose, and plasma level assays may be helpful in dosage selection. Antidepressant medication should be continued after remission of the depressive symptomatology the first 6–12 months following a depressive episode – switching to placebo is associated with 50 per cent relapse rates within 4–6 months. The maintenance dose should be the effective dose; previous practice of using a half dose is now known to be associated with significantly greater relapse rates.

TREATMENT-RESISTANT DEPRESSION

Treatment with re-uptake inhibiting antidepressants should be continued for at least 6 weeks at full dosage to see the full therapeutic effect. If there has been only a partial response, there are four main options:

1. Adding lithium has the strongest evidence-base, but patient acceptability is less.
2. Adding an atypical antipsychotic – quetiapine, olanzapine or risperidone – appears to have clear augmenting effects as well as useful calming and sedative actions.
3. Switch to venlafaxine and increase dose to maximum.
4. Switch to phenelzine and augment as above as necessary – this requires specialist supervision.

The combination of an MAOI, lithium and the 5HT precursor, tryptophan, has been advocated by some authorities. *Table 8.4* shows the main pharmacological effects and side-effects of antidepressant drugs.

100

Table 8.4 *Antidepressant drugs*

Older	Newer (1990s)	Pharmacology and side-effects
Monoamine re-uptake inhibitors		
Mixed uptake inhibitors (MARIs)		
Amitriptyline	Venlafaxine	Older ones have multiple side-effects due to
Imipramine	Duloxetine	acetyl-choline, noradrenaline and serotonin
Clomipramine		receptor blockade
		Venlafaxine aggravates hypertension
Serotonin selective re-uptake inhibitors (SSRIs)		
Fluvoxamine	Escitalopram	Nausea, sexual dysfunction, initial agitation
Paroxetine		
Sertraline		
Citalopram		
Noradrenaline re-uptake inhibitors (NARIs)		
Dosulepin (dothiapin)	Lofepramine	Urinary retention, insomnia
	Reboxetine	
Dopamine – noradrenaline uptake inhibitor		
	Bupropion	Main use as adjunctive to SSRI
		Effective in smoking cessation
Monoamine receptor active drugs		
Mianserin	Mirtazepine	α_2-noradrenaline and 5HT2c blocker
		sedative, weight gain
		Probable dual action increasing noradrenaline
		and 5HT release
Trazodone		5HT2 receptor antagonist, weak uptake
		inhibition, poor evidence of efficacy
	Buspirone	5HT1A receptor agonist
		Marketed as anxiolytic
		Used as adjunctive treatment
Monoamine oxidase inhibitors (MAOIs)		
Phenelzine		Irreversibly bound to MAO
Tranylcypromine		Side-effects as for older MARIs
	Moclobemide	Competitive inhibitor of MAO-A

3. Mood stabilizers

LITHIUM

Lithium is a unique drug that has no psychotropic effect in normal individuals. However, it has remarkable effectiveness in bipolar (manic-depressive psychosis) illness, both in reducing mania and in stabilizing mood – preventing relapse into depression or mania. There is evidence it has a specific effect in reducing suicide. Like sodium, it is a monovalent cation that is available for clinical use in the form of carbonate or citrate salts.

Pharmacology

Lithium has several actions:

1. Competition with sodium ions for the sodium pump: interference with the maintenance of membrane potential and action potential generation in neurones.
2. Increased synthesis and release of 5HT.
3. Decreased effectiveness of second messengers linked with the 5HT2c receptor.
4. Increase in the uptake of catecholamines into nerve terminals.
5. Reduced effectiveness of the activation of central α_1-adrenoceptors and muscarinic receptors.
6. Inhibition of the activation of adenylate cyclase
   - by antidiuretic (ADH) in renal tubules
   - by thyroid-stimulating hormone (TSH) in the thyroid gland.

It is very uncertain how these actions mediate the anti-manic and mood-stabilizing properties of lithium. The effect on adenylate cyclase activation seems to be the basis for some side-effects (nephrogenic diabetes insipidus; hypothyroidism).

The elimination of lithium from the body is almost entirely through the kidneys. In steady state, the serum lithium concentration is determined by the ratio of the daily lithium intake and the renal lithium clearance. Renal lithium clearance is the product of the fractional tubular excretion of lithium and the glomerular filtration rate. The elimination of lithium through the kidneys can be impaired if either of these components is reduced: fractional tubular excretion of lithium will be reduced if the serum sodium concentration declines (e.g. as a result of thiazide diuretics, Addison's disease); glomerular filtration rate can be reduced as a result of dehydration, cardiac failure, or kidney disease.

Indications

- *Prophylactic maintenance treatment.* Relapse in both bipolar (manic and depressive) and unipolar (recurrent depressive) illnesses can be prevented, or their frequency and/or intensity reduced, by maintenance treatment. Patients with frequently alternating mood states (rapid cycling manic-depressive psychosis) need additional or alternative mood stabilization with an anticonvulsant stabilizer. Patients on lithium maintenance treatment need regular blood checks. This is done monthly until a steady state has been achieved; three-monthly thereafter. The recommended plasma level is 0.5–1.0 mmol/l for maintenance treatment. Abrupt withdrawal of lithium can trigger rebound mania, so it should be done gradually. There is evidence that lithium may be less effective if re-instituted after discontinuation. For these reasons, patients should be clear that it is a long-term treatment before starting it.
- *Anti-manic effect.* The therapeutic (anti-manic) effect of lithium does not appear for about a week, therefore the additional use of antipsychotics is often required. The plasma concentration aimed at is higher than in maintenance treatment (0.8–1.0

mmol/l); thus there is an increased risk of lithium toxicity. In general, an anti-psychotic is more effective and safer for the management of acute mania.

- *Adjunctive use in depression*. There is good clinical trial evidence that the addition of lithium to an antidepressant has antidepressant efficacy.
- *Mood stabilization in other disorders*. Lithium may help the marked mood instability seen in borderline personality disorder, and may have a role in the management of aggressive behaviour in schizophrenia.

Contraindications

Lithium maintenance treatment is contra-indicated in the following conditions:

- Renal and cardiac insufficiency.
- Addison's disease.
- Hypothyroidism.
- Pregnancy – lithium is associated with teratogenic defects in about 10 per cent of births.

It is usual to do blood urea, creatinine, and thyroid function tests before starting lithium. A pregnancy test in women of reproductive age is advisable. Lithium has a low therapeutic index, and toxicity quickly appears as the plasma concentration rises above 1.2 mEq/1.

Side-effects

Side-effects can occur even at therapeutic plasma levels:

- Thirst, polydipsia, and polyuria resulting from nephrogenic diabetes insipidus are usual but generally only mildly inconvenient.
- Weight gain is common and should be monitored.
- Precipitation and exacerbation of psoriasis and other skin disorders may occur.
- Gastrointestinal side-effects are common, especially early in treatment, and include nausea, vomiting, indigestion, metallic taste, diarrhoea.
- Of the neurological side-effects, a fine static tremor is the most common; the appearance of coarse tremor, ataxia, fasciculations are the signs of intoxication.
- An important endocrine side-effect is the development of hypothyroidism.

Drug interactions

- Thiazide diuretics – they can lead to sodium loss and thus to lithium toxicity.
- Antipsychotics – they can increase the neurotoxicity of lithium.

ANTICONVULSANT MOOD STABILIZERS

Valproic acid (sodium **valproate**)

Valproate is thought to exert its anticonvulsant effect through increasing GABA neurotransmission in the brain. There is strong clinical trial evidence that valproate is as effective as lithium in treating mania and it is licensed for this purpose in the UK as a first-line treatment. It is more frequently prescribed than lithium in the USA but there have been no proper comparative studies. There is some evidence valproate may be effective in prevention of relapses and have weak efficacy in bipolar depression. Women of child bearing age should not be prescribed valproate because of the high risk of fetal abnormality and polycystic ovary syndrome.

Carbemazepine

Like valproate, carbemazepine enhances GABA neurotransmission in some poorly understood way. It too has clinical trial evidence for efficacy in acute mania, but it is licensed for prophylaxis of bipolar disorder unresponsive to lithium. It has a reputation for efficacy in rapid cycling bipolar disorder (more than four relapses a year). Oxcarbazepine is closely related to carbemazepine but better tolerated because it is not metabolized in the same way. However, there is less clinical trial evidence but it appears to be anti-manic.

Lamotrigine

In contrast to the anti-manic anticonvulsants, valproate and carbemazepine, lamotrigine is only weakly anti-manic but is clearly effective in treating and preventing bipolar depression, where it is more effective than lithium. Furthermore, whereas valproate and carbemazepine enhance GABA function, lamotrigine is thought to work by decreasing glutamate release. This is an indirect effect of its primary action, which is to block one of the many varieties of sodium channel that exist.

Side-effects

All three agents are prone to hepatotoxicity and skin rashes. Lamotrigine can provoke the Stevens-Johnson syndrome and for this reason there is a standard slow titration regimen. Valproate and carbemazepine can cause blood dyscrasias and have teratogenic effects.

Carbemazepine is a liver enzyme inducer so some drugs including lamotrigine are metabolized more rapidly. The dose of concurrent lamotrigine has to be increased.

Valproate is a liver enzyme inhibitor so some drugs including lamotrigine may reach toxic levels at therapeutic doses. The dose of concurrent lamotrigine has to be decreased.

Indications

- Acute mania – valproate as an alternative or adjunctive treatment to lithium.
- Unstable bipolar disorder – any of the anticonvulsants, usually added to lithium to improve control.
- Bipolar depression – lamotrigine.

ANTIPSYCHOTIC MOOD STABILIZERS

All antipsychotics are effective in treating acute mania, and probably in preventing mania. However, it is increasingly clear from double-blind controlled trials that the atypicals, especially quetiapine, olanzapine and clozapine are effective in treating and preventing bipolar depression.

4. Anxiolytics

GENERAL

There are three main pharmacological treatments for anxiety: antidepressants (including buspirone, see above), benzodiazepines, and beta blockers. Formal clinical trial evidence exists for the effectiveness of antidepressants in panic disorder, generalized anxiety disorder and obsessive compulsive disorder, even in the absence of co-morbid depression. Like the antidepressant effect, anxiolytic actions take a week or two to begin to emerge and treatment needs to be sustained for some weeks before the degree of response can be gauged. 5HT uptake inhibition is essential for efficacy in obsessive compulsive disorder, and response is slower and may continue over many weeks. Benzodiazepines have an immediate anxiolytic action but it is probable that tolerance develops, with rebound exacerbation up on the withdrawal of treatment. Beta blockers are useful in the treatment of anxiety states, particularly when associated with somatic symptoms.

BENZODIAZEPINES

Pharmacology

These drugs used to be called 'minor tranquillizers' and they are effective in reducing pathological anxiety, tension and agitation at doses that do not cause sedation or sleep. They have only one pharmacological action and they differ only in their duration of action. They act to enhance the effect of GABA at GABA receptors. GABA receptors are ion channels that open when GABA binds to its recognition site. Benzodiazepines bind to another part of the GABA receptor complex and prolong the opening of channels when GABA acts at their receptors. Benzodiazepines thus potentiate GABA-induced inhibition in the CNS. The GABA-benzodiazepine receptor complex is widespread throughout the brain. The anti-anxiety effect may be a result of enhancement of

GABA-mediated inhibition of specific 5-hydroxytryptamine and noradrenaline-containing neurones, whereas enhancement of GABA-mediated neuronal inhibition in the cerebral cortex has been related to the anticonvulsant and central muscular relaxant effects of benzodiazepines. Each benzodiazepine possesses, to a greater or lesser extent, five important pharmacological effects: (1) anxiolytic, (2) hypnotic (3) muscle relaxant (e.g. in spasticity) (4) anticonvulsant, and (5) amnestic.

Indications

- *Anxiety states*. Benzodiazepines are effective and relatively harmless in the short-term treatment of anxiety, but tolerance and dependence (see below) limit their long-term usefulness. They should be used for only a limited period (2–4 weeks) during which time the patient will become more amenable to other (e.g. behavioural, social, medical) forms of treatment. Drugs with a longer half-life such as diazepam are preferred over short-acting drugs such as lorazepam and oxazepam with dependence potential – see below.
- *Sleep disturbance*. Several benzodiazepines with shorter half-lives are used as hypnotics but again dependence limits their usefulness. Some drugs such as zopiclone are marketed as non-benzodiazepine, but this merely refers to their structure, they act at the benzodiazepine site and they do not have major clinical advantages.
- *Alcohol detoxification*. Long-acting benzodiazepines are part of the standard management of alcohol detoxification not only because of their sedative-anxiolytic action but also because their anticonvulsant action reduced the risk of seizures.

Side-effects

Day-time sedation, drowsiness and impairment of psychomotor performance can occur in conjunction with both anti-anxiety treatment and the use of long-acting hypnotics ('hangover effect'). Increased hostility and aggressive behaviour can occur as a rare but unpleasant complication.

Physical dependence and withdrawal can occur and it is difficult for regular users to give up the medication. Tolerance and withdrawal symptoms can be demonstrated as rapidly as 2 weeks after initiation, and tolerance can be demonstrated for as long as 2 years after cessation of chronic use. Short-acting drugs may be particularly prone to dependence because withdrawal symptoms after a few hours trigger the need to take another dose. For this reason, it is thought helpful to switch to a long-acting drug such as diazepam and then very gradually reduce the dose. Withdrawal symptoms include increased anxiety, rebound insomnia, dysphoria, anorexia; rarely more severe symptoms (severe agitation, panic, depression, delusions, hallucinations, convulsion) can occur. These withdrawal symptoms can take some weeks to resolve, and specialist addiction treatment may needed.

The benzodiazepines are relatively safe drugs in over-dosage; fatalities are usually a result of the concomitant use of CNS depressants (ethanol, barbiturates).

5. Cognitive enhancers

These drugs are used to improve cognitive (intellectual) performance in the treatment of dementia. Alzheimer's disease involves degeneration of acetyl-choline neurones in the midbrain that innervate the cerebral cortex. There are several drugs that inhibit the metabolism of acetyl-choline by acetyl-choline esterase, thereby prolonging the effect of remaining acetyl-choline. Three are licensed in the UK – **donazepil**, **rivastigmine**, and **galantamine**.

Glutamate neurones make up most of the grey matter of the cerebral cortex and they also degenerate in dementia. Drugs that weakly block the NMDA glutamate receptor ion channel show promise in improving cognition and in slowing progression through a neuroprotective effect.

There is good clinical trial evidence these agents are effective both on psychological test performance and also in improving daily living skills. However, diagnosis, assessment and prescribing should be carried out in specialist clinics.

PHYSICAL TREATMENTS: ELECTROCONVULSIVE TREATMENT ('ECT')

The use of electroconvulsive therapy has been the cause of much controversy, both in psychiatry and among the general public. This is partly because the treatment has been used outside those situations where its use is appropriate and partly because there has been difficulty in performing accurate research. Several large studies have established that ECT is superior to antidepressant drugs, and far superior to placebo, in the treatment of depression. The necessity of the seizure has now been proven by studies comparing the effects of ECT with 'simulated' ECT (administration of the anaesthetic and muscle relaxant but without the electric shocks).

The relative effects of treatments for severe depressive illness were demonstrated in a study some years ago:

> After four weeks over 70 per cent of those receiving ECT had few or no symptoms (they had received four to eight treatments during this time). Just over one half of those receiving imipramine had made a similar response, to be compared with 39 per cent of the placebo group and only 30 per cent of the phenelzine group.

Mode of action

It is highly probable that grand mal seizure activity is necessary for the antidepressant effect, and there is some evidence that seizures elicited by higher currents have greater antidepressant activity than those elicited by lower currents. Thus, attempting to minimize confusion and memory loss by minimizing the current may reduce the therapeutic efficacy. However, unilateral ECT to the non-dominant hemisphere evokes a bilateral seizure with much less confusion but with reduced efficacy: it requires on average between two and four additional treatments.

ECT potentiates behaviour mediated by serotonin (5HT) and there is neurochemical evidence from work with experimental animals that this is because of an increase in post-synaptic 5HT receptor numbers. Behaviours mediated by dopamine are also enhanced by ECT, and there are also influences on noradrenergic functions similar to those described for antidepressant drugs (see p. 96). In particular, it has been shown that ECT has an effect in down-regulating β receptors. The neurochemical and behavioural effects of ECT parallel its antidepressant actions since the changes emerge after several treatments and sub-seizure currents are ineffective.

Clinical uses

The principal use of ECT is in severe depressive illness. Features of that illness that predict a good response to ECT are:

1. Severe weight loss.
2. Pronounced early morning wakening.
3. Psychomotor retardation.
4. Psychotic features – especially depressive delusions.

In clinical practice ECT is used:

1. **When depressive illness fails to respond** to antidepressant treatment.
2. In psychotic depression with **depressive delusions**.
3. In **depressive stupor**.
4. In **catatonic stupor**.
5. In **puerperal psychoses**, especially those with clouding, perplexity, and marked affective features.

More controversial indications include:

6. *Acute schizophrenia* with clouded consciousness and perplexity.
7. *Schizophrenia* where there are pronounced depressive features.
8. *Mania* when neuroleptic and lithium have failed to control persistent over-activity.

Administration of ECT

ECT requires a general anaesthetic and the usual precautions are observed. The treatment is usually given early in the morning so the patient is starved from midnight. Atropine is administered as pre-medication to dry up bronchial and salivary secretions and also to prevent an extreme bradycardia. A short-acting anaesthetic is administered together with a muscle relaxant to modify the fit. Following ventilation with oxygen (this has been shown to reduce amnesia afterwards), the electrodes – moistened to ensure good contact with the skin – are placed one on the temporal region and one near the vertex of the side of the non-dominant hemisphere for unilateral ECT. (For bilateral ECT the electrodes are placed on each temporal region.) Treatment is given twice a week with 2 clear days between treatments until a satisfactory response has been obtained: this is usually after six to eight treatments.

Unwanted effects

ECT is a safe treatment. The mortality rate is similar to that of a brief anaesthetic when used for dental or investigative procedures. The largest series demonstrates a mortality of one death per 20,000 treatments.

Physical side-effects following ECT are rare. However, *physical problems following the anaesthetic* may include:

Myocardial infarction.
Cardiac arrhythmias.
Pulmonary embolism.
Pneumonia.

If the *muscle relaxant has not been properly given* the following may occur:

Dislocations and fractures.

Increased blood pressure during the fit itself may occur, causing:

Cerebral haemorrhage.
Bleeding from peptic ulcer.

PSYCHOLOGICAL SEQUELAE

Mania is precipitated by ECT in approximately 5 per cent of cases. This figure is similar to that found with tricyclic antidepressants and occurs in those patients known to have, or be vulnerable to, bipolar manic-depressive illness.

A post-ECT **confusional state** usually lasts for about half an hour, a headache may also occur but is usually short-lived.

Memory loss is a more important side-effect. There is a short and rapidly dwindling amnesia for the time preceding each treatment (retrograde amnesia) and a longer post-ECT (anterograde) amnesia. Patients may also complain of *subjective difficulty in remembering* previously well-learned material, like telephone numbers or addresses. These problems are usually hard to demonstrate with objective tests of memory. However, the following factors will reduce the memory problems:

1. Unilateral shock to the non-dominant hemisphere.
2. Not giving too many treatments (more than 12).
3. Not giving treatment too frequently (more than three per week).

4. Oxygenating the patient well before the shock.
5. Not using an unnecessarily big shock.

CONTRAINDICATIONS TO ECT

The treatment causes *alteration of pulse rate, a rise in blood pressure* and *a great increase in cerebral blood flow*. The contraindications are therefore illnesses affecting the cardio-vascular and central nervous systems:

Cerebral and aortic aneurysms.
Recent cerebral haemorrhage.
Myocardial infarction.
Cardiac arrhythmias.
Raised intracranial pressure and brain tumour.

Acute respiratory infections form a contraindication to the anaesthetic and require treatment before ECT is given.

COGNITIVE AND BEHAVIOURAL TREATMENTS

These treatments involve the manipulation of the patient's thought processes (cognitions), overt behaviour, physiological responses (autonomic functions) and environment in order to bring about positive change and alleviation of the identified problem. These manipulations or therapeutic tactics can vary depending on the problem and the results of the behavioural analysis, but will make up a treatment programme or therapeutic strategy that will have predefined goals. Cognitive-behaviour therapy is not necessarily antagonistic to physical approaches to treatment: rather the two approaches can be complementary. Many patients derive benefit from a combination of the two types of treatment.

Theoretical foundations

The fundamental principles of change in psychological treatments based on cognitive-behaviour therapy are:

1. **Classical (Pavlovian) conditioning**. This is the process by which a neutral stimulus (the 'conditioned' stimulus, or CS) acquires the ability to elicit an involuntary response (a CR) as a result of association with a stimulus (the 'unconditioned' stimulus, or UCS) that normally evokes that response. Pavlov's famous experiments on gastric acid and salivary excretion in dogs exemplify this form of learning. Thus the sight of food (UCS) usually evokes salivation, and by initially pairing this with a bell (CS), Pavlov was subsequently able to make the dog salivate (CR) when the bell rang in the absence of food.

110

A clinically relevant example of classical conditioning would be the hypothetical explanation of the origin of phobic anxiety, whereby the phobic object (for example, a spider) acts as a CS eliciting a fear response because of earlier pairing with such responses.

2. **Operant (instrumental) conditioning**. This is the process whereby voluntary behaviours are strengthened ('reinforcement') or weakened ('punishment') because of their consequences. Skinner's experiments in which rats pressed levers for food reinforcement typify this type of learning in animals, while a clinically relevant example in humans would be the engendering of temper tantrums in a young child when he discovers that such behaviour is particularly effective in obtaining his parents' undivided attention.

3. **Vicarious learning**. This refers to the process by which learning occurs through symbolic representations by exposure to instructional, observational or imaginal material. Learning is thought to occur through the informative and instructional function of reward. For example, many childhood fears are thought to be acquired through the child observing other people's reaction to the feared situation, and hence building up expectations about the situation. This process is known as modelling and can be used as a powerful therapeutic tool as well as a process through which disorders are acquired. The action of the therapist modelling appropriate coping responses during a stressful situation, or appropriate management strategies with a difficult child, are good examples of these.

4. **Cognitive processes**. These refer to the way that information is detected (perception and attention) and then organised, stored and retrieved from memory. This flow of information is manifest in conscious thought, processes of attention and interpretation, and in underlying beliefs and attitudes. There is a subtle interplay between such cognitive processes, physiological processes and overt behaviour in all human actions, but they are especially important in abnormal behaviour and emotional disorders. For example, certain types of information may be more accessible and hence come to the fore under certain conditions such as low mood or high levels of physiological arousal. A clinical example would be the patient who suffers panic attacks because they over-attend to minor physical sensations that when detected are catastrophically interpreted as being the sign of a major illness. Small changes in heart rate or difficulty breathing because of tension are interpreted as an indication of an imminent heart attack, resulting in the sudden upsurge of anxiety characteristic of panic attacks.

Both classical and operant conditioning tend to be situationally specific (that is to say, the learned responses occur most readily in situations similar to those prevailing when the conditioning took place). Both types of conditioning are deemed to be reversible. Thus a classically conditioned fear of crowded places would be expected to extinguish as a result of repeated visits to busy shops, while tantrums cease when they no longer elicit the same parental attention.

Many pathological behaviours involve a complex interplay between classical and operant conditioning. For example, although phobic anxiety may arise from a classical learning experience, phobic behaviour is more likely to be maintained by operant conditioning – that is, the reinforcement of avoidance behaviour by anxiety reduction.

Contemporary thinking incorporates all of these principles into explanations of abnormal behaviour and psychological disorders although the emphasis given to the balance of the different contributions of each can vary across different disorders.

General principles of cognitive-behaviour therapy

All cognitive and behaviour therapies start with a cognitive-behavioural analysis. The objective symptomatology or problem area is clearly defined, and details of the frequency, duration, and intensity of the symptoms are recorded, together with events that occur at the time when symptoms are experienced. This is usually accomplished by asking the patient to keep a diary for a week or so before any formulation is attempted. It is frequently helpful to describe the patient's problem in terms of their thoughts (cognitions), actions (overt behaviour) and physical sensations (physiological reactions). Practical considerations usually mean that it is the patient's subjective account of these cognitions, behaviour and physiological reactions that is used in the cognitive-behavioural analysis. However, if possible the patient's behaviour should be observed and their physiological responses measured directly through non-invasive methods. Such a formulation must take account of:

A. The **A**ntecedents   – the environmental context in which the symptom occurs.
B. The **B**ehaviour   – the problem itself.
C. The **C**onsequences – events which may contribute to the maintenance of the behaviour.

The formulation constitutes a **hypothesis** about the nature and origin of the symptom. The hypothesis will usually suggest appropriate treatment strategies: for example, the hypothesis that a patient's withdrawal from social contact is maintained by anxiety reduction might suggest a different type of intervention from the hypothesis that it stems from an inadequate repertoire of social skills. The treatment thus constitutes a test of the hypothesis, which itself may require modification in the light of success or failure of the treatment.

Cognitive-behavioural treatment invariably involves a clear objective goal based on the formulation derived from the cognitive-behavioural analysis and agreed on by the patient. Most therapists also use **intermediate goals** or 'targets', the attainment of which provides an important source of reinforcement for the patient.

Specific Techniques

RELAXATION

Since the conditioned response in so many of the above states is one of anxiety, the patient must first be trained to produce the opposite response, relaxation. This is done initially well away from any anxiety-provoking stimulus. The patients are first taught to recognize the signs of tension in their body and how these can be altered by voluntary control. They are then taught a series of exercises by which they can learn to reduce physiological arousal, and they may also be given an audiotape of these exercises that they can use for regular home practice. The technique of relaxation must become sufficiently rehearsed so that it can be applied even in situations that have previously caused anxiety. There are a number of different methods of relaxation, such as **progressive muscle relaxation** (PMR) in which the patient is taught a series of exercises during which muscle blocks are alternatively tensed then relaxed to achieve a relaxed state, or **autogenic relaxation** in which muscle tension is released without the muscle block first being tensed. Other variations include the speed in which training in relaxation progresses, and the application of relaxation skills to stressful situations. It is generally accepted that learning to relax is a skill and will also include cognitive aspects such as a sense of control over difficult situations. It is also worth noting that some patients find it very difficult to relax or even find it anxiety-provoking because the feeling of 'letting go' of tension fuels their fear of 'being out of control'.

Breathing exercises are also important, especially for patients who hyperventilate, such as some who have panic attacks.

EXPOSURE

Many of the treatments used in cognitive-behaviour therapy require an exposure to the feared or conditioned stimuli. This is to allow the **habituation** of the emotional response conditioned to that set of stimuli. It is thought that exposure may also serve the function of disproving the expectations or beliefs held by the patient about specific situations and their consequences. There are a number of variations to exposure-based treatments that depend on the mode and speed of exposure (i.e. whether exposure is carried out gradually or not and whether it is carried out in imagination or in vivo). In some circumstances such as exposure to traumatic memories, as in the treatment of post-traumatic stress disorder (see p. 228), by the nature of the disorder exposure has to be imaginal. Similarly, in cognitive-based treatments irrational thoughts are challenged by the patient exposing themselves to situations which indicate that these thoughts are untrue or unrealistic. Some examples of exposure-based treatments are given below.

DESENSITIZATION

With the therapist's help, the patient constructs a hierarchy of anxiety-provoking stimuli. These stimuli are then presented to the patient, starting with the most innocuous. As each stimulus is mastered, the patient progresses to the next one. The stimuli may be presented in one of two ways.

1. **Desensitization in imagination** consists of the patient imagining anxiety-provoking scenes while in a relaxed state.

2. **Graded exposure** (or 'in vivo' desensitization) This treatment consists of the patient having to encounter anxiety-provoking stimuli in real life, starting with those that provoke least anxiety. This procedure is favoured by most therapists since confrontation with stressors in real life is always the eventual goal of treatment, and it is more effective.

Here is an example of graded exposure:

Mrs X presented with a moderately severe fear of wasps. On occasion this resulted in her running away leaving her baby and pram unattended in the street. A 12-step hierarchy of increasingly anxiety-provoking wasp-related stimuli was constructed and this determined a programme of graded exposure, starting with reading about and looking at pictures of wasps in books, and ending with killing a wasp trapped against a window. Initial exposure to each item took place in the clinic, the patient then being encouraged to complete similar assignments at home without the therapist. The duration of each exposure to an item was dependent on the rate of habituation of the anxiety response: exposure was discontinued when the patient described a significant reduction in anxiety. In practice this was rarely more than 15 minutes per item. Usually more than one item was completed at the same appointment. After only five treatment sessions, the patient completed the hierarchy, and remained anxiety-free in the presence of wasps at a 6-month follow-up point.

FLOODING

Whereas desensitization is a 'little-by-little' approach, flooding plunges in at the deep end. The patient is confronted with a situation at the top of her hierarchy (for example, shopping in a crowded department store, or travelling on a bus in the rush hour), and is required to remain in that situation until her anxiety has spontaneously dissipated ('habituation'). Although it is often difficult to persuade patients to undergo flooding, it is a rapid and a generally more effective treatment than desensitization:

Mrs Y had not ventured more than one quarter of a mile from her home and had completely avoided all shopping areas for more than a year, because of agoraphobic anxiety difficulties. The patient and therapist travelled by car into the city centre on a Saturday afternoon and spent two and a half hours in a crowded shopping mall. Initially the patient complained of extreme panic, the therapist both reassuring and prompting her to remain in spite of an intense desire to exit from the situation. These feelings began to subside after about 30 minutes, and by the end of the session the patient was euphoric. Two further sessions of the same type took place, and these were characterized by even more rapid habituation of anxiety. Subsequently, Mrs Y was encouraged to travel alone to the same shopping centre, and this was accompanied by a generalization of the treatment effect to other public situations. After only 3 weeks from the commencement of treatment she was able to travel to and shop in local supermarkets and city centre departmental stores.

BIOFEEDBACK

Many visceral and neuromuscular activities of which we are normally unaware can be brought into consciousness by providing an auditory or visual 'feedback' signal (for example, a tone whose pitch varies with frontalis muscle tension). This technique is often used as an adjunct to relaxation training, but can also by used in the treatment of specific symptoms such as tension headache, or in the treatment of hypertension.

SOCIAL SKILLS TRAINING

Sophisticated social behaviour is largely acquired by learning. Many people cope poorly with social situations because they have never acquired a full repertoire of appropriate social responses. Social skills training is usually undertaken with groups of patients, and aims to provide explicit training of such social responses. Mock social situations are set up, and the patients practise by **role-playing**, after the therapist has provided a model of the appropriate behaviour ('modelling'). The patient's performance may be videotaped, so that particular problems can be discussed and corrected in debriefing sessions.

BELL AND PAD TRAINING

This is a behavioural treatment for nocturnal enuresis. A pad containing electrical contacts is placed under a sheet on the patient's bed. If the patient urinates in the bed a circuit is completed, setting off an alarm bell that wakes the patient. This is one of the most effective treatments for enuresis, although the underlying psychological processes remain obscure. Simple classical conditioning cannot provide a full explanation for the treatment's efficacy, because the alarm bell (CS) occurs after the unconditioned reflex of micturition. It seems likely that as a result of extensive practice the patient learns to become more aware of stimuli associated with bladder distension.

RESPONSE PREVENTION

This is used in the treatment of compulsive rituals. The patient feels compelled to perform some act such as washing hands but is firmly persuaded from doing so. This must be maintained for prolonged periods to be effective. It is best performed while the person is repeatedly faced with a situation in which the compulsion occurs, such as touching dirt. In this way it is similar to flooding – the patient is faced with intense anxiety that gradually wanes as it is not relieved by the habitual means of giving in to the compulsion.

Mr Z presented with an obsessional preoccupation with dog excrement. After returning home from walking in the street, he would be compelled to engage in a decontamination ritual beginning with scrubbing his shoes with disinfectant (these were not normally soiled to the objective observer). He would then take all his clothes off, and place them in the washing machine, then scrub his hands, and bath himself. The ritual took more than 2 hours to perform. Treatment involved the patient being encouraged to deliberately soil his shoes with dog excrement and return home, leaving his contaminated shoes on the door step. The therapist then spent an hour or more with the patient, preventing any cleaning ritual from occurring and distracting him with other activities. After 2 months of twice-weekly visits by the therapist the patient was able to venture out alone and return without performing the ritual, apart from washing his hands in a normal fashion.

Cognitive-behavioural approaches to severe mental disorders

DEPRESSION

In depressive illnesses cognitive approaches can be used in conjunction with pharmacological treatment, and are especially useful in milder or long-standing depressive conditions where antidepressant drugs are either ineffective or undesirable. They are based on the observation that depressed patients often have erroneous and highly pessimistic beliefs about themselves, their circumstances and their future (the 'negative triad').

Cognitive therapy aims to correct these gloomy thoughts, and at the same time to demonstrate to the patient that he is capable of surmounting problems that because of his pessimistic beliefs he would not normally undertake. Although the primary focus of this type of therapy is the patient's beliefs, it can be included with behaviour therapies because of the emphasis on practical goals, and because thoughts appear to be subject to the same laws of reinforcement as acts.

Mr A who 6 months previously had failed to obtain an important job promotion, was diagnosed as suffering from a moderately severe depressive illness. He was preoccupied with thoughts of incompetence at work and in the home, worries that nobody liked him, and ideas of low self-esteem. He was asked to keep a diary in which he recorded recurrent negative thoughts and their underlying assumptions. Treatment sessions focused on reality-testing these assumptions. For example, one recurrent thought suggested that he had been passed over for promotion because he was incompetent in his current position.

Underlying assumptions included:

1. *His manager paid particular attention to every error that he had made over the years, no matter how insignificant.*
2. *Because of (1), the manager believed Mr A to be the most incompetent person in the firm.*
3. *It was because of (2) that Mr A had not been promoted.*
4. *Mr A would not be promoted at any future date.*

As a result of treatment sessions and reality-testing assignments, the patient began to realize that most of these assumptions were incorrect. This led to adjustments in his attitude towards his work and his career, and after 3 months of treatment the depression was ameliorated.

SCHIZOPHRENIA

Besides the use of social skills training, which has long been a part of rehabilitation programmes for the severely mentally ill, recent cognitive-behavioural approaches to schizophrenia have shown great promise. These have taken two forms. First, based on a recognition that stress is frequently a precipitant of psychotic relapse, interventions have focused on helping the families, relatives or carers of schizophrenic patients to cope better with stress, especially by modifying the manner in which they interact and deal with problems and difficulties within the home situation. These methods have been termed **family management** or **family intervention**. The other approach, which is becoming more prevalent, is the cognitive-behavioural treatment of **positive symptoms** of schizophrenia, such as delusions and hallucinations. In cases in which medication is failing to further improve residual symptoms, or when the patient does not comply with their medication, or there are reasons why medication is contra-indicated these methods have proved useful.

Indications for cognitive-behaviour therapy

It can be seen that behavioural treatments are helpful in a very wide range of psychological disorders. In **affective disorders** like anxiety, phobias, post-traumatic stress disorders or depression; in **maladaptive behaviours** such as obsessional states and sexual problems; in **abnormal illness behaviours**; in deficient social skills and nocturnal enuresis, and as an adjunct treatment in the severe mental illnesses.

Some brief psychological skills based on cognitive-behaviour therapy

PROBLEM-SOLVING

Problem-solving is a brief psychological treatment that has been adapted for particular use in primary care. The underpinning theoretical assumption is that the psychological symptoms of anxiety and depression are often caused by the practical problems that people face in their everyday lives. People readily recognize this link, so the treatment makes good sense to them. Problem-solving is a very practical, collaborative and structured approach to resolving problems and setting achievable goals for the future. It has been effective in treatment of depression and in the management of people who self-harm. The steps involved in problem-solving are shown in *Box 8.2*.

It is important that the patient does the work in generating the list of problems and brainstorming the potential solutions, as they need to 'own' the work as their own ideas (see 'Providing information and advice' below). The problem can be worked through in stages, with some steps carried out as homework – for example generating the list of problems, or brainstorming the possible solutions.

Box 8.2 Steps of problem-solving

1. Draw up a list of problems
2. Choose a problem to manage
3. Form a clear definition of the problem – break down complex problems into smaller, manageable problems
4. Establish achievable goal(s)
5. Brainstorm potential solutions
6. Evaluate and choose the best solution by considering the pros and cons of each of the alternatives
7. Implement the chosen solution: What exactly needs to be done to put it into practice? What are the steps?
8. Evaluate the outcome

MOTIVATIONAL INTERVIEWING

Motivational interviewing is a specific approach to interviewing that has been found to be effective in helping people to change their behaviour, specifically in the fields of addiction (drugs and alcohol) and eating disorders. The principles behind the approach to the interview are that people learn what they think about a problem as they hear themselves talking about it, and, when they feel ambivalent about a problem, they will tend to respond to direct advice by assuming the opposing position. Therefore, a person who is told too forcefully to 'give up drinking' might reply *but all my friends drink exactly the same amount as me and none of them have any problems'*.

Again, as in problem-solving, it is essential to get the patient to do the work. For example:

'Can you tell me what the good things are about drinking alcohol . . . what do you enjoy about it?'

'Well, it helps me to relax, and to sleep.'

(doctor summarizes) *'So it helps you to sleep and to relax . . . what about the problems it causes . . . can we look at those?'*

'I've been really ill . . . my wife says she will leave me . . . And I've lost my driving licence.'

(doctor summarizes again) *'So you have been really quite ill . . . and it's causing problems at home and you've lost your licence . . . what problems will that cause?'*

As in problem-solving, the doctor can give information to help the patient to arrive at an informed decision, but he leaves that final decision up to the patient. Paradoxically, the

---

Box 8.3 Stages in motivational interviewing

Explore motivation for change
- Build rapport and be neutral
- Help draw up list of problems and priorities
- Is problem behaviour on the patient's agenda?
- If not, raise it sensitively
- Does the patient consider the behaviour to be a problem?
- Do others?

Clarify the patient's view of the problem
- Help draw up a balance sheet of pros and cons
- Empathize with the difficulty of changing
- Reinforce statements that express a desire to change
- Resist saying why you think the patient ought to change
- Summarize frequently
- Discuss statements that are contradictory

Promote resolution
(If no change is wanted, negotiate if, when, and how to review)
- Enable informed decision-making
- Give basic information about the safety or risks of the behaviour
- Provide results of any examination or test
- Highlight potential medical, legal, or social consequences
- Explain the likely outcome of potential choices or interventions
- Get feedback from the patient

---

ambivalent patient is more likely to change his or her behaviour when this approach is used rather than if given direct advice to do so.

PSYCHOTHERAPY

The doctor–patient relationship is one in which the patient places great trust in the doctor. The patient discusses personal problems that he would otherwise keep private, and he may be prepared to comply with whatever treatment and advice the doctor prescribes. Some knowledge of how this relationship operates is essential to be a good doctor. However, it is important to realize that this relationship can be used in a therapeutic way. This is formalized in psychotherapy, in which the doctor aims to help the patient by recognizing his needs and helping him with them through the medium of the therapeutic relationship.

Psychotherapy may be divided according to the type of recipient: thus **individual**, **marital**, **family** and **group psychotherapy**; or it may be divided according to the kind of technique used. We will now consider, first, the kinds of psychotherapeutic techniques that should be possessed by every doctor; and second, techniques that are used by those with greater experience.

Supportive psychotherapy – techniques necessary for all doctors

Even in a crowded general practitioner's surgery or a busy out-patient clinic there are a number of techniques that a doctor will find helpful. Supportive psychotherapy consists of the following simple components.

ACTIVE LISTENING

Students are often surprised to find that taking a full history in the psychiatric out-patient clinic leads to the patient saying that he feels much better! The patient will probably have never before had such an opportunity to review all aspects of his life and to express emotions associated with events in his life. In addition the student's intense interest in what the patient is saying demonstrates a concern that the patient appreciates.

Active listening is an important part of the therapeutic process. There is no need for such listening to be a time-consuming business – in fact it can save time. The patient with a sexual problem, for example, can spend many fruitless consultations with the doctor who is not skilled in gaining her confidence and listening for clues as to the nature of the underlying worry.

EXPLORING THE PATIENT'S WORRIES AND CONCERNS

It is very important to try and find out exactly what a person is worried about before attempting to offer any reassurance. What is the person worried may be wrong with them? What are their fears and concerns, not just about diagnosis but also about receiving treatment? This is always important, but particularly so when a patient presents with a problem for which there is no clear organic cause. The patient may have different ideas about what is causing the problem. He may be very worried that there is something physically wrong, and want the doctor to take his symptoms seriously and organize investigations, but also suspect that stress or worry may be playing a part. Simply exploring the patient's worries and concerns in detail can itself be therapeutic.

VENTILATION OF FEELINGS

Allowing expression of feeling is an important aspect of the therapeutic relationship. It is especially useful to be able to express anger, frustration or grief that has previously been suppressed. This is particularly important following bereavement, or where the doctor has just had to give 'bad news'. For example, after the birth of a child who unexpectedly has a severe deformity the parents will often feel numb and will not be able to take in important factual information until after they have had a chance to express their feelings of shock, bewilderment, anger, and loss.

REASSURANCE

The patient who correctly suspects that he has cancer may ask the doctor about the diagnosis. He may well be asking for reassurance rather than for information. Even if there is nothing in the prognosis about which the doctor can reassure, listening carefully to the patient may help to understand his particular fears, such as unrelieved pain, incontinence, or the effect on his relatives. On these matters the doctor can reassure and in doing so relieve some of the patient's suffering.

It is important to realize that a properly conducted **physical examination** may be a vital ingredient in the ability to provide reassurance, and that the doctor's own behaviour during a physical examination can serve either to increase or to decrease the patient's anxiety.

A doctor frequently has to reassure a patient (especially an anxious one) that he does not have a serious disease. In spite of these efforts, attempts at reassurance may fail and the patient may seek further tests elsewhere. This is because the doctor has either not fully understood the patient's underlying worries or not explained adequately the cause of the symptoms.

EXPLANATION

The patient who fears that his headaches indicate an underlying brain tumour is less reassured by the doctor's statement *'All the tests show that nothing is wrong'* than:

> *Your headaches are due to the muscles of your scalp tightening; this is why they also affect the back of your neck and occur when you get tense.*

Thus an explanation by the doctor can be very therapeutic, although it uses neither technological investigations nor drugs.

You may observe a patient in the out-patient clinic look greatly relieved by the consultant's authoritative statement that the patient's illness is recognized and appropriate treatment can be prescribed. The 'explanation' may just be a name for a disease whose aetiology is not understood; the 'treatment' something that is known to work, although no one is quite sure why. Yet until this time the patient has been perplexed as to what has been happening to him, and the *doctor's explanation is reassuring*.

PROVIDING INFORMATION AND ADVICE

Patients often turn to the doctor for advice. These may be matters about which the doctor can be precise (such as giving up smoking, or stopping benzodiazepines), or they may be related to problems such as leaving a job, or getting a divorce. The doctor must avoid telling people what they should do, although it is legitimate to tell them what effect a particular change might be expected to have on their health. In other words, information is helpful, but advice may be harmful, even though people often ask for it. It is important to enable people to reach their own decisions (see 'Problem-solving').

Thus the doctor might inform the patient that if she took time off from caring for a sick parent it would help in the treatment of her own depressive illness: but whether the patient does so or not must be her own choice.

Insight-oriented psychotherapy

These techniques are often used in an attempt to reconstruct the possible original causes of a patient's symptoms, or to look for factors that are maintaining them. There are a number of techniques, including:

- Instead of asking questions, use statements to encourage the patient to talk.
- Be prepared to try to understand what the patient is feeling (using empathy), and then make intelligent guesses to prompt further discussion.
- Allow the patient to show their emotions to you, whether they be crying, anger, distress. (You can respond with a supportive comment, such as 'I can see you've been through a difficult time'; but remember that silence can also be supportive.)
- The doctor is not always right. Give the patient the chance to correct you.
- Don't reassure too soon.

It is easier to get an idea of such techniques by looking at what might actually be said during a consultation. We will return to Angela Cooper, and first see how a doctor who has no knowledge of psychotherapeutic techniques might interview her, using a traditional 'question-and-answer' format:

Doctor	Angela Cooper
What's wrong? What is the matter?	*Nothing.*
Why did you take an overdose of tablets?	*I just felt like it.*
Was it because you split up with your boyfriend?	*Yes.*
Well I'm sure you'll get over it eventually	
It just takes time . . .	*How do you know?*
Because people do usually. Really.	
I need to ask some other questions now . . .	
Are you sleeping okay?	*No.*

A more experienced doctor might say:

Doctor	Angela Cooper
You look very sad . . . how have you been feeling?	*Awful.*
Awful . . . (silence) . . . can you tell me what has been happening?	*I took an overdose of tablets (starts to cry).*
I can see it's very upsetting even to talk about it.	*Yes . . .*
You must have felt very sad and upset to do that . . .	*I'm all on my own now.*
All on your own . . .	*And it's all my fault (tears).*
How is that?	*(silence)*

> *Do you feel able to tell me about it?*   *I'll try . . . I don't know.*
> *I understand it's not easy.*   *No – I'll try.*

Angela's response to unsympathetic questioning is anger and hostility. She does not find it easy to trust. In the second example, the doctor tries, gently, to gain Angela's trust in talking about something she finds very painful. He does this by picking up on non-verbal cues, and also demonstrating empathy. He also indicates a familiarity with how difficult it can be to talk about painful experiences, uses silences, and shows patience and understanding.

Formal exploratory psychotherapy

This type of psychotherapy is more intensive and is usually given by those who have received some special training. It aims to help the person modify long-standing aspects of their feelings and behaviour, often by modifying defence mechanisms. It is more formal in the sense that the therapist (who might also be a doctor or another mental health professional with special training) spends a specified time with the patient each week, the therapy may last for some time, and in the longer forms of treatment there is much greater emphasis on analysis of the doctor–patient relationship.

Getting the patient to express their most intimate feelings and to react spontaneously within the therapy requires:

- Careful selection of suitable patients.
- A fixed time each week for the therapeutic session, which is held in a quiet and private office where interruptions are prevented.
- A trusting relationship in which the therapist facilitates the patient's spontaneous expression of emotion, and yet makes the patient feel that it is safe for this to occur.
- Treatment takes place in the framework of a **therapeutic contract**, which makes clear to the patient how much treatment is being offered, and what should be achieved during these sessions. The therapist must be very careful not to break his or her side of the contract, so that if the patient breaks their side the therapist can interpret this behaviour.

INDICATIONS

This type of psychotherapy may be used as an adjunct to other treatments in anxiety disorders, depressive illness, and eating disorders. It is occasionally used alone in any of these conditions and in the management of personality disorder and maladaptive behaviours such as self-harm. Patients are selected who are well-motivated to engage in this form of treatment and who can understand it. They must be able and willing to make some important changes in their lives.

Almost invariably patients who will benefit from exploratory psychotherapy will describe difficulty in relationships and problems of self-esteem, even when other psychiatric disorders are present.

CONTRAINDICATIONS

This treatment is generally not recommended for patients who:

- Are psychotic.
- Show marked paranoid traits.
- Are seriously dependent on drugs or alcohol.
- Are unable to tolerate personal discomfort.
- Are involved with an impossible life situation that cannot be expected to change.
- Have an anti-social personality.

HAZARDS

The principal hazard is **excessive dependency**, so that the patient relies so completely on the therapist that he needs to consult him on every aspect of his life, and termination of treatment is impossible. This should be avoided by careful selection of patients for this form of treatment, by not allowing treatment to be prolonged unnecessarily, and by recognizing the early signs of dependency and dealing with them appropriately.

CONTENT OF TREATMENT SESSIONS

Psychotherapy often starts with the patient asking *'What do I talk about?'* There is usually a presenting problem to initiate the discussion, but the therapist is deliberately non-directive. This is partly to ensure that the patient does the work of exploring his own feelings, and partly so that the patient, not the therapist, leads the discussion.

It is assumed at the outset that the therapist and patient can together make sense of the patient's symptoms and life situation. This requires a theoretical model (for example most *psychodynamic* psychotherapists use a model that is based on the ideas of Sigmund Freud – but there are other models too) around which the material brought up during psychotherapy may be arranged. Any such model must enable the doctor to identify key problems, provide explanations for the present problems, and prescribe a means of change.

A case treated by formal exploratory psychotherapy will now be used to illustrate several general principles.

- **The problem**: A 40-year old man presented to the neurologist with a marked tremor at times of stress. This had been present for 20 years, but was becoming more of a problem as the patient was promoted at work. Previous treatment with propranolol and tranquillizer had been ineffective and he increasingly used alcohol to suppress the tremor.
- **Indications for psychotherapy**: He was treated with psychotherapy in view of the failure to respond to other treatments, and the evidence that the tremor was related to interpersonal conflicts. The patient also showed considerable determination to find a psychological cause for his tremor.

- **The contract**: It was agreed that the patient would attend six sessions of 50 minutes each, and progress would then be reviewed. During these sessions the patient's emotions would be explored to try to understand why he reacted to particular situations.

- **The treatment**: When tackled directly no progress was made: the patient simply went over his habitual thoughts on the matter – saying that his marriage was happy, his friendships normal, and others become nervous in front of a crowd; it was inexplicable that his anxiety was so marked.

  Once the patient began to trust the therapist, however, it became appropriate to point out that the patient repeated this description as though he was trying to hide his true feelings ('denial'). It eventually transpired that he felt a failure in his own eyes and that he felt he had let his parents down. This emotional arousal was accompanied by tears. Rather than try to ignore these, he was encouraged to dwell on the feeling of failure. This sense of failure was profound and extended to another problem that had only been hinted at previously, namely premature ejaculation.

  The therapist suggested that the patient normally kept such feelings well hidden, which meant that he lived in terror of being exposed. But the true fear of exposure did not become apparent until later, when, with great anxiety, he admitted to **dreams** of a homosexual nature. He felt enormous relief that his bisexual feelings could be accepted by the therapist as a normal part of his personality.

  The whole set of problems then began to make sense. The tremor had begun soon after he had left a boys' boarding school (where homosexual activity had been common) and at a time when he was beginning to experience a sense of rejection in his heterosexual relationships. His aspirations to be a great success both socially and in his career were proving unrealistic, and those situations where he felt he was under scrutiny were those in which he developed anxiety.

  He then felt able, for the first time, to tackle the sexual problem that had previously seemed insuperable. The anxiety symptoms did not at this stage disappear but he also felt able to tackle these and a course of behavioural therapy utilizing relaxation and desensitization was successful.

PARTICULAR TECHNIQUES USED DURING PSYCHOTHERAPY THAT ARE ILLUSTRATED IN THE ABOVE CASE HISTORY

Analysis of the **patient's reaction to the therapist**: the patient habitually promoted a self-confident image. When the doctor persistently suggested that this facade hid anxiety and doubt, the patient became annoyed. It was analysis of this annoyance that led to exposure of the feelings of failure.

The **emotional arousal** that occurs during treatment may lead to the patient expressing strong feelings (love or hate) towards the therapist. This is also known as the '*transference*'. The origin of such feelings may be in the patient's past experience and important early relationships, and this can be pointed out. It emerged that sitting with the doctor aroused feelings of being with his father, this elicited feelings of dislike and frustration that were initially directed to the doctor.

Such **linking of the present with the past** is often helpful in psychotherapy, but is most efficacious if the present is actually within the psychotherapy treatment session.

The therapist's **reaction to the patient** – which is also known as the '*countertransference*': in the above case the therapist felt irritated that the patient repeatedly asserted that he was really no different from anyone else. He noted that the patient was using denial too forcefully, and this prevented the treatment progressing. The patient initially refuted the therapist's suggestion that he was using denial, but later said that if he had allowed himself fully to accept the need for treatment he would have crumbled into a nervous wreck.

Interpretation of dreams: this technique is simply a way of gaining access to unconscious material that is usually blocked by defence mechanisms. In the above example there had been little or no hint of the patient's homosexual feelings – he was so ashamed they had been well hidden – and it cost the patient an enormous effort to describe them to the therapist. Yet having described the dreams the patient felt enormous relief. The fact that the therapist could accept these as part of the patient's make-up without expressing the revulsion that the patient himself felt was the starting point of improvement.

Note also that in this case it was possible to move from an initial exploratory phase onto a more task-oriented stage while maintaining the patient's cooperation in treatment.

Group therapy

Some patients benefit from discussing their problems in a group. Groups are especially sensible for those who have difficulty relating to other people, or for people sharing a common problem. Large numbers of specialized groups exist for helping patients with particular problems: for example, groups exist for patients who have had operations such as mastectomy or colostomy; for people with alcohol problems, and for those who have recently been bereaved. Support comes from the knowledge that others are experiencing similar problems, and learning ways of coping from other group members. Groups may simply offer support, or they may be the setting for more formal psychotherapy (group analytic psychotherapy) and be conducted by a trained group analytic therapist.

Family therapy

Working directly with a family or a couple can be particularly helpful when relationships within the family are maintaining or perhaps even causing a psychiatric disorder. For example, the family can play a significant role in anorexia nervosa, especially when the patient is still adolescent, and the parents have used eating as a way of exerting control within the family. The eating problem then draws attention to the conflicts about control and the particular ways in which a particular family might express them. Family therapy is most commonly used where a child or adolescent is the presenting patient, but it can also be used where the identified patient is an adult.

126

FURTHER READING

Drug therapy

Anderson, I.M. and Reid, I.C. (2006) *Fundamentals of Clinical Psychopharmacology*. London: Informa Healthcare.

Cooper, J.R., Bloom, F.E. and Roth, R.H. (2004) *The Biochemical Basis of Psychopharmacology*. New York: Raven Press.

Stahl, S.M. (2007) *Stahl's Essential Psychopharmacology. Neuroscientific Basis and Practical Applications*, 3rd edition. Cambridge: Cambridge University Press.

Psychotherapy

Ashton, Heather (1992) *Brain Function and Psychotropic Drugs*. Oxford: Oxford University Press.

Bateman, A., Brown, D. and Pedder, J. (2000) *Introduction to Psychotherapy: An Outline of Psychodynamic Principles and Practice*. London: Routledge.

Meyer, V. and Chesser, E. (1970) *Behaviour Therapy in Clinical Psychiatry*. Harmondsworth: Penguin Books.

Mynors-Wallis, L. (2005) *Problem-Solving Treatment for Anxiety and Depression*. Oxford: Oxford University Press.

Shaw, D., Kellam, A. and Mottram, R. (1982) *Brain Sciences in Psychiatry*. Oxford: Butterworth.

9   PROGNOSIS

The outlook for a psychiatric illness depends partly on the particular condition under consideration, but also partly on factors that cut across diagnoses, and is considered in this short chapter. If you are trying to predict the future course of a particular patient's illness, read the text on prognosis in the appropriate section and then take the following factors into account as well.

Genetic factors

A patient with a strong family history of an illness known to be partly determined by genetic factors – such as schizophrenia or manic-depressive illness – can be expected to have a worse outlook than one with a slight or no family history. However, do not put much reliance on this factor, because there are exceptions in each direction: those with a strong family history can have a good prognosis, and vice versa.

Early childhood factors

Severe deprivation in early childhood often leaves scars for the rest of a lifetime. If your patient will need to settle down in some stable relationship in order to improve, ask yourself what experience life has so far offered your patient of such relationships. A person who has been bereaved in early childhood will always carry a greater vulnerability to losses in later life.

Pre-morbid personality

Don't forget that personality characteristics are by definition relatively constant, so you must not expect your patient to improve much in these respects. For example, a person who has always had depressive traits in their personality is unlikely suddenly to cheer up in middle age.

Similarly, the damage done to anti-social personalities has been inflicted in childhood, and cannot be undone. If your patient is aged over 30, the best level of their pre-morbid adjustment probably indicates the limits of what can be expected of them in the future.

Maturity and immaturity

If your patient is under 30, ask yourself to what extent they can still be expected to mature. Emotionally healthy people in our society, who have not experienced deprivation and upheaval in childhood, can be expected to have completed the greater part of maturation before the age of 20: in developing countries, it is much earlier than that.

However, those who have had disrupted childhoods and who have had no good parental role-models, may take much longer to grow up. Thus a young woman from a miserable home, who has endured divorce of her parents and has been poorly parented, may present in her twenties with episodes of wrist-cutting and self-poisoning. With sympathetic and patient handling such patients may settle down in life later on, so that the demands they have made on medical services during the time of their repeated episodes of self-injury appear, in retrospect, to have been a phase in growing up.

Try to assess your young patient's maturity by asking yourself these questions about them:

1. How physically mature do they look?
2. Are they emotionally independent of their parents yet?
3. Are they financially independent of their parents and, if they are, are they earning their own living?
4. Have they succeeded in having a lasting sexual relationship with another adult?

To the extent that your patient is still immature, there is scope for further improvement. With help, maybe they can learn to adapt more successfully.

Level of pre-morbid achievement

Ask yourself what your patient has been able to achieve in their life before they became ill. Those who have achieved much – emotionally and occupationally – have a much sounder basis to build on after an episode of psychotic illness or head injury. Try to identify any ways in which your patient was disadvantaged **before** he became ill: these are his **pre-morbid handicaps**, and it may be very important to help him with them during rehabilitation.

Previous psychiatric history

This is critically important. As any actuary can tell you, if you want to know about the future, look at the past. One saying has it that in psychiatry 'the diagnosis is from the mental state, but the prognosis is from the history'.

If your patient has never been ill before, there is a much better chance that he will recover completely. If a patient tells you that they have been depressed off and on for the past 20 years, the chances are that they will continue to have episodes of depression in the future.

Precipitating factors

To what extent can your patient's illness be understood as a reaction to a stressful environment? To the extent that it can, and provided that the patient has a good record of pre-morbid adjustment, the future is likely to be good.

Current life adjustment

What sort of social environment has your patient got to go back to in the community? Has the patient someone in whom he or she can confide, and how much support does this confidant provide at times of crisis? What are the living conditions like? And is there financial hardship?

These factors seem especially important in determining the course of non-psychotic affective illness.

Mode of onset

How did the illness begin? Generally speaking, psychological illnesses that begin suddenly have a much better outlook than those with a gradual onset. The best combination is to have a severe stress followed by an illness with an acute onset, while the worst is to have an unprovoked illness of insidious onset.

Length of present illness

Once more, on actuarial considerations: the longer, the worse.

Compliance with treatment

Is the patient likely to comply with treatment? Some people with eccentric personalities, and many of those with sociopathic personalities, are less likely to accept any treatment that requires prolonged cooperation.

If they have had previous episodes of illness, to what extent have they complied with treatment in the past?

The nature of the disorder itself

Generally speaking, the majority of patients with psychiatric illnesses will recover, and a substantial proportion may never have another episode of illness. Even major psychoses like schizophrenia and psychotic depression can have wide variability in their course, with some patients getting completely well, some having only a partial recovery, some having a fluctuating course, and others having a progressive course.

Remember that disorders like manic-depressive psychosis are known to be remittent, so that although you can assure your patient that they will get well, they are actually very likely to have further episodes of illness.

Other disorders – like Alzheimer's disease and Huntington's chorea – are progressive and incurable: details will be found in the appropriate sections.

When considering an individual patient's prognosis, avoid such uninformative terms as 'guarded'. Weigh up the different factors that suggest a good or bad outcome for that particular patient. Remember that the expected outcome may vary according to which aspects of the case we are considering: for example, we might predict:

Complete recovery from florid symptoms, but will probably fail to return to work and there is a high probability of further episodes.

10   FORMULATION

THE PURPOSE OF THE FORMULATION

The formulation is the method used to integrate all the clinical data that are required in order to treat the patient and evaluate the outcome: it is not a case summary. It follows a logical sequence that we have dealt with in turn in the preceding chapters. The purpose of this chapter is to show how these are integrated, and why.

No doubt you will by now be in the habit of making and using diagnoses and may wonder why that isn't good enough for psychiatry, but we have already noted in Chapter 5 that psychiatric diagnoses have important limitations. A diagnosis involves a *nomothetic* (literally 'law-giving') process. This means that all cases included within the identified category have one or more properties in common. For example all those with a diagnosis of pulmonary tuberculosis will have an infectious disease of the lungs caused by the tubercle bacillus. While this is useful information it is quite inadequate as a basis for management. It tells us little about the clinical state, which might range from a chance radiological finding in an apparently healthy person to a fulminating pneumonia, and it certainly won't help us to decide which are the appropriate drugs to use.

In contrast the formulation is an *idiographic* process (literally 'picture of the individual'). This means that it includes the unique characteristics of each patient's case that are needed for the process of management. So, while nomothetic processes are the only way we can advance knowledge about diseases, we use idiographic methods to understand and study the individual.

To pursue the example of pulmonary tuberculosis, the additional information that is taken into account might include the subject's previous state of immunity, nutrition and the state of health of those with whom he lives. It would also take into account the varieties of clinical presentation, sensitivities of the tubercle bacillus, the extent to which the patient is likely to be compliant with medication, and the risk of relapse through cross-infection.

THE FORMAT OF THE FORMULATION

Demographic data

Begin with the name, age, occupation, and marital status.

132

Descriptive formulation

Describe the nature of onset, for example acute or insidious; the total duration of the present illness; and the course, for example cyclic or deteriorating. Then list the main phenomena (i.e. symptoms and signs) that characterize the disorder. As you become more experienced you should try to be selective by featuring the phenomena that are most important, either because of their greater diagnostic specificity, or because of their predominance in severity or duration. Avoid long lists of minor or transient symptoms and negative findings. These basic data are chiefly derived from the history of the present illness, the mental state, and physical examinations, and are used to determine the syndrome diagnosis in the next section. Note that this is not usually the place to bring in other aspects of the history: that comes later. If we know the diagnosis of a previous episode of mental illness, this should also be taken into account, but remember, the present disorder may not be connected and the diagnosis may be different.

Now let's return to Angela Cooper for an example. We have already seen most of the history and examination findings in earlier chapters, but this is how it would be used in the formulation:

> *Angela Cooper is a 29-year-old unmarried woman who works in an office. Eighteen months ago she became depressed following the death of her grandmother with whom she had a close relationship. Over the next year her relationship with her fiancé deteriorated as she accused him of infidelity. Six months ago she discovered that he was indeed having an affair and he broke off their engagement. Since then she has been increasingly low in mood, with associated difficulty sleeping, poor appetite, loss of interest, feelings of guilt and worthlessness, and suicidal thoughts. She recently took an overdose of medication and has been drinking more heavily than usual. On examination there is mild retardation of movement and speech and she appears depressed and anxious. Her thought content is focused on thoughts of guilt about the end of her relationship. She admits to hearing a voice (auditory hallucination) telling her to harm herself. Physical examination reveals small scars on her upper arms and three healing scars on her left thigh.*

Differential diagnosis

List in order of probability all diagnoses that should be considered and include any disorders that you will wish to investigate. These will usually be syndrome diagnoses based on the descriptive formulation above. Give the evidence for and against each diagnosis that you consider. Include any current physical illness that may account for some or all of the phenomena. A common error is to include, for example, thyroid function studies in the investigations without including thyroid disease in the differential diagnosis. If you think a condition is worth investigating, then you are obviously including it in your differential diagnosis; if it's not worth mentioning, don't bother to investigate it.

Remember that in addition to the primary diagnosis you may need to consider a supplementary diagnosis, for example alcoholism in a patient presenting with delirium, or a personality disorder in a patient with an anxiety state. Regarding Angela Cooper:

1. *Depressive illness: morbid grief reaction* (preferred diagnosis). *The symptoms and signs are essentially those of a depressive illness, with depressed mood, depressive thought content and neuro-vegetative features. This has developed in the setting of bereavement, but has been exacerbated by a further recent life event – the end of her relationship. The psychotic symptom is consistent with depressed mood.*

2. *Manic depressive disorder: In view of the psychotic symptom it is necessary to consider the possibility that this is a depressive episode in a bipolar affective disorder. However there is no evidence of manic episodes in the past.*

Additional diagnoses:

1. *Self harm: Recent overdose of medication. Evidence of possible self-injury on physical examination.*

2. *Alcohol misuse or dependence: Recent heavy consumption of alcohol.*

Aetiology

The various factors that have contributed should be evident mainly from the family and personal histories, the history of previous illness, and the pre-morbid personality. Remember you should aim to answer these questions: Why has this particular patient developed this particular illness at this particular time? If necessary, look back to *Table 6.1* for the systematic method used to identify the relevant factors. We have already considered the aetiology of Angela Cooper's case in some detail (p. 77) but this is how it might be presented in the formulation:

> *Predisposing factors include a family history of depressive illness in her mother, and family violence and emotional trauma in childhood. It has been precipitated by the illness and subsequent death of her grandmother, and maintained by the subsequent break-up with her boyfriend to whom she had been engaged.*

Investigations

List all investigations that are required to support your preferred diagnosis and to rule out the alternatives, and also any that you think are required to improve your under-standing of the aetiology. Give reasons for investigations if they are not self-evident. Include all sources of additional information. Have another look at *Table 7.1* to remind yourself about how to plan investigations systematically.

> *Investigations should include contacting her general practitioner to find out more about her past history of mental illness and review her own and her mother's hospital records. She also requires physical examination, full blood count and liver function tests. It will be important to observe her mood state through the day, sleep and appetite, and to keep a weight chart. Insight-oriented psychotherapy may help to determine the aspects of her bereavement that have determined morbid grief.*

Treatment

Outline the treatment plan that you wish to follow. This should stem logically from your discussion of the aetiology as well as from the diagnosis. Consider each stage of management in turn as described in Chapter 8, starting with the preliminary arrangements and finishing with the possible need for prophylaxis.

> **Treatment**: *It is preferable initially to provide treatment on an in-patient basis in view of the severity of Angela's depression and the risk of suicide. This should be on a voluntary basis. If the depressive symptoms persist in hospital following a few days observation she should then be started on an antidepressant (SSRI) for treatment of her depression. She may also require antipsychotic medication. She should be encouraged to attend occupational therapy in order to maintain social and occupational skills. **Psychotherapy** should initially be supportive and, although some insights may be obtained, it should not be interpretive – at least until her depressive symptoms are much improved. However in the longer term she might benefit from more insight-oriented psychotherapy to help her come to terms with the death of her grandmother in the first instance, and possibly to explore deeper issues relating to her low self-esteem and sense of insecurity in relationships that probably relates originally from her early childhood experiences.*

Prognosis

Describe the expected outcome of management of this illness episode, with regard to both the symptoms and also subsequent function, for example self-care and return to the community. Consider the risk of subsequent relapse. Give your reasons for these predictions based on the principles described in Chapter 9.

> **Prognosis**: *Angela is likely to have a protracted recovery from her depressive illness because it has lasted for 18 months and has been complicated by a recent further loss event, and also excessive use of alcohol. The prominence of neuro-vegetative symptoms suggests that she will respond to antidepressant medication, but will also need continuing psychological treatment and social support to help her make sense of events and recover fully. It will be necessary to liaise with the GP for long-term support aimed at preventing future episodes.*

HOW TO USE THE FORMULATION

Aim to write up formulations for each patient you clerk during the psychiatric attachment, and discuss them with the medical staff. The formulation should be written up as soon as you have clerked the patient and written up the record of the history and mental state examination. Of course you will probably want to modify your formulation later on when you have additional information.

The formulation is not an alternative to the history and mental state examination. In many departments you will be expected to present the history and mental state followed by the formulation, but this will depend on local practices.

We have referred in earlier chapters to the hypotheses that are an intrinsic part of the clinical approach, and this requires explanation. In the formulation the clinical data are used to set up hypotheses concerning the diagnosis and aetiology of the case. The investigations, and even more important the response of the illness to the treatment, provide the method for testing them. By observing the outcome of investigations and management we are able to discover whether our initial hypotheses were correct, but we can only do so if we recorded them in the formulation.

If our hypotheses are not supported, for example the patient has failed to improve with the planned treatment, then we have to review the accuracy of the original data. This will require reappraisal of the history and mental state and possibly further investigations.

Now we are going to look at a further formulation to illustrate this process, based on a different clinical problem. This should help you to start to integrate what you have learnt from the previous chapters in this section of the book, and give you an idea of what to aim at when you are writing up your own formulations.

FORMULATION: PSYCHOSIS

Demographic data

Mr Alan Reeves is a 24-year-old unmarried graduate who is unemployed.

Descriptive formulation

He was admitted as an emergency 1 week ago after being taken to the casualty department by his flat-mates. He had shown increasingly disturbed behaviour in the last 3 months, with persecutory delusions of being followed by the CIA and believed that they were using laser beams to control his actions. He had heard voices discussing plans to kill him, and on the day of admission had destroyed most of his possessions while apparently searching for a video camera that he thought had been 'planted' in his room. He had started to become withdrawn socially 4 years previously, in his final year at university, and despite graduating had not worked since. He had cared for himself adequately but showed little motivation or interest except for playing the guitar and taking a variety of non-opiate drugs, including cannabis and amphetamines, regularly since then.

On mental state examination he appeared fully conscious, his clothes were dishevelled, he was suspicious in manner, and he paced the room. There was no spontaneous speech and he appeared secretive when answering questions, but talk was coherent and relevant. His mood was subjectively 'all right' but he appeared tense and frightened, and sweated profusely. He was secretive about the recent destruction of his possessions. During the interview he appeared to be distracted, listening and talking to voices on several occasions, but denied this when asked. He was correctly orientated in time and place. He would not cooperate with formal tests of cognitive function but correctly identified and had learnt the names of the ward staff and gave an accurate account of a recent visit from his parents. He thought he was not ill but needed help – 'probably police protection' – and was willing to remain in hospital because he said he felt safer.

On physical examination he was thin, with evidence of self-neglect, but no other abnormality.

Differential diagnosis

1. **Paranoid schizophrenia**. This is characterized by the persistent delusions of persecution and control and auditory hallucinations discussing the patient. The history prior to this suggests the insidious development of 'negative' symptoms, with apathy, lack of volition and marked social deterioration, and gradual development of hallucinations. There is no evidence at present of clouding of consciousness, cognitive impairment or persistent mood disorder. Drug abuse is likely to be secondary to schizophrenia.
2. **Psychotic disorder due to drug abuse (symptomatic schizophrenia)**. The symptoms that have occurred in the last 3 months are consistent with the acute psychoses that are associated with both amphetamines and cannabis, particularly following heavy or prolonged abuse. The chronic social deterioration during the preceding 4 years may be due to the 'amotivational syndrome' that is associated with chronic ingestion of cannabis. These states commonly occur in clear consciousness. The possibility of other drug and alcohol effects must also be considered despite the patient's denial of abuse.
3. **Psychosis secondary to other organic conditions**. Many other intracranial or systemic disorders (e.g. cerebral tumours, endocrine disorders) can present with a paranoid psychosis, but the absence of physical abnormalities on examination, together with the long duration, makes this less likely. Some evidence of clouding of consciousness or intellectual impairment would be likely and these have not yet been excluded, due to the patient's limited cooperation.
4. **Drug abuse with psychological dependence**. This is an additional rather than differential diagnosis, which does not in itself account for the psychotic features. It is based on evidence of the prolonged use of, and strong desire to continue taking, cannabis and amphetamines; the neglect of other activities; and continuation of the habit despite evidence of harm.

Aetiology

Predisposing. There is a non-specific family history of a maternal uncle who is said to have lived for many years in a mental hospital, and one of his brothers has shown social deterioration similar to the patient's, so there may be a genetic predisposition to schizophrenia. There is no evidence of perinatal or developmental problems, or of personality problems before the last 4 years.

Precipitating. The social withdrawal and deterioration started in his final year at university when he had the stress of impending final examinations and the disappointment of a broken engagement (although the latter may have been secondary to his disorder). The more recent deterioration followed within weeks of the arrival of a new flat-mate who wanted the patient to move out.

Maintaining. Contributory factors are likely to be drug abuse, increasing social isolation, and failure to receive treatment.

Investigations

1. **Medical records** of the uncle and brother.
2. **Further history** from parents, particularly concerning family history, childhood development and pre-morbid personality, and from flat-mates about his recent state.
3. **Psychological**. Observations on the ward of his beliefs, perceptions and behaviour – including possible drug or alcohol ingestion. Examination of cognitive aspects of the mental state and, if performance is impaired, psychometric testing for an organic disorder. Later, it will be necessary to assess his insight into psychosis and drug abuse and his likely compliance with their management.
4. **Physical investigations** should include haematology, electrolytes and liver function tests in view of self-neglect and possible effects of drugs and alcohol; urine drug and alcohol screen. If there is evidence on mental state of a possible organic disorder, then electroencephalogram and computerized axial brain scan.
5. **Social**. Observation of extent of social withdrawal on ward and relationships with his family and flat-mates when visiting – consider whether there is evidence of 'high expressed emotion'. When mental state improves, assess his abilities and strengths in occupational therapy and other settings in order to plan aspects of rehabilitation, including self-care, occupation, and recreation.

Treatment

Initially he should receive in-patient care, in view of his self-neglect and destructive behaviour; and as a voluntary patient as he was willing to be admitted and accept treatment.

Physical. It is best to observe him for 1 to 2 weeks without medication to see if the psychosis starts to resolve spontaneously when he is drug free, although a neuroleptic such as chlorpromazine or haloperidol may be given if he is otherwise difficult to supervise on the ward, for symptomatic control. If there is no obvious improvement then he should be started on regular doses of an oral neuroleptic, the dose of which will have to be adjusted depending on response and possible unwanted effects. In view of chronicity, it is very likely that subsequently he will require long-term neuroleptics, preferably with depot injections to improve compliance. He will need counselling regarding the effects of drug abuse, and encouragement to remain abstinent.

Psychological and social. Initially he should be allowed to avoid pressures of involvement in group activities, but as psychotic symptoms settle down there should be increasing emphasis on rehabilitation. This should include individual and group activities, which build on past interests and achievements, and encourage self-care and social activities, initially in hospital and then increasingly in the community. He will then need help to find suitable accommodation, possibly in a supervised hostel or sheltered housing for the mentally ill. Alternatively it may be possible for him to return to live with his family, who will need information about his disorder and how they can contribute. He will also need arrangements for day-care, either in a day hospital or social services day-centre. Subsequently it may be possible for him to do voluntary work, or retraining for work might be arranged through the disablement resettlement officer.

Long-term care may involve follow-up at the psychiatric out-patient clinic and/or clinic for depot medication, or this may be provided by close collaboration with the general practitioner or community psychiatric nurse to ensure long-term support

Prognosis

Factors suggesting a poor outcome include insidious onset, prolonged duration, and 'negative symptoms'. However, there are also some favourable factors – the lack of problems in his pre-morbid personality, his good educational record and continuing contact with and support from a caring but not over-involved family. If drug abuse has been an important cause and he becomes abstinent this will greatly improve the outcome.

FURTHER READING

Greenberg, M., Szmukler, G. and Tantam, D. (1986) *Making Sense of Psychiatric Cases*. Oxford: Oxford Medical.

PART 2

SYNDROMES
OF DISORDER

11   PSYCHIATRIC ASPECTS
OF PHYSICAL DISEASE

This chapter first considers the kinds of relationships that can exist between psychological and physical ill-health, and then considers the psychological manifestations of various physical illnesses, including psychiatric aspects of epilepsy. A final section deals with acute and chronic pain.

Numerous studies have shown that there is a strong relationship between physical and psychological illness, which cannot be accounted for by chance association. All too often, doctors in hospital practice consider the possibility that there is something psychologically wrong only when they have failed to find a physical cause for their patient's symptoms. This is a very bad policy since most psychologically disturbed patients on the medical wards *have a physical disorder* as well. Nor is it true that patients in whom we have failed to make a physical diagnosis necessarily have psychological disorders! *Psychiatric diagnoses should be made on positive evidence of disorder, and not by exclusion.*

At one time it was usual to divide physical diseases into those in which psychological factors were thought to be relatively unimportant, and others called 'psychosomatic diseases', which were thought to be partly caused by psychological factors. Eczema, asthma, coronary heart disease, diabetes, and ulcerative colitis were thought to be examples of such diseases. However, the term is no longer used since no one now supposes that diseases can be divided up in this way. It is impossible to think of a disease that is not affected in some way by psychological factors – even a virus wart can be removed by hypnosis.

RELATIONSHIPS BETWEEN PHYSICAL DISEASE AND PSYCHIATRIC ILLNESS

There are in fact five kinds of relationship between psychiatric disorders and physical symptoms that account for the high rates of psychiatric illness seen on surveys in general medical settings:

1. **Psychiatric disorder may provoke or release physical disease**. Depression is the illness most likely to do this. In surveys of psychiatric illness in medical in-patients, a proportion of cases will be found where the sequence is:

    stressful life event → episode of depression → physical ill-health

It is possible that these apparently causal sequences are just part of the tendency for illnesses to come in clusters in people's lives, rather than at random time points. There is no doubt that 'functional' illnesses like asthma and migraine are more likely to occur when patients are psychologically unwell, and there is some evidence that the same is true for conditions such as eczema and carcinoma of the cervix.

2. **Psychiatric illness may be the direct consequence of a physical disease**. If the physical disease had not occurred, the psychiatric illness would not have done so – at least, not at that particular time in the patient's life. This is a common relationship, and is perhaps the easiest one to understand. A patient who has noticed a potentially serious symptom like a breast lump or an episode of rectal bleeding may become anxious about the possible cause; a patient who knows he has cancer may become depressed. Physical illnesses that are associated with disability in previously healthy people are also likely to lead to depression, which in turn exacerbates the disability. Allow the patient to ventilate his anxieties, and be sure to correct any fears that are unrealistic or just wrong. If it is not possible to reassure the patient, give information about the investigations that are to be carried out, and promise to keep the patient informed. If the patient has a depressive illness an antidepressant should be prescribed. SSRIs are better tolerated by patients with physical illnesses, since they have fewer side-effects than tricyclic antidepressants. Sedating antidepressants are also effective in anxiety, and will not lead to dependence, but females do not tolerate them very well.

3. **Psychiatric disorder may exacerbate the pain of a physical disease**. Patients who are depressed experience pains and discomforts more severely than when they are well, and the experience of anxiety has been shown to lower the pain threshold. This general relationship holds for any chronic pain, from sciatica to malignant disease. When a patient who is known to have some chronic disease complains of an exacerbation of their pains it is tempting to conclude that the underlying disease has deteriorated: but it is often not true. Treatment of such affective illnesses is an extremely important part of your general management plans for the patient's illness. However, the principles are the same as those described already: see page 225 for anxiety states, and pages 217–220 for depressive illnesses with anxiety.

4. **Psychiatric illness may present to doctors with physical symptoms that have no organic basis. Anxious people experience pain – often abdominal – from increased muscle tension; depression lowers the pain threshold**. This phenomenon is called the 'somatization' of psychological distress, and its existence explains why some clinicians consider psychological causes only when they have failed to make a physical diagnosis. However, as we shall see, somatization can be expanded to cover cases where there is undoubted physical disease, but this disease does not really account for the patient's physical symptoms. Treatment here is directed at the psychiatric disorder. The patient needs to understand how emotional disturbance may result in physical pain, so that they can 're-attribute' the pain they experience, and discuss the problems that are related to their distress. We give an extended account of somatization in Chapter 16 (see pp. 234–249).

5. **The psychiatric symptoms may be the presenting symptoms of a physical disease**. This is not all that common, but it happens. Thyrotoxicosis may present as an anxiety state, myxoedema and pernicious anaemia may present as depression, myasthenia gravis may be mistaken for neurosis. Treatment will of course be directed at the underlying disease. However, do not forget to explain to your patient that their disease has been responsible for the psychiatric symptoms described to you, and ask the patient to let you know if these symptoms do not remit. A full account of such disorders follows in the next section.

PSYCHIATRIC PRESENTATIONS OF PHYSICAL DISEASE

Many physical diseases have psychological symptoms as part of their presentation. This is true of most endocrine disorders, many metabolic disorders, and some neurological diseases.

ENDOCRINE DISORDERS

Hypothyroidism

Mental symptoms are as prominent as physical symptoms in myxoedema, and take the form of memory loss, somnolence, and depressed mood. The cognitive changes may be so severe that the patient is thought to have a **chronic brain syndrome**: since the condition is reversible in its early stages, **thyroid function tests** should be done in all cases of **pre-senile dementia** (see pp. 174–177). The patients complain of lethargy: they feel slowed up, are disinclined to undertake even familiar tasks, and are unable to concentrate. Patients are often diagnosed as depressed, and the hypothyroidism is missed. Major psychotic illness may also occur.

Hyperthyroidism

Patients are over-aroused, distractible and anxious. The presentations may be irritable, show easy startle responses, and be intolerant of frustration. They can therefore closely resemble **anxiety states**, but the additional feature of hyperthyroidism should allow the correct aetiology of the anxiety to be diagnosed.

There may be histrionic disturbed behaviour, and sometimes excitement is such that the patient satisfies the criteria for a **manic illness**. As with myxoedema, other psychotic illnesses, including agitated depression and schizophreniform illnesses, have also been reported. The thyroid disease is presumably releasing psychosis in vulnerable people.

Cushing's syndrome

Depression is easily the commonest psychosyndrome seen, ranging in severity from mild to severe with paranoid features. Well over 50 per cent of patients with Cushing's syndrome may be expected to have depressive symptoms. These symptoms are a direct result of the increased level of corticosteroids, since treatment of the hormonal disorder causes the depressive symptoms to disappear, yet they re-appear if the Cushing's syndrome relapses. In theory one might expect manic syndromes since exogenously administered steroids produce euphoria, but such syndromes are rare.

Hypopituitarism and hypoadrenalism

The psychosyndrome consists of weakness, lack of energy, tiredness with defective memory and poor concentration. The patient may be somnolent and self-neglectful, so the condition can be misdiagnosed either as depression or as dementia.

Sheehan's syndrome

This is a post-partum necrosis of the pituitary. There is chronic ill-health with lack of energy, depression and sensitivity to cold: think of it if lactation did not occur and menstruation did not resume after the post-partum haemorrhage: confirm by the absent pubic and axillary hair followed by appropriate biochemical investigations.

Acromegaly

Earliest symptoms often include apathy and loss of initiative. Some patients become depressed and irritable, while others show lability of mood.

Parathyroid disease

The commonest psychological disorder is **depression**, which tends to be both marked and early. It occurs in both hypo- and hyper-parathyroidism, and appears related to calcium rather than to parathormone levels.

Diabetes mellitus

Listlessness, irritability, and confusion may usher in diabetic coma. Late complications include some degree of chronic brain syndrome if there have been cerebrovascular accidents, or if there has been damage secondary to prolonged hypoglycaemia.

Hypoglycaemia

This may occur with diabetes mellitus, with an insulinoma ('spontaneous hypoglycaemia'), or it may be provoked by alcohol. Early psychological symptoms are anxiety or panic, weakness, and sometimes depersonalization. This may be followed by ataxia or clouding of consciousness, or by peculiar and uncharacteristic behaviour. The patient may be aggressive and noisy, and there is usually some degree of motor incoordination. If treatment is delayed, irreversible brain damage will result. When hypoglycaemia is provoked by alcohol, a malnourished person takes a large quantity of alcohol and lapses first into stupor, then coma. Surrounding drinkers assume he is 'dead drunk'. Unless the true diagnosis is made, death is indeed a possibility.

Renal failure

Mental clouding, poor concentration, and listlessness lead to drowsiness and disorientation. 'Uraemia' may thus present as **delirium**, or it may aggravate a mild dementing illness in an elderly patient. Depression can be marked and require treatment. Symptoms are not due to urea itself, but to electrolyte imbalance and toxic levels of drugs.

RENAL DIALYSIS

This is associated with three psychological problems: patients often complain of *anxiety and depression*; rapid reduction of urea may lead to *headache, muscular twitches, fits* and *confusion* – perhaps because of cerebral oedema; and a *progressive dementia* has been described associated with high brain aluminium concentration ('dialysis encephalopathy').

Hepatic failure

The features of hepatic pre-coma are psychological and motor, and are a result of nitrogenous substances derived from food. The patient may be noted to have a fixed, staring appearance with a reduction of spontaneous movements.

There are periods of clouded consciousness with perplexity, forgetfulness, dysarthria and ataxia. Hypersomnia occurs, and the characteristic flapping tremor can be elicited. There is sometimes a fatuous personality change similar to a frontal lobe disorder (see p. 171).

Acute intermittent porphyria

This is a rare disorder, but psychotic symptoms may be prominent, in association with unexplained abdominal pain. Histrionic behaviour and emotional lability are common. It is beginning to look as though George III did not suffer from it.

TOXIC DISORDERS AND DEFICIENCIES

Carbon monoxide poisoning

This is a cause of a severe amnestic syndrome. Extrapyramidal damage may also occur: personality changes include impulsiveness, moodiness, and aggression.

Thiamine

Depression, irritability, lassitude, and anorexia occur in those deprived of dietary thiamine. Vague somatic complaints and forgetfulness occur as the deficiency becomes

147

more severe; finally Korsakow's syndrome (see pp. 179–180). Acute depletion will cause Wernicke's encephalopathy (see pp. 179–180).

Nicotinic acid

Pellagra has prominent psychiatric abnormalities, of which the most dramatic is a *paranoid hallucinatory psychosis*. However, other psychological manifestations include disorientation and confusion, excitement with outbursts of violent behaviour, and depression.

Vitamin B₁₂ and folic acid

Amnestic syndrome, subacute delirium, and chronic brain syndrome may either antedate or accompany the megaloblastic anaemia, and are reversible with treatment. *Vitamin B_{12} deficiency* has been said to lead to depressive symptoms, but the evidence is unclear.

Folic acid deficiency is associated with depressive symptoms accompanied by low drive and anergia, and also with chronic dementia in the elderly (see p. 175).

ACQUIRED IMMUNE DEFICIENCY SYNDROME (AIDS)

AIDS is caused by infection with *human immunodeficiency virus* (HIV) and at present is a fatal illness. The virus is thought to be neurotropic and symptoms can arise from any site in the central nervous system. In addition to the direct effect of the virus, there may be effects on the central nervous system, caused by intercurrent infections and neoplasia. The organic effects, the psychosocial consequences, and the anticipated fatal outcome all contribute to the high psychiatric morbidity.

Epidemiology

The world-wide distribution of HIV infection and AIDS is thought to vary considerably. In the United Kingdom high-risk groups include intravenous drug abusers, homosexual men, and haemophiliacs, and infection may be increasing in heterosexual men and in women. A high risk for mental disorders arises as a result of AIDS and also to the increased psychiatric morbidity associated with substance abuse and homosexuality.

Psychiatric syndromes

CHRONIC BRAIN SYNDROME

Chronic brain syndrome occurs eventually in at least two-thirds of patients with AIDS, in whom it has been called *AIDS dementia complex* (ADC). The early stages may not be obvious on routine clinical examination, but defects on complex mental and motor tasks

148

are evident on psychological testing. The disorder usually develops gradually over months, with increasing cognitive impairment, focal neurological signs, and sometimes psychotic symptoms. More rapid deterioration may be caused by infection or malignancy. Computerized tomography or magnetic resonance imaging usually show cortical atrophy.

ACUTE BRAIN SYNDROME

Acute brain syndrome results commonly from the various physical disorders that occur in the course of AIDS, and from their treatments. It presents in the same way as in other medical disorders.

AFFECTIVE DISORDERS

Depressed and anxious mood are common in all the groups that are at high risk for HIV infection, even if they are HIV negative, but tend to be increased in those who are HIV positive. There are many factors that contribute. Depressed mood is often found in patients with ADC and is also thought to occur as a *symptomatic mood disorder* as a result of HIV infection, in the absence of cognitive impairment. Suffering from a socially stigmatizing, terminal illness often leads to *major depressive disorders* or *generalized anxiety states*, and in others there are *adjustment disorders* with depressive and anxiety symptoms, anger, and hostility. Most patients are likely to go through a process of *grief*. Investigation of haemophiliac men has demonstrated the effect of *predisposing factors* in addition to the effects of infection, diagnosis, and their consequences. Those who are HIV positive are particularly susceptible to disorders of mood if there is a past or family history of mental disorder, poor social support, or recent life events involving loss.

Treatment

Antiviral treatment, for example with zidovudine, can result in improved cognitive function in those with ADC. *Neuroleptic drugs* may be needed to control psychotic symptoms, but should be used with particular caution because HIV appears to result in supersensitivity to the dopamine blocking effects and there is particular risk of extrapyramidal symptoms as well as neuroleptic malignant syndrome. The use of *tricyclic and heterocyclic antidepressants* should be based on the same criteria as in other disorders, although there are reports of increased sensitivity to anticholinergic side-effects so that it is preferable to start with relatively small doses that should then be increased. Heterocyclics may be better tolerated than tricyclics.

Psychosocial approaches to treatment should be made available to all patients, and contributions to compassionate care can be provided effectively by voluntary and self-help organizations as well as by professional multi-disciplinary services. Individual and group support can help patients and carers, and some patients may benefit from psychological approaches to anxiety management.

Prevention of spread of infection is a major priority. Measures include education and counselling for sexually active heterosexuals and homosexuals about 'safe sex', and also the availability of uncontaminated syringes and needles for intravenous drug users.

NEUROLOGICAL DISEASE

We deal with cerebral tumours and dementia in Chapter 12. Two neurological illnesses are strongly linked with *affective illness*.

Parkinson's disease

There is an important association with **depression**, which often follows the onset of Parkinsonian symptoms. Treatment of the depression may dramatically alleviate the motor symptoms.

Multiple sclerosis

At one time students were taught that patients tended to develop euphoria. This can happen when there is general cerebral impairment, but it is not common. Most patients will describe symptoms of **anxiety and depression**, and such symptoms can greatly add to the burden that their disease imposes.

EPILEPSY

Most of those patients prone to epilepsy are psychiatrically normal, and are not at particular risk for chronic brain syndromes, for major mental illness, or for personality disorder. However, there is an increased risk for such disorders in those whose epilepsy is symptomatic of some organic cerebral disorder, and pathology in the temporal lobe seems especially important in this respect.

Nevertheless, most epileptic patients experience prejudice from others, and this may cause both social handicaps and depressive symptoms that are more disabling than the fits.

Definition

A *seizure* is an attack of sudden onset and usually brief duration that becomes clinically manifest through sensory, motor, psychic (affective, cognitive), or autonomic symptoms. It is associated with spontaneous abnormal electrical activity in the brain as measured by the EEG.

Every brain has a *threshold* for the development of seizures. Given the right type of stimulus, anyone could develop a seizure. These triggers include metabolic derangements, febrile illnesses, cerebral inflammatory or infectious illnesses, acute stroke or head injury, intoxication with certain drugs, and acute drug or alcohol withdrawal syndromes. The occurrence of such *symptomatic seizures* does not indicate a diagnosis of epilepsy.

150

Epilepsy may be defined as the occurrence of *recurrent* seizures. Although patients are not usually started on anti-epileptic drugs after an isolated spontaneous seizure, the other factors that are taken into account in estimating the risk of further seizures are: age of onset (children and old adults being more at risk), partial seizures, structural or congenital brain lesions, neurological disorder, and an abnormal EEG. However, an abnormal EEG is not by itself sufficient for a diagnosis of epilepsy, since 'epileptiform' EEG abnormalities may also occur in seizure-free individuals.

Epidemiology

The prevalence of epilepsy in the general population has been estimated to be between four and six per thousand at risk, with an equal sex incidence. The lifetime risk of developing seizures is about 5 per cent, and about 30 per cent of those with epilepsy will develop a mental disorder.

The incidence of epilepsy is highest in childhood and adolescence and is approximately equal in both sexes. There is a small tendency, thought to be genetically determined, for epilepsy to run in families. Among children, psychiatric disorders occur in around 7 per cent of those without epilepsy, 30 per cent of those with uncomplicated epilepsy, and 60 per cent of those with epilepsy complicated with brain damage.

Clinical features and classification

The most important basis for the classification of seizures is whether or not they start focally in the brain. This has implications for choice of anti-epileptic drugs. *Partial seizures*, as their name implies, start focally, most commonly in the temporal lobes. *Generalized seizures* have no focal onset when recorded on the EEG.

PARTIAL SEIZURES

Partial seizures are divided into *simple* or *complex*: the former do not involve impairment of consciousness, whereas the latter do. Partial seizures may spread and become generalized, a process known as *secondary generalization*. It is important to note that a partial seizure may only manifest itself clinically at the time of generalized spread, so that its focal nature may only be realized when recorded on the EEG.

In **simple partial seizures** the ictal manifestations include sensory or motor phenomena, depending on the part of the cortex involved. Spontaneous movements may spread along a limb and then recede, while the subject retains full awareness – a sequence called a 'Jacksonian march'. The focal symptoms of which the patient is aware are called *auras*, and they may or may not be followed by a generalized seizure with impairment of consciousness. Auras last only a few seconds. This, together with their sudden onset and intense, stereotyped characteristics, helps to differentiate them from other types of mental phenomena such as anxiety attacks or other neurotic symptoms.

In **complex partial seizures** the aura is followed by impairment of consciousness, as the attack originates in areas of higher cerebral organization. In complex partial seizures of *temporal lobe* origin (previously called temporal lobe epilepsy or psychomotor epilepsy) the aura may include hallucinations of hearing, vision, taste, or smell. There may be an 'epigastric aura' experienced as a central abdominal churning feeling that spreads upwards through the chest, and there may also be feelings of flushing, tachycardia, fear, and dizziness. Particularly memorable are sudden feelings that unfamiliar surroundings are familiar (*déjà vu*) or the reverse (*jamais vu*), but similar experiences occur commonly in the absence of epilepsy. Automatic behaviours, such as grimacing, lip-smacking, **automatisms** (*p. 369) and **fugues** (*p. 370) may occur in a state of clouded consciousness.

GENERALIZED SEIZURES

The two commonest types of generalized seizures are *tonic-clonic* and *absence attacks*, also known as 'grand mal' and 'petit mal'.

Tonic-clonic attacks are subcortical in origin, and therefore start without warning. However, there may be ill-defined prodromata such as malaise, nausea, or headache that build up in the days before an attack. There is sudden loss of consciousness and generalized increase in muscle tone. This tonic phase is shortly followed by a clonic phase of generalized, rhythmic, muscle spasms involving all parts of the body symmetrically from the same moment. During the fit the tongue may be bitten and there may be incontinence of urine. This stage usually lasts for minutes but can last for hours ('status epilepticus'). Clinical examination during this stage reveals fixed pupillary dilatation, absent corneal reflexes and extensor plantar reflexes. The post-ictal phase lasts for about an hour, during which time the patient may be disorientated, incoherent or drowsy, and may complain of nausea or headache.

In **absence attacks** the patient suddenly loses touch with his environment and appears dazed. Posture and balance are maintained, but the pupils will dilate and the patient appears pale and immobile to an observer. Sometimes the head may slump forward slightly and there may be twitches round the eyes. Consciousness is deeply impaired during the attack, which typically lasts only 5 seconds or so, but can last longer. Attacks typically occur at least daily, and there is usually no evidence of a brain lesion.

Other types of generalized attacks include *myoclonic* and *atonic attacks* ('akinetic attack'). The former is characterized by generalized myoclonic jerks, and the latter by an abrupt loss of muscle tone. All generalized attacks are associated with sudden loss of consciousness at the onset of the attack.

Epilepsy in childhood

Epilepsy presents in distinctive ways:

1. **Neonatal seizures** are often the presenting symptoms of serious congenital abnormalities or meningitis. Unless they are a result of hypocalcaemia, the prognosis is grave.

2. **Febrile fits** are the commonest form of epilepsy, affecting 3 per cent of children at some time. They accompany fevers and are generally bilateral, brief, and benign. If they take their onset in the first year of life, last for more than half an hour, or are lateralized, the prognosis is more serious.
3. **Infantile spasms** take the form of recurrent forward flexion of the trunk ('Salaam epilepsy') coming perhaps three times a day. The onset is between 4 and 18 months, there is an association with early infantile autism (see p. 307), and there may be failure of normal intellectual development.
4. **The Lennox–Gastaut syndrome**, or 'atypical petit mal', is associated with four kinds of attack: generalized seizures, drop attacks, tonic attacks, and atypical absences. The EEG shows atypical, 'notched' spike and wave discharges.
5. **Petit mal** occurs in childhood: the child maintains posture, but is unconscious during attacks (which may be referred to as 'absences'). The EEG shows three per second spike and wave during an absence, and the child may have generalized seizures at other times.
6. **Petit mal status** ('status of minor epilepsy') is commoner in childhood and old age than in adult life: it can persist for prolonged periods (several months) and although the child is conscious there is clouding accompanied by inability to concentrate and motor incoordination: school work usually suffers, and the EEG shows continuous three per second spike and wave.
7. **Generalized epilepsy** ('grand mal') is sporadic throughout childhood.

Differential diagnosis

Epileptic seizures must be distinguished from other organic causes of sudden loss of consciousness, such as simple faints (syncope), transient ischaemic attacks, and spontaneous hypoglycaemia.

Psychiatric and behavioural disorders include: temper tantrums and breath-holding attacks and night terrors in children; hyperventilation, panic attacks, aggressive outbursts in explosive personalities, and pseudo-seizures in adults.

PSEUDO-SEIZURES

Finally, epileptic seizures must be distinguished from psychologically determined simulations of fits, or pseudo-seizures. Although pseudo-seizures tend to occur in young females they can present in anybody, *including those who also have epileptic seizures*. The simulation may be unconscious (usually classified with dissociative symptoms – see pp. 241–245) or conscious (i.e. malingering – p. 244).

Pseudo-seizures are usually characterized by non-stereotyped motor activity, which does not follow closely any of the recognized patterns of epileptic fits. They tend to occur when other people are present, and may involve emotionally laden cries or sexualized movements. The patient may tend to fight the examiner off, but fixed pupillary dilatation, absent corneal reflexes, and extensor plantar reflexes are not found if the examiner persists. It is rare for the patient to void urine and bite her tongue during the attack. However, they appear to be unconscious during the attack, and to thrash their limbs about in ways that can be quite convincing if they have seen others with genuine seizures. They tend to be in a bad temper when 'coming round', but they share this characteristic with patients recovering from tonic-clonic attacks.

The importance of a past history of sexual abuse is increasingly being recognized in some of these patients. These episodes are not accompanied by the typical EEG changes of epilepsy, nor is a raised serum prolactin level found subsequently.

Aetiology

In about 66 per cent of cases no cause can be found for epilepsy even after full investigation ('idiopathic'); in such cases genetic factors appear to have some importance. In the remainder the epilepsy can be shown to be secondary to some known cerebral disease: birth injury, congenital malformations, exanthemata, and metabolic disorders in children; cerebrovascular disease, head injury, and degenerative disorders in the elderly.

Drugs may cause epilepsy in two ways: sudden withdrawal of agents known to have anti-convulsant properties such as benzodiazepines or barbiturates; or administration of agents known to lower the convulsive threshold, such as phenothiazines and, to a lesser extent, tricyclic antidepressants.

Withdrawal from large doses of alcohol also causes generalized seizures (see p. 151). Alcohol or drug abuse should therefore always be considered in a patient with no previous history of epilepsy who has a fit following admission to hospital.

Psychiatric aspects of epilepsy

PERSONALITY CHANGES

Attitudes of dependency and insecurity may be engendered by over-protection during childhood, or by the social and occupational problems that must be faced. These may increase vulnerability to depressive illness.

Patients with temporal lobe epilepsy can exhibit explosive irritability and aggressiveness, and also may report sexual problems: either hyposexuality or deviant practices such as fetishism or transvestism.

ANXIETY AND DEPRESSION

The most common psychiatric disorders that occur in those with epilepsy are anxiety states and depressive disorders. There is an increased risk of suicide. An over-protected existence and the social handicaps that often accompany epilepsy may contribute to feelings of worry and low self-esteem, although these do not necessarily amount to psychiatric disorder.

Depression, anxiety, and low self-esteem are common, perhaps because of the social handicaps experienced by most epileptics.

PSYCHOTIC ILLNESSES AND EPILEPSY

Post-ictal psychosis is uncommon. Typically it develops following a period of lucidity, about 24 hours after a major attack. A florid psychosis, with schizophreniform or affective symptoms, or a mixture of these, then develops and lasts around 3 weeks, sometimes longer. It may take the form of a *paranoid hallucinatory state* accompanied by some clouding of consciousness ('epileptic twilight state').

Inter-ictal psychoses are uncommon but tend to develop many years after the onset, particularly of complex partial epilepsy arising from the temporal lobe. They usually present as *symptomatic schizophrenia* of chronic paranoid type. There is no clouding of consciousness. It takes its onset a decade or more after the onset of the complex partial seizures. It is thought that this is more likely to develop in patients with a dominant (usually left-sided) epileptic focus in the temporal lobe. The expectation of schizophrenia in first-degree relatives is not increased, nor is there increased expectancy of schizoid personality, suggesting that the psychosis is indeed secondary to the epilepsy. *Forced normalization* refers to the normalization of the EEG or the improvement in seizure frequency that occurs in some patients when they develop recurrent psychotic episodes.

EPILEPSY AND CHRONIC BRAIN SYNDROME

There are two possible relationships: a dementing illness may present as epilepsy; or hypoxia associated with long-standing epilepsy may cause a chronic brain syndrome. In old age *petit mal status* may present as an apparent dementing illness of sudden onset. Diagnosis is on the EEG.

MANAGEMENT OF EPILEPSY

A full history, including an interview with anyone who has witnessed the seizures, is essential. A physical examination followed by laboratory and brain imaging investigations are necessary to exclude the possibility of symptomatic seizures. Inter-ictal EEG studies are used for the classification of epileptic seizures. Video-telemetry consists of video-recording of seizures in parallel with EEG recordings. A post-ictal EEG is invaluable in the diagnosis of post-ictal psychosis, which demonstrates generalized post-ictal slow wave changes.

Serum prolactin rises immediately after a tonic-clonic seizure and reaches a peak about 20 minutes after seizure onset. It does not, however, rise after status epilepticus and it may be equivocal following complex partial seizures.

The vast majority of patients with epilepsy can be managed with *single anti-epileptic agents*. In a minority with recalcitrant seizures, combinations of drugs may be useful,

155

although this increases the likelihood of drug-interactions and side-effects. The drugs are described on pages 101–106.

Counselling on social aspects, such as driving law, and on practical steps to avoid injury, must not be forgotten. Relatives must be advised to ensure the safety of patients during a seizure, but to avoid restraining movement as much as possible. In particular, they should be asked not to insert spoons or any other sharp objects into the mouth in misguided efforts to open the airways. Inappropriate disability is common, and advice for the patient and carers is needed to avoid its development, or to reduce disability after it is established.

Neuroleptic drugs or antidepressants may be needed for the treatment of mental disorders associated with epilepsy, but many psychotropic agents *lower the convulsive threshold*.

The treatment of **pseudo-seizures** follows the same principles as other forms of abnormal illness behaviour (Chapter 16, see pp. 246–249). (This may include suggestion coupled with a cognitive-behavioural programme and, in suitable cases, family therapy.)

PAIN

Pain is a perception and as such is a part of the mental state. It is commonly associated with tissue damage, and peripheral nerves then play an important part in its transmission. However, central neural mechanisms play a predominant part in pain perception: pain can be caused by CNS lesions, and is also modified by CNS activity, serving both to exacerbate it (as in depressive illnesses) and to relieve it (as exemplified by the use of hypnosis for dental analgesia).

Frequency and diagnosis

Pain is the commonest symptom of which patients complain, accounting for between 50 per cent and 95 per cent of presentations in medical out-patient clinics. Frequently it remains undiagnosed: approximately half of all patients presenting with pain to neurologists, cardiologists, and gastroenterologists show no evidence of relevant organic pathology after intensive investigation and long-term follow-up. Of patients with diagnosed mental illness in general practice and psychiatric out-patient settings, about 60 per cent complain of pain. It seems likely that pain is associated as much with mental as with physical illnesses, and occurs particularly in the setting of affective disorders. However it has little diagnostic specificity and can occur as a symptom of any mental illness. As usual, diagnosis is based on the nature of associated symptoms.

Psychological mechanisms of pain

1. The physiological effects of anxiety are widespread. Increased muscle tension is believed to result in 'tension headache'; increased intestinal motility may be experienced as abdominal pain; palpitations may lead to chest pain.

156

2. Pain is often experienced at a site where there is, or has been, some minor organic pathology, which has not previously caused the patient distress, but serves as a focus once the patient becomes anxious or depressed.
3. Depression and anxiety result in reduced tolerance of pain, whatever its origins.
4. Somatization frequently presents as pain and may result from the use of other defence mechanisms, such as introjection. It is a common feature of anxiety states, depressive disorders and morbid grief reactions (see pp. 229, 230).
5. The awareness of pain becomes more intense and the associated illness behaviours more frequent as a consequence of reinforcement by others who respond to the patient more positively when he shows such behaviours.

Acute pain

The intensity of pain associated with organic disease and trauma, including post-surgical pain, is related particularly to anxiety. Patients in hospital may experience anxiety for many reasons, but much is often due to lack of familiarity with investigation and treatment procedures and the extent to which pain should be anticipated. Pre-surgical preparation which includes careful explanation of the procedures that the patient will experience and the availability of post-surgical analgesia, has been shown to reduce both the post-surgical pain experienced and the need for analgesia.

Female patients and those with higher scores on measures of neuroticism tend to complain more about post-surgical pain and receive more analgesics from ward staff; others suffer pain of similar intensity but complain less, and consequently suffer more because staff are unaware of their pain and fail to give analgesics. It is important to ask patients routinely about pain in order to determine the appropriate management.

Chronic pain patients

Patients with chronic pain (usually defined as of more than 6 months duration) may suffer from a wide range of physical and mental disorders. It is a common error to suppose that such patients can be divided into those with 'real' or 'organic' pain and those with 'imaginary' or 'psychogenic' pain': first because both organic and psychological factors often play a part in the same patient, and second because pain is primarily a subjective experience and, if perceived, is always 'real', whatever its origins. Any combination of the mechanisms described above may play a part, and many aspects of illness behaviour associated with the pain may appear inappropriate. Drug abuse is often an important secondary problem that may be iatrogenic.

Surveys of patients attending pain relief clinics show that at least half are suffering from mental illness, diagnosed using standardized methods, but few of these disorders are recognized by the anaesthetists who run the clinics and few are referred to psychiatrists. About two-thirds of those with mental illness have depressive disorders, most of the remainder having primary hypochondriasis.

FURTHER READING

Eastwood, M. (1975) *The Relationship between Physical and Mental Illness*. Toronto: University of Toronto Press.

Kleinman, A. (1980) *Patients and Healers in the Context of Culture*. London: UCLA Press.

Williams, P. and Clare, A. (1979) *Psychosocial Disorders in General Practice*. London: Academic Press.

12   ORGANIC BRAIN SYNDROMES

Organic brain syndromes may either involve the entire cortical canopy, in which case they are said to be **generalized**; or they may involve only a specific part of the cortex, in which case they are said to be **focal**. These conditions are further described by their clinical course – acute illnesses are described as **delirium** and chronic illnesses as the **dementias** (the terms acute and chronic brain syndromes are no longer used). These are all syndromal diagnoses, and they will always require further investigations to establish the cause in a particular case.

DELIRIUM

Terminology

You may be confused by a variety of terms for delirium, all meaning almost the same thing. Older people are often said to present with an *'acute confusional state'* (see discussion on page 343). A *toxic confusional state* refers to an acute brain syndrome secondary to toxic causes such as those listed in *Table 12.1*. Many clinicians use the word delirium to mean an acute brain syndrome with pronounced psychomotor agitation often accompanied by hallucinations and illusions, but others do not make this distinction.

Epidemiology

This is a common condition occurring in 5–10 per cent of general medical and surgical in-patients. It is common in the elderly and up to 30 per cent of the population have been estimated to suffer from this syndrome at some time in their lives. It is the most common cause of a psychotic state that occurs in the general wards.

Clinical features

Despite the plethora of aetiologies shown in *Table 12.1* the clinical picture is relatively constant. It is characterized by:

Table 12.1 *Causes of delirium*

	Systemic	Intracranial
Trauma		Head injury
Degenerative	Dementia with acute illness	
Epileptic		Post-ictal states Petit mal status
Vascular	Myocardial infarction Anaemia Heart failure Hypertensive encephalopathy	Cerebral thrombosis or embolism Subarachnoid haemorrhage Transient ischaemic episode Internal haemorrhage
Infections	Exanthemata Septicaemia Pneumonia Influenza Typhoid Typhus Cerebral malaria Trypanosomiasis	Encephalitis Meningitis Rheumatic chorea Cerebral abscess
Metabolic	Uraemia Liver failure, Alkalosis, acid–base disorders Acidosis, hypercapnia Electrolyte disturbances Remote effects of carcinoma Anoxia CVS, chest disease and anaemia	
Endocrine disorders	Hyperthyroid crises Myxoedema Addisonian crisis Diabetic pre-coma; hypoglycaemia Parathyroid disease	
Toxic	Drugs: see text, p. 162 Alcohol: delirium tremens Wernicke's encephalopathy Heavy metals: lead, arsenic, mercury	

1. **Clouding of consciousness** (see p. 26) that has an acute onset and a fluctuating course – being worse at night, better during the day, and improving as the underlying pathological process resolves. Minor degrees of clouding of conscious-ness may be difficult to detect unless the patient is examined at night or when he is fatigued. Poor attention and impaired thinking may only be evident with persistent cognitive testing. In severe cases it may be impossible to gain the patient's attention at all as he is responding only to hallucinatory experiences and his speech is an

incoherent rambling totally incomprehensible to the observer. Clouding of consciousness can be a difficult concept to grasp and so this symptom is now regarded as mainly a disorder of attention.

2. **Disorientation in time** (see p. 37) occurs first, followed by that of **space and person**. The disorientation fluctuates with level of consciousness, and the person may be orientated by day and disorientated by night.

3. **Impaired thinking** ('confusion') occurs in conjunction with clouding of consciousness. Thinking may be slowed initially but progressively reasoning becomes less clear and incoherent.

4. **Disturbance of registration, retention, and recall** occur.

5. **Perceptual abnormalities** often make the staff first aware of the patient's abnormal mental state. *Illusions and misinterpretations* may dominate the picture. Unfamiliar objects and people are at greatest risk of being misinterpreted. Members of staff may be regarded by the patient as enemies or involved in a plot. Drugs may be misinterpreted as poison and these will be refused. *Visual hallucinations* are common though *auditory and tactile hallucinations* also occur. The hallucinations may form complex scenes in which the patient feels he is involved and by which he may be terrified.

6. **Emotional changes**. Anxiety, irritability, depression, and apathy occur first but frank fear may occur with or without the hallucinatory or persecutory phenomena described above. The patient may attempt to leave the ward in order to escape the frightening scenes he is experiencing.

7. **Psychomotor changes**. Either change may occur: *psychomotor retardation* may be evident with apathy and withdrawal from the patient's surroundings; but in the more severe forms *restless over-activity* is more common, with the patient plucking at the bedclothes or attempting to get out of bed. The latter pattern is seen in *delirium tremens* (see p. 165).

The failure to learn new material is usually evident on recovery when a dense amnesia for the duration of the delirium is evident. Occasionally there have been lucid intervals when the patient's conscious level returns to normal and there may be fragmented but vivid memories of emotionally charged scenes.

Diagnostic criteria

The following criteria may be used for research purposes:

A. **Clouding of consciousness** of acute onset, accompanied by *reduced capacity for attention*,

B. and TWO or more of following:
  1. **Disorientation** or **memory impairment**.
  2. **Perceptual disturbance** (misinterpretations, illusions or hallucinations).
  3. **Incoherent speech**.

4. Disturbed **sleep–wakefulness cycle** with insomnia and daytime sleeping.
5. Increased or decreased **psychomotor activity.**

Aetiology

The syndrome is produced by any cause that disrupts total brain functioning, and is the same irrespective of whether the exciting cause is intracranial (such as encephalitis or subdural haematoma) or systemic (such as pneumonia or uraemia). More than one factor may be present, and factors may contribute to the aetiology that have not been listed as 'main causes'. For example, following an operation residual anaesthetic, pain, mild respiratory problems, toxins from blood transfusion, opiate analgesic drugs, dehydration, anxiety, and unfamiliar surroundings may each be insufficient in themselves, but together account for delirium.

Examination of the time of onset of the condition may provide a clue to the principal factor; this may coincide with the onset of a pyrexia, the changing of a drug, or development of dehydration.

TOXIC EFFECTS OF DRUGS

A wide range of drugs are capable of causing an acute brain syndrome, particularly:

1. **Dopamine agonists** (especially in combination):
   Benzhexol.
   L-dopa.
   Amantadine.
2. **Antidepressants.**
3. **Tranquillizers and hypnotics**:
   Barbiturates.
   Benzodiazepines.
   Neuroleptics.
4. **Anticholinergic drugs**:
   Atropine.
   Hyoscine.
5. **Antituberculous drugs**:
   Isoniazid.
   Cycloserine.
6. **Cytotoxic drugs**.
7. **Anticonvulsants** (especially in high dose).

Alcohol and **barbiturates** can cause toxic symptoms either by acute intoxication or by withdrawal. Thus, an acute brain syndrome developing 24 to 72 hours after admission may result from the sudden cessation of regular alcohol intake, or of a drug upon which the patient is dependent.

Differential diagnosis

DEMENTIA

A previously undetected dementia can present for the first time as a delirium if the person develops some intercurrent infection that produces a state of acute cerebral decompensation. As the infection resolves, dementia becomes apparent. The same can happen if there is some sudden change in the patient's environment, such as the death of a spouse or moving to a new house. In either case, such a transient acute brain syndrome is sometimes referred to as a *decompensated dementia*.

FUNCTIONAL ILLNESS

Depression in the elderly (see pp. 345, 346) may present with clouding of consciousness and impaired ability to concentrate. The acute onset of *mania* or *schizophrenia* may be accompanied by perplexity, clouding, and impaired ability to think in addition to more typical schizophrenic phenomena.

In these functional conditions, clouding, disorientation, and impaired concentration will generally be less pronounced than other features of the mental state. Thus in severe depressive illness depressed mood and psychomotor retardation will predominate over the cognitive changes, and in schizophrenia the psychotic features will become clear with time.

Investigations

These will be ordered according to the abnormal physical findings present. Unless a likely cause is evident from your physical examination:

A useful first round of investigations would be:

Full blood count
ESR

Urea and electrolytes
Liver function tests

Thyroid function tests
Blood sugar
Serology for neurosyphilis

Urine for microscopy and culture
Urine for drugs

Chest X-ray

To distinguish between delirium and functional illness:

> EEG – shows slow waves in delirium

The following may be necessary:

> Serum B$_{12}$ and folate
> Lumbar puncture
> CT or MRI scan

Treatment

Investigations are best carried out in hospital in all but the mildest of situations.

TREATMENT OF THE UNDERLYING CAUSE

Correction of the underlying physical abnormality is the primary goal of treatment. It may be necessary to correct a number of factors. Any abnormalities of fluid or electrolyte balance, or haematological and nutritional factors should be corrected. *Any drugs that are not essential should be stopped.*

SYMPTOMATIC AND SUPPORTIVE MEASURES

Tranquillizers may be necessary if the patient is otherwise unmanageable. Since such medication can itself cause delirium it should be kept to a minimum and only used if the nursing procedures described below are unsuccessful.

Any of the second-generation antipsychotics (*risperidone, olanzapine, quetiapine, aripiprazole*) can be helpful in the treatment of delirium. Doses should be adjusted according to the frailty of the older person. Haloperidol is an effective drug when the disturbance is severe. *Chlomethiazole* is useful in delirium from any cause in which epileptic fits might occur, such as delirium tremens.

These drugs are particularly useful at night, as sleep deprivation can exacerbate the delirium.

In order to minimize misinterpretations the patient should be nursed in a room that is *well lit during the night* and by a small number of staff whom the patient can easily recognize. The patient will require *frequent reassurance* because of his fear, and *repeated explanation* by calm members of staff can reduce the need for sedation.

Early detection of delirium may avoid the necessity for sedation, so any reports by the night staff of mild degrees of clouding or disturbed thinking in seriously ill patients should be investigated fully.

Course and prognosis

Following resolution of the underlying disorder, the delirious state may linger for days. In one study of delirium the majority of patients had either cancer or serious heart disease and the mortality rate during the index admission was 20 per cent and by 1 year nearly 50 per cent. However, the prognosis in cases caused by drug intoxication or withdrawal is much better than for those in whom an underlying potentially fatal illness causes the delirium.

SUBACUTE DELIRIUM

This is a state intermediate between an acute and a chronic illness: the onset will have been less sudden than is usual in delirium; there will be a combination of features of the two; and the course is also intermediate. Wernicke's encephalopathy (see pp. 179, 180) often presents in this way.

DELIRIUM TREMENS

About 5 per cent of patients admitted to hospital with physical complications of alcoholism will display delirium tremens. Typically it occurs in middle-aged men who have been drinking heavily for some years, but it can also occur after only a few months of heavy drinking.

The first 12 hours:

Mild withdrawal phenomena such as tremor and agitation occur.

Twelve to 48 hours after withdrawal:

Generalized epileptic seizure may occur.

Three to 4 days after withdrawal:

The clinical picture in delirium tremens occurs, and is similar to that in acute brain syndromes of other aetiologies, but the following features are marked:

1. Dramatic, sudden onset with restlessness, insomnia, and fear.
2. Clouded consciousness and disorientation.
3. Startle reactions, nightmares, and panic.
4. Face terror-stricken.
5. Ataxia and tremor present.
6. Perspiration, tachycardia, low pyrexia; flushing or pallor.

Later:

1. Profuse visual and tactile illusions and hallucinations (pink elephants rare; rats, snakes and nameless small animals common, vivid, and terrifying).

2. Auditory hallucinations may be threatening or persecutory.
3. Disorientation and confusion.

Treatment

This is an urgent matter, the patient is **admitted to hospital** and:

1. **Sedation** is essential with chlormethiazole or diazepam, which have **anticonvulsant properties** in addition to being tranquillizers. These can be given 4-hourly and intravenously if necessary. They should be given on a reducing regime and stopped after, at most, 14 days.
2. Parenteral administration of **B vitamins** can prevent Wernicke's encephalopathy if instituted early.
3. **Fluid replacement** may be necessary as dehydration can be severe. Electrolyte balance must be obtained: hypokalaemia and hypomagnesia are common.
4. **Hypoglycaemia** is common and can cause serious cerebral damage. The infusion fluid should therefore include **dextrose**.
5. Concurrent **infection or head injury** often accompanies the delirium and treatment is instituted as necessary.
6. Once the acute phase is over the patient will require continuing **sedation at night** when vivid nightmares result from REM rebound. To avoid dependence on the sedative drug a *reducing regime lasting for approximately 10 days* is used.
7. On recovery, the patient must be examined for all the *effects of alcohol* including evidence of chronic alcoholic brain damage (see p. 171). Assess motivation for treatment of alcoholism.

Course

Delirium tremens usually resolves in 3 days, but continuing high levels of anxiety may continue for weeks or months afterwards. These require treatment as they contribute to the risk of the patient rapidly returning to alcohol.

Mortality of DTs has been 10–15 per cent, with death resulting from epileptic fits, heart failure, infection, or self-injury during the most disturbed phase.

DEMENTIA

Epidemiology

It is estimated that 10 per cent of the population over 65 years of age are affected by dementia. This figure rises to 22 per cent in the over 80 year-olds. The majority remain in the community and less than one-fifth of the severe cases are admitted to hospital or live in an old people's home.

Clinical features

The manifestation of the clinical syndrome of dementia can be divided into three parts. First, a neuropsychological element consisting of **amnesia** (loss of memory); **aphasia** (either a receptive aphasia or expressive aphasia, the latter being more apparent in conversation, and nominal aphasia tested by direct questioning of naming of objects); **apraxia** (the inability to carry out tasks despite intact sensory and motor nervous systems, manifest in dementia most usually by an inability to dress often described as putting on a shirt or coat back to front, or the inability to use a knife and fork correctly); and **agnosia** (the inability to recognize things such as one's own mirror reflection or a family member – remember this is different to forgetting the name of someone).

Second, a neuropsychiatric component with associated symptoms such as psychiatric disturbances and behavioural disorders that are present in a substantial proportion of patients. The commonest are (approximate frequencies in brackets): **depression** (up to 66 per cent at some point during their dementia); **paranoid ideation** (30 per cent); **misidentifications** (usually based on agnosia, 20 per cent); **hallucinations** (most commonly auditory, suspect an intercurrent delirium or *Lewy body dementia* if **persistent visual hallucinations** are present, 15 per cent); **aggression** (20 per cent); **wandering** (20 per cent).

Third, deficits in **activities of daily living**. Towards the later stages of dementia these are manifest by obvious problems in dressing, eating, and going to the toilet. In the early stages they may be manifest by a failure to wash or dress to a person's usual standard, and in people living alone, self-neglect of the diet can lead to weight loss and neglect of household tasks to comments about the cleanliness of the house.

This triad of presentation is common to all types of dementia, the differentiation being based on the clinical presentation, the presence of other features, and other aspects of the history and examination.

Presentation

Failure of memory may be so insidious that it does not attract medical attention until it is very pronounced. There may be progressive failure to cope with social situations, or matters may come to a head when normal routines are disturbed, and the patient is unable to cope.

1. **Memory impairment (amnesia)** without clouding of consciousness is the hallmark of the syndrome. This is often first noticed by relatives and workmates rather than the patient himself, who may even deny the impairment. It may be so gradual that it is difficult to date the onset. Minor forgetfulness, and failure to remember names and appointments, lead on to more definite evidence of amnesia. The patient may lose his way in familiar territory, a decline in performance at work may become evident, and the patient may become hopelessly mixed up with complex tasks at home such as cooking from a recipe. Leaving the gas on, wandering at night and forgetting the day are common ways in which the memory loss is brought to the

attention of others. The impairment of memory is global, but loss of short-term memory is a conspicuous early sign with relative preservation of long-term memory initially. Recall is affected and the person may need prompts even for previously well-established memory traces. Some patients conceal their memory loss by using lists and sticking to a strict daily routine. A spouse or other close relative may have tolerated and helped to compensate for the patient's memory loss, in which case the death or move of the relative will bring the difficulties to light.

2. **Personality deterioration** reflects both intellectual deterioration and changes in social awareness. The earliest change may be an exacerbation of personality traits producing obsessional or hypochondriacal symptoms. Loss of manners may occur, the person ignores the feelings of others and becomes increasingly stubborn, irritable and withdrawn. In later stages personal care and hygiene deteriorate, with food stains on clothing and chaotic living conditions resulting. Eventually urinary and faecal incontinence occur, but the patient may have become so apathetic that he appears unconcerned by this.

3. **Thinking** becomes slowed and restricted with a tendency to brood on a few themes from the past. Perseveration occurs. The dementing person cannot cope with new ideas and abstract thinking is lost. Concentration is impaired and the person becomes easily fatigued. Judgement is impaired, and ideas of reference or even delusions develop because the power to reason is lost. Thus an item that is lost through forgetfulness and later found is regarded by the person as evidence that an intruder has been in the house. In later stages thinking is confined to very few themes and may become incoherent. These abnormalities of thinking are reflected in the speech of the dementing person, which is slow, impoverished and may eventually become a series of incomprehensible words and phrases.

4. **Psychiatric symptoms**, traditionally associated with the functional psychoses, can occasionally occur as the presenting sign of an organic brain syndrome. Between one-third and one-half of patients with Alzheimer's disease will have such a symptom at some stage in their illness. They include: delusions, paranoid ideas, hallucinations (mainly visual or auditory), misidentifications (of other people, of themselves in a mirror, of events on television or a belief others are in the house), affective disturbance (usually depression but occasionally mania), and behavioural disturbances (such as aggression, wandering, sexual disinhibition, and eating disorders). Some changes may be understandable in the light of amnesia (accusing a relative of stealing a handbag when in reality it has been lost). Irritability occurs and occasionally emotional lability (unprovoked outbursts of anger, distress, or laughter) but these are said to be commoner in vascular dementia. Occurring during cognitive testing, an outburst of frustration and tears is deemed a **catastrophic reaction**.

5. **Aphasia, apraxia, agnosia**. These are signs of cortical dysfunction:
   - **Aphasia** is usually a mixture of receptive and expressive, and may be manifest as an inability to name objects on confrontation (anomia).
   - **Apraxia** indicates an inability to carry out a motor task, despite intact motor and sensory symptoms, and is manifest by an inability to dress properly or to use a knife and fork.

- **Agnosia** reflects an inability to recognize people or objects. Occasionally, the presenting symptom of dementia may be an inability to recognize a close friend or relative.

Alzheimer's disease

This is the commonest form of dementia.

Familial cases have been described with autosomal dominant inheritance, but generally a multifactorial inheritance is suggested. The morbid risk of first-degree relatives of patients with Alzheimer's disease is increased four times.

NEUROPATHOLOGY AND NEUROCHEMISTRY

Cortical atrophy is generalized but most marked over the frontal and temporal lobes. Loss of neurones in the neocortex, together with proliferation of astrocytes, senile plaques, and neurofibrillary tangles are striking, and in greater number than in the normal aged brain. Clinical manifestations of dementia appear when the plaque count and neurofibrillary changes reach a certain threshold. In normal ageing the brain seems to have sufficient reserve capacity to withstand a limited amount of such changes and yet maintain normal function.

There is a **loss of cholinergic neurones** innervating the neocortex: the loss of these neurones is indicated by marked reductions in the concentration of the enzymes *choline-acetyltransferase* and *cholinesterase*. Much of the cholinergic innervation of the neocortex originates from the nucleus basalis of Meynert located at the base of the forebrain; neurones in this nucleus degenerate in Alzheimer's disease. The importance of cholinergic mechanisms has been demonstrated: cholinergic drugs, such as the cholinesterase inhibitor *physostigmine*, cause a transient improvement in memory functions in patients suffering from Alzheimer-type dementia, whereas anticholinergic drugs, such as the muscarinic receptor antagonist scopolamine, have the opposite effect. Since cortical postsynaptic muscarinic receptors remain relatively unaffected in Alzheimer's disease, attempts have been made to stimulate these receptors by *cholinomimetic agents* (choline, lecithin) administered to the patients: these efforts, however, have remained unsuccessful.

Apart from cholinergic neurones, noradrenergic and 5-hydroxytryptaminergic neurones innervating the neocortex can also degenerate, resulting in reductions in cortical noradrenaline and 5-hydroxytryptamine levels. Consistent decreases have been shown in the cortical levels of *somatostatin*, indicating the degeneration of nerve cells containing this neuropeptide transmitter.

Vascular dementia

This results from chronic cerebrovascular disease and often occurs in the absence of an identifiable cerebrovascular accident. Other evidence of arteriosclerosis is found throughout the cardiovascular system, and focal signs such as **pseudo-bulbar palsy**, **increased reflexes, extensor plantar responses**, and **extrapyramidal features** occur more often than in Alzheimer's disease. Marked cerebral softening occurs in this type of dementia and this differentiates it from Alzheimer's disease, where senile plaques predominate.

Onset is uncommon before the age of 50, and the sex ratio is approximately equal. The most striking difference between this type of dementia and Alzheimer's disease is the step-wise progression, and the presence of the evidence of arteriosclerosis on physical examination. Patients may complain of **somatic symptoms** such as headache, dizziness, tinnitus, and syncope in addition to problems with memory. There may be transient attacks of hemiparesis, dysphasia, or visual dysfunctions that are at first followed by restitution, but that eventually lead to the dementia becoming more profound.

Pick's disease

This is less common than Alzheimer's disease, but a familial pattern is also well recognized. The frontal and temporal lobes are particularly atrophied. **Personality changes** and **dysphasia** therefore occur early in the disease. Neuronal loss occurs with gliosis, but plaques and tangles do not and the EEG may be normal.

Huntington's disease

This disorder is characterized by a combination of **dementia**, **extrapyramidal features**, and **choreic movements**. The transmission of this disease by a single autosomal *dominant gene* is well recognized, with half the offspring of an affected person being affected. It is now becoming possible to identify some of the carriers of the gene. Reduced levels of GABA in the basal ganglia and substantia nigra are thought to be responsible for the choreiform movements. The dementia often appears slowly, and later in the disease than the neurological or psychotic features. The latter start with personality changes, such as becoming quarrelsome, slow, and apathetic, but schizophrenic symptoms and marked mood changes occur.

The frontal lobe shows greatest atrophy, along with the caudate nuclei, and marked dilatation of the ventricles.

Creutzfeld-Jacob disease

Cerebral atrophy is less marked in this form of dementia, but a characteristic spongy appearance of the grey matter is seen microscopically along with neuronal loss and proliferation of astrocytes. This may occur in different parts of the brain accounting for the different clinical presentations. The *EEG is always abnormal* with increased slow-wave activity and bilateral spike-wave discharges that accompany the characteristic **myoclonic jerks**. It has been demonstrated that this disease can be transmitted from man to primates experimentally, and some instances have occurred when 'natural' transmission has occurred. It is therefore believed that a slow virus or virus-like particle is responsible, and the illness has been related to Kuru. It is probable that the virus-like particle fails to invoke the usual inflammatory response in the brain, and a similar aetiological factor is being sought in other forms of pre-senile dementia.

Lewy body dementia

In the last 10 years, Lewy body dementia has been increasingly recognized as a cause of the dementia syndrome. It draws its name from the fact that the pathological changes consist of Lewy body (an intercellular protein deposit named after the describer) found in the neocortex.

CLINICAL FEATURES

These are fluctuating cognitive impairment affecting memory and higher cognitive functions, visual or auditory hallucinations (usually accompanied by paranoid delusions), spontaneous extrapyramidal features, or evidence of extreme sensitivity to neuroleptics, and repeated unexplained falls. The fluctuating pattern lasts months rather than weeks (in the case of delirium), and other physical causes (including cerebrovascular disease) have been excluded. As with vascular dementia, Lewy body disease can co-exist with Alzheimer's disease. The important issue in relation to dementia of Lewy body type is the tendency for patients to be very sensitive to the effects of neuroleptics, and injudicious use of these drugs can lead to extreme sensitivity of reactions and an increased mortality rate.

Dementia of frontal lobe type

Dementia of frontal lobe type is characterized by atrophy of the frontal lobe in the absence of Alzheimer-type pathology. There seems to be an overlap between this type of dementia and Pick's disease. Clinical and pathological criteria for fronto-temporal dementia have been published, with the main features being insidious onset and slow progression. There is early loss of personal and social awareness, early signs of disinhibition, hyperorality, stereotyped behaviour, distractibility, and emotional changes. Spatial orientation and praxis are relatively preserved.

Alcoholic dementia

There is increasing evidence that cerebral atrophy occurs in a proportion of those who have drunk heavily for many years. In the early years the chronic brain syndrome associated with alcoholism appears to be reversible. Four *neurological diseases* are worth highlighting.

NORMAL PRESSURE HYDROCEPHALUS.

This is a form of hydrocephalus in which there is an obstruction in the subarachnoid space to the free egress of CSF from the ventricles. **Memory impairment**, a stiff-legged

171

shuffling gait, urinary incontinence, and slowness develop over weeks or months. The EEG is frequently abnormal; but the diagnosis is confirmed by CAT scan, which shows symmetrical ventricular enlargement but no enlargement of the subarachnoid space above the basal cisterns. Treatment is by insertion of a shunt with a low-pressure one-way valve, between the lateral ventricle and the superior vena cava. Results are variable, but sometimes impressive.

NEUROSYPHILIS

General paralysis of the insane (GPI) has become something of a rarity, but was at one time an important cause of a chronic brain syndrome accompanied by highly characteristic neurological signs (Argyll-Robertson pupils, trombone tremor of tongue, dysarthria, ataxia and upper motor neurone signs). *Meningo-vascular syphilis* presents with headache and lethargy, which proceeds to a dementia: there may be a basal meningitis with cranial nerve palsies and a wide variety of other neurological signs depending on the area involved.

PARKINSON'S SYNDROME

Arteriosclerosis may underlie both the dementia and movement disorders in Parkinson's syndrome. But dementia has also been reported in cases of idiopathic Parkinsonism, the aetiology of which is uncertain.

MULTIPLE SCLEROSIS

Minor cognitive impairment can be detected in the majority of patients with multiple sclerosis. Profound global dementia is uncommon but is rarely the presenting feature of the illness.

When investigating a case of chronic brain syndrome it is especially important to detect conditions that may be either arrested or partially reversed, and these have been asterisked in *Table 12.2*.

Differential diagnosis

DEMENTIA MUST BE DIFFERENTIATED FROM FUNCTIONAL ILLNESSES

1. **Depressive pseudo-dementia.** Old patients who are depressed may appear to be demented, in that they complain of defective memory, appear disoriented, have a poor knowledge of current events, and perform poorly on cognitive tests. A detailed history from an informant should differentiate the initial depressed mood, leading to later disturbance of memory from the picture of dementia that starts with memory and behavioural impairments but leads on to depression at a later stage. A past history of a depressive episode, depressive symptoms antedating other symptoms, and a more acute onset should put one on the right track.

Table 12.2 *Non-degenerative causes of dementia*

	Systemic	*Intra-cranial*
Degenerative		See text p. 174 Boxing encephalopathy
Space-occupying lesions	Secondaries	Cerebral tumours* Subdural haematomas* Normal pressure hydrocephalus*
Infections		Neurosyphilis* (GPI or meningovascular) Chonic encephalitis
Anoxic	Anaemia* Congestive cardiac failure* Chronic respiratory failure	Carbon monoxide poisoning Post-cardiac arrest
Metabolic	Uraemia* Liver failure* Remote effects of carcinoma	
Endocrine	Myxoedemia* Addisons disease* Hypoglycaemia* Parathyroid disease*	
Toxic	Barbiturates* Bromides* Manganese Carbon disulphide	Alcohol atrophy
Vitamin deficiency	B_{12} and folic acid deficiency* Thiamin deficiency* Nicotinic acid deficiency*	

Note: * Potentially reversible cause for chronic brain syndrome.

2. **Hysterical pseudo-dementia**. A patient may be brought to a casualty department having been found wandering and unable to give his name and address (see **hysterical amnesia**, p. 241). Alternatively a patient may be admitted with suspected dementia, but close observation reveals inconsistencies between his poor performance on formal cognitive testing and his ability to find his way around the ward. The **Ganser syndrome** consists of 'talking past the point' and giving 'approximate answers':

> *How many legs does a horse have?*
> *Five*
> *What colours are the lights on a traffic light?*
> *Red, yellow and blue.*

173

The patient's answers are markedly inaccurate, yet they indicate that the question has been understood. The absurd responses are given deliberately and with apparently serious intent. The playful, childish quality of some of the patient's answers is also seen in the 'buffoonery syndromes' associated with hebephrenic schizophrenia or chronic hypomania. The patient may also report hallucinatory experiences, have a fluctuating level of consciousness and demonstrate other hysterical phenomena. Such states are most likely among those with low IQ and a history of previous head injury. Either hysterical mechanisms or conscious simulation (malingering; see p. 244) may be involved.

3. **Psychotic illness**. *Hypomania* may appear as a picture of dementia, especially as formal cognitive testing is difficult or impossible. Chronic schizophrenics with prominent defect symptoms may also appear demented. The other characteristics of the illness should be clear from the history.

DEMENTIA MUST ALSO BE DISTINGUISHED FROM OTHER ORGANIC ILLNESS

1. **Korsakow's syndrome** (see p. 179). Here the disorder is confined to short-term memory and disorientation in time; whereas chronic brain syndrome is a global syndrome involving ability to think, lability of emotion, and changes of personality.
2. **Delirium** (see p. 160). Here the onset is more acute, and there is clouding of consciousness. In chronic brain syndrome the patient is more in touch with his surroundings, and attempts to cooperate despite cognitive difficulties. In acute brain syndrome the patient fluctuates, and can sometimes be shown to be cognitively intact in lucid intervals. Severe perceptual disturbances are more likely in acute brain syndrome.
3. **Focal brain syndromes**. Focal neurological signs are of great importance in localizing disease within the brain. In the degenerative pre-senile dementias neurological signs are usually symmetrical. If dysphasia is produced by focal disease, patients have as much difficulty recalling objects from sight as from memory, whereas patients with diffuse chronic brain disease do much better if they can handle and see the object.
4. **Learning disability**. A careful history will reveal that the patient's problems are not of recent origin, and psychometric tests will show a vocabulary in keeping with verbal and performance IQ, whereas in dementia there will be relative preservation of vocabulary.

Investigation of dementia

CONFIRMATION OF THE DIAGNOSIS

Psychometric testing (see p. 180) when the patient is not physically ill, in pain, unduly depressed, or anxious.

INVESTIGATIONS

Interview an informant to obtain the following information:

1. Possible family history of dementia or Huntington's chorea.
2. Previous head injuries: even slight ones may be important.
3. Recent history of faints, fits, or episodes of collapse.
4. What drugs have been taken? Is there possible dietary neglect?
5. What is the patient's usage of alcohol?
6. Obtain description of the personality before illness. Ask about previous episodes of depression.
7. What is the duration of the patient's symptoms? (Short duration suggests tumour, covert infarction or extra-cranial causes.)

PHYSICAL INVESTIGATIONS TO DISCOVER REMEDIABLE CAUSES

All patients should have the following:

1. Haemoglobin, full blood count, viscosity.
2. Wasserman reaction or equivalent.
3. Blood urea, electrolytes, calcium, and phosphate.
4. Liver function tests, cholesterol, and plasma proteins.
5. B_{12} and folate.
6. Thyroid function tests.
7. Urine should be examined microscopically, and cultured if necessary.
8. Chest and skull X-ray.
9. EEG.
10. CAT scan (if available).

Neuroimaging

There are two main types of brain imaging: structural imaging, which reflects the anatomy of the brain, and functional imaging, which assesses cerebral function in relative or absolute terms. This division is useful in attempting to understand the two types of brain imaging, but increasingly there is an integration of the two methods (e.g. by functional magnetic resonance imaging, fMRI). Structural imaging includes CT and MRI, whereas the two examples of functional imaging are single photon emission computed tomography (SPECT) and positron emission tomography (PET).

COMPUTED TOMOGRAPHY (CT)

The main use of CT is to exclude intracranial lesions such as tumours (primary or secondary), cerebral infarctions, subdural or extradural hematomata, cerebral abscess, and normal pressure hydrocephalus. Two other features of the CT scan are of particular

175

interest: cerebral atrophy and ventricular enlargement, both as a result of brain shrinkage. Cerebral atrophy (also referred to as sulcal, surface, or cortical atrophy) represents a diminution of the cortex, whereas ventricular enlargement (subcortical or central atrophy) indicates swelling of the ventricular system. The CT scan in dementia can provide useful information on the following: (1) the distribution of cerebral atrophy (frontal atrophy may suggest frontotemporal dementia); (2) the size of the caudate nuclei (gross shrinkage would support a clinical diagnosis of Huntington's disease); and (3) white matter changes (indicative of small vessel vascular disease).

Many people mistakenly regard the failure to find a treatable structural lesion as indicating that the scan is superfluous. However, it is important to exclude small vascular lesions such as lacunar infarctions. It is also important to evaluate the distribution of cerebral atrophy and observe the presence of leukoariaosis, which may indicate small vessel disease.

MAGNETIC RESONANCE IMAGING (MRI)

MRI scanning has several advantages: no radiation is involved, resolution is superior to CT, and there is no bone artefact. There is prolongation of the T1 relaxation in patients with Alzheimer's disease and multi-infarct dementia compared with non-demented age-matched controls. However, the ability of this technique to differentiate Alzheimer's disease from multi-infarct dementia is poor and it is possible that prolongation times represent small infarcts or white matter changes that can occur in both disorders. White matter changes have been investigated extensively in Alzheimer's disease and normal ageing. The exact nature of white matter changes or leukoaraiosis is still uncertain. Subcortical white matter lesions appear to be age related whereas periventricular lesions are more associated with cognitive decline and are found in Alzheimer's disease.

SINGLE PHOTON EMISSION COMPUTED TOMOGRAPHY (SPECT)

SPECT involves the administration (usually intravenously) of single photon emitting elements (e.g. Technetium-99, Xenon-133, iodoamphetamine-123) attached to compounds (e.g. hexamethylpropyleneamineoxime) that are distributed in the brain according to cerebral blood flow. The compound crosses the blood–brain barrier and is trapped within functioning brain cells. The amount of radioactivity present can be measured by a rotating gamma camera (which can be used for any nuclear medicine examination), or by multiple scintillation counters in a machine dedicated to brain imaging. Image reconstruction allows sagittal, coronal, and transverse planes to be viewed, enabling localization of radionucleotide distribution to be made.

POSITRON EMISSION TOMOGRAPHY (PET)

PET can be used to measure regional cerebral metabolism (as opposed to purely blood flow) in vivo. However, the practicalities of performing a PET scan have thus far precluded use in clinical diagnosis in psychiatry and the value is still primarily as a research tool. The two most common positron emission compounds are ^{15}O and ^{18}F-deoxyglucose.

Electroencephalography

The EEG is usually normal in very early stages of Alzheimer's disease, but diffuse slowing of the tracing can occur thereafter. As the disease progresses there is progressive slowing of the tracing, with alpha and beta activity decreasing symmetrically and delta and theta waves increasing.

THE FOLLOWING MAY BE CARRIED OUT IF INDICATED

1. Lumbar puncture (if no cause has been found from other tests).
2. Anti-nuclear antibodies.
3. ECG.

Treatment

GENERAL MEASURES

Any physical illness that is present (this is common in the elderly) must be treated, and **hearing or visual deficits** corrected as far as possible. **Antidepressant treatment** is indicated if depression is severe. **Sedation** may be required for behavioural disturbance, but should only be prescribed if the patient is disruptive or is a danger to others. It may make matters worse.

Continuation of normal life at home should be aimed at if it is possible, since this provides sufficient stimulus and the familiar surroundings that help to preserve functions. Increased social support will become necessary, and attendance at a day centre or day hospital can provide further systematic assessment and stimulating daily routine. The needs of relatives at home must be considered if they are to be able and willing to continue the care of an increasingly dependent person.

DRUG TREATMENT OF ALZHEIMER'S DISEASE

The neurotransmitter system most studied in Alzheimer's disease is that involving acetyl choline, and the rationale for the treatment of cognitive deficits in Alzheimer's disease focuses on cholinergic strategies in an attempt to potentiate the central cholinergic function that is deficient in Alzheimer's disease, being most pronounced in the basal forebrain and neocortex. Diminished synthesis of acetyl choline and higher breakdown result in a large decrease in central acetylcholinergic activity, which correlates with the degree of cognitive impairment. Research has focused on cholinergic strategies and

177

pharmacological agents that increase cholinergic activity. This is an excellent example of a disease treatment based firmly on knowledge of the pathophysiology of the condition.

In the UK, three anticholinesterase drugs are approved for the treatment of Alzheimer's disease – **donepezil** (Aricept®), **rivastigmine** (Exelon®) and **galantamine** (Reminyl®).

Donepezil (Aricept®) was released for marketing in the United Kingdom early in 1997 and has probably had the greatest impact so far on the treatment of Alzheimer's disease. Its characteristics include its high oral bioavailability, being unaffected by food, and a long plasma half-life of 70 hours, permitting once-daily dosing. The most common side-effects of donepezil are gastrointestinal, and include nausea, vomiting, diarrhoea, and anorexia. Some patients develop muscle cramps, headache, dizziness, syncopy, or flushing. Haematological side-effects include anaemia and thrombocytopaenia, and cardiac side-effects include bradyarrythmia and syncope. CNS side-effects include headache, dizziness, insomnia, weakness, drowsiness, fatigue, and agitation.

Rivastigmine (Exelon®) was licensed in the United Kingdom in 1998, a year after donepezil. It has an effect both on acetyl-cholinesterase and butyril-cholinesterase. It has a half-life of 2 hours, but cholinesterase inhibition in the brain is thought to last for up to 10 hours. The main drawbacks of rivastigmine are its short half-life, the consequent twice daily dosing, and the necessity for slow titration to minimize the cholinergic side-effects. The trial data suggest these effects are no worse than donepezil, but include nausea, vomiting, and anorexia.

Galantamine has two sites of action: nicotinic receptors and acetyl-cholinesterase. It has a half-life of about 8 hours and thus needs to be given twice daily and has an optimal dose of between 16 and 24 mg a day. It can be given with food due to its greater than 90 per cent bioavailability.

Memantine (Ebixa) acts on the glutamate receptors to alleviate the toxic effect of that neurotransmitter. It is licensed for the treatment of more severe Alzheimer's disease.

There are currently no licensed treatments for vascular dementia.

Drug treatments for behavioural disturbances

These treatments are for symptomatic relief, regardless of the cause of the dementia associated with them. **Neuroleptics** are the agents that are most commonly used for treating behavioural disorders, and they are generally regarded as being moderately effective. It is well documented that they improve anxiety and mood, reduce aggression and agitation, and reduce hostility and uncooperativeness. The primary efficacy is similar for all neuroleptics, but the side-effects and induced tolerance of these drugs are variable. They are certainly effective in treating agitation and restlessness; there have been a number of meta-analyses of the literature showing that in patients with Alzheimer's disease, neuroleptics are effective in controlling agitation, and that about 20 per cent of patients will benefit from these. More recent studies have concentrated on Alzheimer's disease, whereas many earlier studies also included patients with acute confusional state. There are no absolute rules on dosage – generally one should use a lower dose than one might in a psychotic patient who does not have cognitive impairment. The side-effects are well known and are probably more exaggerated in patients who have dementia – extrapyramidal signs, tardive dyskinesia (in up to 50 per cent of patients), postural hypotension, sedation (due to blockage of histamine receptors), anticholinergic effects, agranulocytosis, liver and cardiac toxicity. *Neuroleptics can cause higher mortality and morbidity in patients with Lewy body dementia.* With regard to the specific agents that can be used, there may be little to choose between the main neuroleptics and, as with other drugs, choice is determined often on the basis of familiarity. A number of non-neuroleptic drugs are also used in the management of patients with dementia. **Antidepressants** can control agitation and restlessness, not necessarily in patients with obvious depressive features, although obviously they are specifically effective when depression is present. Trazodone seemed to be particularly helpful in controlling screaming. Some anticonvulsants are used to control agitation. A few case reports suggest that **lithium** improves agitation, but because of its relative toxicity and the need for monitoring it is not likely to become a treatment of first choice. **Buspirone**, which is a GABA antagonist, is said to have some effect on agitated patients. Other antidepressants, such as MAOIs and SSRIs have been used and may be beneficial. **Beta blockers** have traditionally been used to control aggression in younger patients with brain damage. **Benzodiazepines** should not be forgotten: in cases where there is a clinical suspicion of Lewy body dementia, a combination of benzodiazapines and **chlormethiazol** can be effective.

Course and prognosis

The course of dementia is variable. Creutzfeld-Jacob disease leads to the most rapid deterioration, with half the patients being dead within 9 months. Alzheimer's disease usually leads to death within 2 to 5 years. With multi-infarct dementia the course is variable, with many patients dying within 5 years of the diagnosis. The latter dementia often has a step-wise deterioration determined by further cerebrovascular accidents.

FOCAL BRAIN SYNDROMES

Wernicke's encephalopathy and Korsakow's syndrome

Wernicke's encephalopathy is a subacute brain syndrome caused by a deficiency of thiamine. **Korsakow's syndrome** is a chronic brain syndrome with the same cause. The acute symptoms of the former syndrome may incompletely resolve, leaving the clinical picture of the latter.

EPIDEMIOLOGY

The condition is found throughout adult life, most often in the 40s and 50s and is twice as common in men as in women.

CLINICAL FEATURES

Wernicke's encephalopathy is a subacute brain syndrome accompanied by **ocular palsies** (especially abducent palsies, conjugate deviation gaze palsies, and nystagmus), and **ataxia of gait**. There may be prodromal nausea and there will usually be a **marked memory disorder**.

It is not confined to alcoholics, and can occur with thiamine deficiency from any cause (i.e. dietary, carcinoma of the stomach, toxaemia of pregnancy, pernicious anaemia).

Korsakow's syndrome refers to the selective memory disturbance that is revealed once the generalized cognitive impairment of the acute state clears. Immediate recall (registration) is intact, but the **ability to form new memories** is grossly deficient. The patient is usually **disorientated in time**, but other modalities may also be affected.

Long-term memories are relatively well preserved. The patient may provide plausible but incorrect answers to questions that he cannot answer – **confabulation**. There is also an apathy or air of **blandness** and **lack of concern** about the failure to answer the questions correctly. Other aspects of cognitive functioning are preserved, and the patient does not show clouding of consciousness. **Peripheral neuropathy** occurs commonly with these disorders.

DIFFERENTIAL DIAGNOSIS

Acute brain syndrome of other causes

The history of alcoholism is helpful, but in Wernicke's encephalopathy the neurological signs confirm the diagnosis, while in Korsakow's syndrome there will be absence of clouding. The neurological signs also help to distinguish the condition from delirium tremens, another acute brain syndrome resulting from alcoholism, which is four times more common than Wernicke's encephalopathy.

Chronic brain syndrome

The specific nature of the memory defect is the principal differentiating feature. Chronic alcohol ingestion may lead to a chronic brain syndrome because of cerebral atrophy (see p. 171).

INVESTIGATIONS

Psychometric testing will identify the specific memory impairment necessary to make the diagnosis. Take blood for pyruvate assay as soon as possible, and before giving intravenous parenterovite. Only if the expected history of heavy drinking is not obtained need the other causes be considered. A lumbar puncture, EEG, and CAT scan would then be helpful. Investigations to identify other damage resulting from alcohol are appropriate.

TREATMENT

Wernicke's encephalopathy requires urgent treatment with large doses of **thiamine**, with the intention of treating the acute symptoms and modifying the memory impairment. The vitamin is given together with other vitamins of the B group intravenously initially ('Parenterovite' contains 250 mg of thiamine in each ampoule), then intramuscularly. Other aspects of management include attention to infection, dehydration, and electrolyte balance. Bed rest is required initially. Sedation may be required and is similar to that used for delirium tremens.

COURSE AND PROGNOSIS

Sixth nerve palsies clear rapidly with prompt treatment, ataxia clears over a few months in many patients but the neuropathy resolves slowly if at all. The subacute brain syndrome sometimes clears rapidly without lasting amnesia. Otherwise it clears over 1–2 months leaving the amnesia, which only shows any subsequent improvement in half of the patients. In this chronic state the retrograde amnesia is pronounced, there is apathy but confabulation is rare.

Temporal lobe lesions

Lesions of the *dominant temporal lobe* produce sensory dysphasia together with alexia and agraphia if the lesion extends posteriorly towards the parietal lobe. *Non-dominant temporal lobe lesions* may be relatively asymptomatic though visuospatial difficulties may occur. *Bilateral lesions of the medial parts of the temporal lobes* are those that cause severe memory deficits in the absence of other intellectual impairment.

Of special interest to the psychiatrist are temporal lobe lesions that present with **personality change**, unpredictable **aggressive behaviour** and 'symptomatic schizo-phrenias' associated with chronic lesions. These have been recognized principally in relation to temporal lobe epilepsy (see p. 152).

Frontal lobe syndrome

Frontal lobe tumours may present to the psychiatrist because of the predominance of behavioural and mood changes over neurological signs. Lateral lesions have been associated with disturbances of volition and psychomotor activity, whereas lesions in the medial and orbital areas affect the limbic system and reticular formation leading to disinhibition and mood changes.

The patient typically shows **lack of spontaneity** and initiative, and a general diminution of motor activity, although when others provide the stimulus he may behave quite normally. The mood is one of rather inappropriate mild **euphoria** – sometimes described as a 'fatuous jocularity' – alternating with apathy, irritability, or even depression. **Over-familiarity** occurs, sometimes progressing to sexual disinhibition. The patient seems unaware of his unsocial behaviour and irresponsible attitude. Judgement and foresight

181

are impaired. Cognitive functions are largely unimpaired, although specific tests for frontal lobe function are available. Neurological signs include combinations of **optic atrophy** and **papilloedema** if the lesion involves the optic nerves, or contralateral spastic paresis, grasp reflex, increased tendon reflexes, and a positive Babinski response if the lesion extends posteriorly onto the motor cortex.

Parietal lobe lesions

There are changes in the cognitive and visuospatial spheres: *agnosia* is a disturbance of recognition without sensory disturbance or intellectual impairment. *Apraxia* is the inability to carry out motor activity when motor and sensory systems are intact. Lesions of either parietal lobe produce visuospatial difficulties.

Right (non-dominant) hemisphere lesions produce:

1. Neglect of contralateral sensory field and **anosagnosia** (Failure to recognize disabilities on that side).
2. Disturbance of **body image**.
3. **Dressing apraxia**.
4. **Visuospatial agnosia** (constructional apraxia).
5. Inability to follow a route on a map ('**topographagnosia**').

Left (dominant) hemisphere lesions produce:

1. **Motor aphasia** (anterior lesions).
2. **Sensory aphasia** (posterior lesions).
3. Difficulty writing and drawing ('**dysgraphia**').
4. Difficulty reading ('**dyslexia**').
5. **Right–left disorientation**.

HEAD INJURY

The severity of brain damage

A patient who has sustained a closed head injury will report a loss of memory from some time before the injury to the time of the injury itself – called the *retrograde amnesia*, or RA – and a loss of memory from the time of the injury to some time afterwards when consecutive memory resumes – called the *post-traumatic amnesia*, or PTA. The RA is usually considerably shorter than the PTA, and does not in any case give a very reliable indication of brain damage. The two factors from the history that best correlate with the severity of organic damage are the *duration of unconsciousness* and the *duration of the post-traumatic amnesia*. Most of those who report a PTA of more than 24 hours will be fortunate if they recover without some degree of intellectual impairment.

182

The location of brain damage

The effects of location of brain injury on subsequent psychological dysfunction can be examined by studying soldiers who have suffered penetrating injuries to the brain. *Frontal lobe damage* causes severe effects on both mood and behaviour; with injuries to the orbital surface producing severe effects on the personality such as lack of perseverance, inability to maintain relationships, and disinhibition especially affecting sexual and aggressive impulses, while those on the convex lateral surface producing lack of drive, indifference, and incapacity for decisions.

Left hemisphere lesions are associated with global intellectual impairment as well as dysphasias and impaired memory; while injuries to the *right hemisphere* are followed by affective and behavioural disorders and by somatic complaints. Injury to the *parietal or temporal lobes* is associated with intellectual impairment and dysphasia.

Long-term psychological sequelae of closed head injury

Since there are many possible sequelae, we organize our account by starting at the top of our hierarchy (see pp. 62–65) and working downwards.

CHRONIC BRAIN SYNDROME

In very severe head injuries the chronic brain syndrome will be accompanied by dysphasias and quadriparesis, and the patient may be apathetic, slow, or even mute. Control of affect will be poor, and loss of libido is the rule. Such severe disabilities present formidable problems for rehabilitation, although assessment is usually straightforward. The main problems of assessment are presented by minor degrees of global damage involving minimal degrees of intellectual impairment and claims for compensation.

POST-TRAUMATIC EPILEPSY

This develops in about 5 per cent of closed head injuries and over 30 per cent of injuries involving penetration of the dura mater. After closed head injury, temporal lobe epilepsy (see pp. 62–65) is the commonest form, and is the form most likely to be followed by psychiatric disability. Epilepsy developing in the year following injury is particularly likely to be associated with psychiatric disability.

PSYCHOTIC ILLNESS

A **post-traumatic psychosis** refers to a psychotic illness manifest as soon as consciousness is resumed after injury: these usually remit with treatment. There is an increased incidence of all types of psychotic illness after head injury, although the available evidence suggests that there is a constitutional predisposition in cases of schizophrenia and affective psychosis, so that the role of the head injury is to increase the likelihood of the disorder being manifested.

DEPRESSIVE ILLNESS

Symptoms of affective illness are very common after head injury, and all combinations of non-psychotic symptomatology occur. Indeed suicide accounts for 14 per cent of all deaths following head injury. A triad of persistent headache, dizziness, and irritability is sometimes described as a **post-concussional syndrome**, although the longer it lasts the more it tends to merge with non-specific patterns of psychiatric disorder, and the less likely are such symptoms to be a pure expression of brain damage. Abnormal illness behaviours, such as hypochondriacal symptoms (see p. 240) and hysterical symptoms (see p. 242) commonly accompany such illnesses. Obsessional neuroses (see p. 231) have also been shown to be more common after head injury.

One theoretically important study compared head-injured twins with their normal co-twins some 10 years following the injury. Although the head-injured twin was found to be inferior to the normal co-twin on a variety of tests of intellectual function, such differences were subtle and unobtrusive in everyday life. The MZ twins were more concordant than the DZ twins for the 'post-concussional' symptoms described above; and those twins thought to have shown a 'change in personality' consisting of tension, fatiguability, and lessened ability to work, were found to have co-twins with the same traits. Once more, it is clear that constitutional predisposition to such symptoms must play a major role, with the function of the head injury being to release the symptoms in the short term.

PERSONALITY DISORDER

The personality changes that go to make up the **frontal lobe syndrome** (see p. 171) have already been referred to, while another pattern consists of **explosive aggressive outbursts** on minor provocation. As you have seen from the twin study reported above, constitutional factors are likely to play a decisive role in the development of non-specific 'neurotic' symptoms.

FURTHER READING:

Lishman, A. (1998) *Organic Psychiatry*, 3rd edition. Oxford: Blackwell Scientific.

13 SCHIZOPHRENIA AND DELUSIONAL DISORDERS

SCHIZOPHRENIA

Schizophrenia and delusional disorders make up the so-called 'serious mental illnesses' that are associated with neither a severe mood disorder nor an organic brain condition.

Epidemiology

Approximately 1 per cent of adults receive a diagnosis of schizophrenia at some point in their lives. The inception rate is around 20 per 100,000 and the prevalence is about 200 per 100,000 in the United Kingdom. Schizophrenia is a chronic illness usually lasting many years, but the course of the illness varies greatly. While some never fully recover and need institutional care, others make a full recovery and lead normal lives. The incidence of schizophrenia is similar across most parts of the world, although there may be important local differences within the same country. The course of the illness appears to be less persistent in the developing countries compared to the developed countries. The peak incidence in males is between 18 and 25 years and in females between 25 and 30 years. Delusional disorders may appear in younger age groups, but may arise for the first time in the over 65 year age group.

There is a tendency for people who eventually develop schizophrenia as a young adult to display more withdrawn, eccentric, or clumsy behaviour in childhood by at least age 11 years. Often there is a prodromal period lasting weeks to years before the full illness appears, with non-specific symptoms such as loss of interest, social withdrawal, neglect in self-care, depression, anxiety, or brief psychotic symptoms. The longer the prodromal period and the longer the time to the correct diagnosis without treatment, the poorer is the long-term prognosis. Currently services in United Kingdom and in many other countries in the world are being set up to recognize the prodromal phases and earliest stages of the first or second episodes of schizophrenia to try to improve the long-term course of the illness.

A higher prevalence of schizophrenia is found in inner-city areas and lower social classes because there is a downward social drift as patients with schizophrenia move into cheaper, temporary or supported accommodation that tends to be found in the inner city. The social class of patients tends to be lower than the general population, but the social classes of their parents are similar to the general population, illustrating this downward social drift.

Symptoms and diagnosis of schizophrenia

In schizophrenia, there is a disturbance in the person's individuality and self-direction in relation to their thinking, sensory perception, motivation, and emotion – but not their alertness. Many intellectual functions are retained but some deficits in intellectual function emerge. Sometimes even movement is affected. There is a disruption in the clear boundaries between the self and the external world, so for instance thoughts, feelings, and acts seem to be known by others or controlled by others. The symptoms and experiences of the person with schizophrenia seem to be predominantly concerned with the self, who may seem preoccupied, perplexed, or frightened during exacerbations of their symptoms. The core symptoms of schizophrenia are called **positive** and **negative** symptoms. There are frequently symptoms of low or elated mood, anxiety, or abnormal behaviour but they are accompanied by the core symptoms of schizophrenia.

POSITIVE SYMPTOMS

Box 13.1 describes how positive symptoms of schizophrenia may be elicited. The symptoms in bold may be used to diagnose schizophrenia. Usually these are frightening experiences for the person who has them because so much seems out of their control. Psychosocial stress, criticism, hostility, and situations inducing anxiety tend to make these symptoms worse.

Auditory hallucinations are possibly the most common and easiest symptom to elicit. Auditory hallucinations are voices that are heard through the person's ears but they do not have a real cause, and would not be audible to anyone else. They occur while the person is wide awake and usually the same voices are heard wherever the person moves to. Typically the person with schizophrenia hears **auditory hallucinations in the third person** ('*Now he's eating his breakfast*'), a voice or voices talking about the person, giving a running commentary on what he is doing, or having a conversation with each other as if he is not there. The voices sound real and are often loud, critical, and derogatory so they can be distressing to the person with schizophrenia. With treatment, the voices may not go away but usually they become quieter and the content of the voices is usually more pleasant, even complimentary. Another typical but rare auditory hallucination is called **thought echo** or 'echo de la pensée'. The person thinks something and then hears their thought spoken aloud, either simultaneously or after a brief delay.

Other hallucinations commonly occur in schizophrenia and may be used to diagnose the condition, provided they are persistent and in clear consciousness. However they also occur in many other mental disorders. Examples include **second-person auditory hallucinations** ('*Are you going to eat your breakfast?*') where the voices talk directly to the person, and hallucinations that are experienced in other senses such as those that are seen through the person's eyes (**visual hallucinations**), tasted, smelt, or felt on the skin

186

Box 13.1 Ten-minute history and mental state examination for positive symptoms of schizophrenia

History
I would like to ask about unusual experiences that people sometimes have.
Have there been people who were talking about you or taking special notice of you? (*Delusions of reference*)
(IF YES: Were you convinced that they were talking about you? What about receiving special messages from TV, radio, computer, or newspaper?)
Is anyone trying to harm you in anyway? (*Persecutory delusions*)
(IF YES: Please tell me more about it)
Do you have special powers to do things that others can't do? Are you especially important in some way? (*Grandiose delusions*)
Do you ever feel that someone or something is controlling you in some way? (*Passivity experiences*)
(IF YES: Please tell me more about it)
Have any thoughts been put in your head that are not your own and you didn't want in your head? (*Thought insertion*)
(IF YES: Please tell me more about it)
Have any thoughts been taken out of your head against your wishes? IF YES: Please tell me more about it. (*Thought withdrawal*)
Have you felt that your thoughts were being broadcast out loud? Do other people actually hear what you are thinking? (*Thought broadcast*)
(IF YES: Please tell me more about it)
Have you heard things that other people couldn't hear, such as noises or the voices of people talking to each other? (*Auditory hallucinations*)
(IF YES: What did you hear? How often did you hear it? Did the voice comment on what you were doing or thinking? How many voices did you hear? Did they talk to each other?)

Mental state examination
1. *Appearance and behaviour.* Poor self-care (cleanliness, tidiness, hydration, and nutrition), odd appearance (e.g. clothing, make-up, hair, restlessness or lack of movement, abnormal movements, preoccupied).
2. *Speech.* Tangential speech (one thought unrelated to the next thought), or disorganized speech or incoherence, poverty of speech, or poverty of content of speech, neologisms.
3. *Mood.* Perplexed, suspicious.
4. *Thought.* Delusions. Ideas of reference or persecution. Thought disorder.
5. *Perception.* Auditory hallucinations.
6. *Cognition.* Poor attention or concentration. Concrete thinking.

or under the skin. **Visual**, **gustatory**, and **olfactory hallucinations** are seen in schizophrenia but they are more common in organic mental conditions and require further investigations to rule out medical and substance use causes. In delusional disorders in the elderly, auditory hallucinations may only occur in the person's own home and nowhere else. (Auditory and visual hallucinations involving a two-way conversation with the voice responding to the person's comments directed to the voice are *not* typical of schizophrenia; they may be a sign that the person has been emotionally traumatized, or that the person is making up their symptoms).

Another common symptom in schizophrenia is a **delusion** (see p. 201), an unshakeable belief unamenable to reason that is out of keeping with the person's cultural, social, and educational background. **Primary delusions** arise new without any clear explanation. They are sometimes preceded by a period of time lasting a few days to a few months when the person seems bewildered and perplexed. The perplexity passes as the primary delusion is formed. A special example of a primary delusion is **delusional perception** (see p. 201). **Persistent delusions** that are culturally inappropriate in clear consciousness can also be used to diagnose schizophrenia if accompanied by other features of schizophrenia, or delusional disorder if they are not. For instance a person may believe that their home has definitely and unquestionably been taken over by aliens. Many delusions reported by people suffering from schizophrenia are **secondary delusions** that are understandable given their other experiences as a result of schizophrenia. For instance a person with auditory hallucinations providing a running commentary that is critical of everything he thinks, says or does, may also believe that there is a conspiracy to torture him mentally by placing bugs and cameras to monitor everything he does, and a transmitter implanted in his ear.

The person with schizophrenia may experience problems with possession of their own thoughts. In **thought insertion**, the person has the experience that someone or something has placed one or more thoughts into their mind that do not belong there. The experience occurs against their will and to their displeasure, unlike telepathy and other experiences where the person wishes to receive and welcomes the thoughts of other people or other things in their mind. In **thought broadcast**, the person's own thoughts are shared with other people or things against their will and to their displeasure. In **thought withdrawal**, the person's own thoughts are removed from their mind against their will and to their displeasure, leaving the mind blank and empty.

Equally distressing a person with schizophrenia may have the experience of their movements, will, impulses, or emotions being under the control of other people or things against their will. These are called **passivity experiences**.

The person with schizophrenia may experience or display **incongruity of affect**, where they have outbursts of laughter or anger without any clear stimulus or reason, or when the emotion is inappropriate, such as laughing uncontrollably at sad news.

A person with schizophrenia may find that the logic of their thinking and speech is disturbed. It may fragment altogether (**word salad**), or more often in **thought disorder** sentences are merged together or one line of thought is followed by a completely different train of thought that is not logically connected to the first. The speech becomes incoherent or irrelevant to the topic of the conversation. Sometimes a new word is invented (**neologism**), which has a unique, idiosyncratic meaning to that person but is unintelligible to anyone else (e.g. *'my mind is spired'*).

Patients with schizophrenia sometimes show repeated bizarre and purposeless movements called **mannerisms**. There are often grimaces of the face in addition. Occasionally, people with schizophrenia show particular movements, postures, and behaviours called **catatonia**, although modern studies show that these features may occur in any mental health condition, especially mood and organic brain disorders. The patient may show **stupor** (alert but unable to speak or move except their eyes), extreme excitement, negativism (does the opposite to what is asked), automatic obedience, posturing (takes up positions that are difficult to hold normally), and waxy flexibility (an abnormal tone to the joints that allows the observer to put the person with catatonia into unusual postures).

NEGATIVE SYMPTOMS

Negative symptoms are present in many but not all people suffering from schizophrenia. They are a poor prognostic sign in terms of function, and can lead to a variety of deficits in self-care, occupational, educational, interpersonal, and social domains. A lack of stimulation tends to make these symptoms worse.

Negative symptoms of schizophrenia (*Box 13.2*) are sometimes difficult to distinguish from symptoms of depression, excessive sedative or neuroleptic medication, and social withdrawal in the presence of frightening positive symptoms that are also common in schizophrenia. Sometimes the presence of negative symptoms of schizophrenia can only be determined by a process of exclusion, as the patient does not have other features of severe depression such as sleep and weight loss, or cognitive symptoms of low self-worth, guilt and hopelessness, the loss of alertness and side-effects from high doses of medication, or the presence of distressing positive symptoms.

Alogia is the term used for impoverishment in thinking and takes two forms. **Poverty of speech** is present when the person gives very brief answers to questions and is unable to elaborate their thoughts. The person has the experience of their mind being empty of thoughts. **Poverty of content of thoughts** occurs when the person gives normal length answers but there is little of substance in the reply. The person's thinking has lost its complexity and richness.

A person may show **blunting of affect (affective flattening)**, an absence of emotional expression in the voice, facial expression, or emotional responsiveness.

There is a **loss of volition (avolition)**, a lack of interest, motivation and drive, leading to social withdrawal, lack of activity and poor self-care. There may also be **slowness of thought and movement**.

Other features of schizophrenia

Depression, anxiety, irritability, agitation, and withdrawal are all commonly seen in schizophrenia. Sometimes other behaviour problems arise that can cause great problems in terms of the person's housing and social care, such as hoarding of belongings, inappropriate and sometimes disgusting eating behaviour (e.g. eating **excessively then**

Box 13.2 History and mental state examination for negative symptoms of schizophrenia

History
The history of negative symptoms generally comes from the report of others. There are a few questions that can be asked but most of the information that can be obtained from the patient directly will be from observation of the mental state.
You may find these questions useful:
How do you spend the time?
What are you interested in doing? (*Avolition*)
What has made you feel sad, happy, anxious or irritable? Have you felt like this recently? When? What happened? (*Affective flattening*)
What have you just been thinking about?
Do you get many thoughts in your mind? (*Alogia*)
A person with negative symptoms will struggle to answer these questions giving positive and detailed answers.

Features indicating negative symptoms in mental state examination:
Appearance and behaviour. Lack of self-care or care over appearance (cleanliness, tidiness, hydration, and nutrition). Slow movement (generally and facially). Alert but lacking drive.
Speech. Slow. Says little and sometimes delayed answers. Little emotion in voice. Conveys little information – responds using single words and does not initiate conversation, or speech is repetitive, rigid in content, concrete (lacking abstract connections), or exceptionally vague and circumstantial (does not address the point of conversation).
Mood. No emotional expression – blunted or flat emotion.
Thought. Slow. Few thoughts or repeated, vague, circumstantial thought, or concrete thinking.
Perception. No abnormality.
Cognition. Poor attention and concentration.

---

vomiting food in front of others), **incontinence, self-harm, destruction of possessions**, or **water intoxication**. The last behaviour is a cause of hyponatraemia, which can lead to delirium, convulsions, coma, and death. The person will drink as much water as they can get hold of, including water out of toilets and baths.

Sometimes a prolonged **depressive episode** can arise in the aftermath of schizophrenia ('post-psychotic depression') and there may be an increased risk of suicide or self-neglect as a result. In post-psychotic depression, the symptoms of depression increase without a change in positive or negative symptoms of schizophrenia, in contrast to the acute schizophrenia episode when depression symptoms increase and decrease in line with the intensity of positive symptoms of schizophrenia. In post-psychotic depression, the patient often feels trapped by their illness, condemned to a lower status and hopeless about the future. Only by a process of elimination can the cause of the depression be identified and the correct treatment be started; it may be a symptom of schizophrenia requiring higher doses of neuroleptic medication, an understandable emotional response to having such a devastating illness requiring counselling and support, an emotional response to distressing side-effects of neuroleptic medication requiring a reduction in neuroleptic medication, or a separate mood episode requiring conventional treatment for depression such as antidepressants.

Diagnosis

Because schizophrenia is a stigmatizing diagnosis it is only diagnosed when the features of the condition have been present for 1 month or more, in order to distinguish it from brief, transient psychotic symptoms.

One or more of the following are required throughout the month in clear consciousness, without severe mood disorder or organic cause:

- Third-person auditory hallucinations.
- Thought echo.
- Thought insertion.
- Thought broadcast.
- Thought withdrawal.
- Passivity experiences, delusional perception.
- Primary delusion or any persistent delusion.

Alternatively, two or more of the following features are required without severe mood disorder or organic cause:

- Persistent hallucinations in any modality.
- Incoherent or irrelevant speech (including neologisms).
- Mannerisms.
- Catatonia.
- Negative symptoms.

Differential diagnosis

Brief psychotic disorder is diagnosed when the symptoms are present for less than a month and then subside completely. They often have a sudden onset. Sometimes a cause such as a severe psychosocial stressor can be identified, but often the cause is never known.

For **delusional disorder** see the end of this chapter, page 201.

In **organic psychosis** the symptoms appear similar to schizophrenia but are a result of psychoactive substances or medical (usually neurological) disorder. Stimulant and/or hallucinogenic drugs such as amphetamines, cocaine, ecstasy, LSD, psilocybin ('the magic mushroom'), mescaline, or phencyclidine can precipitate an organic psychosis. Steroids and high doses or potent forms of cannabis can produce a clinical picture very similar to schizophrenia. Neurological causes for an organic psychosis include complex partial epileptic seizures ('temporal lobe epilepsy' – at the same time or separately from the seizures, can increase or decrease in intensity and frequency as the frequency of seizures increases or decreases), as a feature of the extra-pyramidal disorder such as Huntington's disease or Wilson's disease, as a feature of a space-occupying lesion in the brain such as tumours or neoplasms (primary or secondary, especially involving the temporal lobe, hippocampus, entorhinal, or areas disrupting or involving frontal–subcortical brain structures), brain injury, encephalitis, or as a cerebral complication of HIV infection. Medical causes include some forms of porphyria and immediately after delivery. In organic psychosis, symptoms are often pleomorphic, transitory, and frequently changing. An organic psychosis should be considered when there is a known organic cause of psychosis, the organic cause precedes or coincides with the start of the first symptoms of psychosis, and the symptoms of psychosis subside within 2 weeks of subsidence of the organic cause.

Alcoholic hallucinosis occurs for a few days or weeks when heavy drinking reduces or ceases and is experienced as second-person auditory hallucinations (see Chapter 17).

In **schizoaffective disorder**, there are separate episodes of schizophrenia and severe mood disorder, or the person meets diagnostic criteria for an episode of schizophrenia and severe mood disorder at the same time. Negative symptoms of schizophrenia are uncommon in schizoaffective disorder, which in general has a better prognosis than schizophrenia.

Mania and bipolar disorder: Mania with psychotic symptoms and schizophrenia can generally be distinguished because the former is associated with elation, increased purposeful activity, grandiosity, decreased need for sleep, and pressure of speech and thought. Bipolar disorder is associated with discrete episodes of mania and depression, with sometimes residual depressive symptoms or recovery without continuing psychotic symptoms; schizophrenia is usually associated with accumulating amounts of negative symptoms and often some continuing psychotic symptoms.

Unipolar depressive episodes with psychotic features can be distinguished from schizophrenia because of the severity of the depressive symptoms. The psychotic symptoms will tend to dissipate in unipolar depression, but in schizophrenia they may continue with accompanying negative symptoms.

Risks

Suicide occurs at the same rate as other serious mental disorders. The presence of suicidal plans and persistent suicide ideas puts a person with schizophrenia at risk of suicide, as do auditory hallucinations suggesting suicide. The actual degree of suicide risk can be difficult to predict in a patient with schizophrenia with a lot of positive symptoms, particularly when there are also many depressive symptoms and/or a history of impulsive behaviour (reckless acts carried out with little planning or consideration of the consequences). In these circumstances it is wise to assume that the patient is at a high risk of suicide. Patients with many distressing positive symptoms, depression, or negative symptoms of schizophrenia are at risk of self-neglect that can be sufficient to lead to their own death or physical harm. While the risk of serious violent attack on other people is relatively low and unlawful killing by people with schizophrenia has not changed much over the years, a person with a history of violent acts and schizophrenia needs careful assessment by a psychiatrist or other experienced health professional. Certain positive symptoms of schizophrenia are associated with violence to particular individuals, such as passivity experiences, morbid jealousy, and the presence of specific persecutory delusions centred on a person where there is a risk of violence to their supposed persecutor. Morbid jealousy as a feature of delusional disorder, any other mental disorder such as unipolar depression, or arising without mental disorder is dangerous to the person who is the target of the jealousy, and anyone suspected to be in a sexual relationship with them. Treatment is of the underlying condition, and there should be geographical separation between the person with morbid jealousy and the target of the morbid jealousy.

Neurochemistry, neuroimaging, and neuropathology

The dominant neurochemical theory is that schizophrenia reflects *excessive dopaminergic transmission*. This is based on two main observations: first, most conventional antipsychotic drugs block dopamine receptors to a degree that is proportional to their efficacy. Second, dopaminergic drugs such as amphetamine are psychotomimetic, Transient central D2 blockade, obtained with many atypical antipsychotics such as clozapine, quetiapine, or a mixture of pre-synaptic and post-synaptic effects on D2 receptors, for example with amisulpride, are sufficient to obtain an effect on positive symptoms of schizophrenia. Permanent blockade of central D2 receptors only results in extrapyramidal symptoms without any extra benefit on the symptoms of schizophrenia.

Other neurotransmitters are clearly implicated in schizophrenia, especially the excitatory amino-acid glutamate. Phencyclidine, a drug acting on glutamate receptors, causes a schizophrenia-like psychosis, and some benefits on both positive and negative symptoms have been demonstrated when agonists at the glutamate NMDA receptor such as glycine are given in addition to antipsychotic agents. In post-mortem studies of the brain in schizophrenia, more glutamate receptors and markers for glutamate nerve endings are found in the pre-frontal cortex, but they are reduced in the medial temporal area, suggesting an abnormality of the neural pathways involving glutamate between frontal and temporal lobes of the brain. Serotonin modulates dopamine in the frontal regions of the brain in schizophrenia, and this has been related to negative symptoms and cognitive deficits in schizophrenia. It is also likely that other neural pathways involving dopamine type 1, acetylcholine, and GABA receptors are involved as well.

Neuroimaging studies have shown increased lateral ventricular size present in adolescents at the time the disorder develops, and also in unaffected adolescents who are at high genetic risk for the disorder. There is a small but significant reduction in total brain size, particularly near the temporal lobes. Many symptoms of schizophrenia have been linked to lesions in particular brain regions. In particular hallucinations have been linked to the areas of the brain associated with normal sensory processing, so auditory hallucinations are related to reductions in the size or changes in blood flow to the superior temporal gyrus, while visual hallucinations seem to be associated with changes in blood flow or lesions in the parietal and occipital lobes of the brain. Affective flattening, deficits in the processing of emotional information, and abnormal emotional investment in insignificant perceptual stimuli (as would be expected in the formation of a delusional perception) have been related to abnormalities of the amygdala and other frontal–subcortical connections. Negative symptoms of schizophrenia have been associated consistently with decreased blood flow, deficits in glucose uptake, or abnormal neuropsychological tasks associated with decreased frontal function. There are widespread disturbances of interconnectivity between different brain regions on EEG and functional imaging. This disconnectivity is consistent with relative disorganization of neuronal cells and their dendritic connections within certain layers of the brain in key areas such as the frontal lobe. The findings are relatively small in effect size and at present are unusable clinically to make a diagnosis of schizophrenia or to monitor the effects of treatment.

Aetiology

PREDISPOSING FACTORS

There is compelling evidence of vertically transmissible genetic factors in the aetiology of schizophrenia. The risk in the general population is around 1 per cent, but is 9 per cent in siblings and 13 per cent in the children of schizophrenics. The risk in parents is somewhat lower at 6 per cent, but in general there is a tenfold increase in first-degree relatives. If two schizophrenics produce children, the risk is about 46 per cent. Studies comparing concordance between MZ and DZ twins provide heritability estimates of about 82 to 84 per cent. Adoption studies show that children of schizophrenic mothers adopted away are at the same increased risk as those remaining at home: overall, various adoption studies show that it is shared genes, rather than shared environments, that underline the increased risk.

Schizophrenia may be a neurodevelopmental disorder, with the brain abnormalities developing before the person is born, or in early life before the first symptoms. Evidence supporting this theory includes the following observations: there is epidemiological evidence of increased obstetric complications and childhood neuropsychological deficits in those who will eventually develop the disorder. Children who later develop schizophrenia show abnormalities in pre-morbid personality, social interaction, eccentric behaviour, intelligence, and social adjustment compared to their peers by age 11 years or younger, and structural brain abnormalities are not associated with gliosis, as would be expected if degenerative processes were present. However, there is some evidence for a neurodegenerative disorder that is progressive over 10 to 15 years, with a deterioration in symptoms and function in many patients. Sometimes these changes are reflected in changes in brain function, at least in some patients

Sensory deficits such as blindness and deafness predispose individuals to persecutory disorders such as delusional disorder in the elderly, but there is no evidence of a relationship between sensory deficits and schizophrenia. Some people have personalities that are extremely sensitive to criticism, or they perceive criticism in comments that were never intended to be critical. Under psychosocial stress, people with such sensitive personalities can develop delusional disorders.

PRECIPITATING FACTORS

Environmental stress in the preceding weeks or months may precipitate the onset of an acute episode of schizophrenia, characterized by positive symptoms. Both **positive and negative events** in the person's life, such as passing an examination or the loss of a job, respectively, can lead to an acute episode. Any situation that increases anxiety, worry, tension, or excitement has the potential to cause an acute episode. Exposure to a **high degree of criticism** and/or hostility from other people, usually the family, for more than 35 hours per week can lead to an increased risk of acute episodes of schizophrenia in the following year. This clinical phenomenon is called **expressed emotion**. The importance of this is demonstrated by the effectiveness of family therapy to reduce the hostility and criticism and thereby reduce the frequency of schizophrenia episodes, also achieved by spending less time in the hostile or critical environment, and use of neuroleptic medication. Conversely, exposure to a lack of stimulation for much of the time in the week increases the frequency of negative symptoms.

Other important precipitating factors are hallucinogen or stimulant drugs such as ecstasy, LSD, cocaine, and amphetamines. Cannabis can precipitate schizophrenia. Stopping long-term neuroleptic drug treatment may also precipitate an acute recurrence of schizophrenia.

MAINTAINING FACTORS

Maintaining factors for an acute episode of schizophrenia include situations that continue to generate anxiety, tension, excitement, hostility, and criticism, continuing to imbibe hallucinogens, stimulants, cannabis, or alcohol, and non-adherence to neuroleptic medication.

Management

INITIAL PRESENTATION AND ACUTE PHASE OF MANAGEMENT

Patients with schizophrenia should receive a physical examination, including a neurological examination, and investigations to eliminate organic causes for psychosis, and elucidate aetiological factors, the consequences of the illness, and prognostic factors. Another important task is to monitor the patient for the development of side-effects from medication. A history from carers, other relatives or informants is obtained to confirm the history of illness, and to assess environmental stress, evidence of self-neglect or extreme behaviour, and expressed emotion in the home environment.

On the first presentation with schizophrenia, a **drug screen** for amphetamines and cannabis, an **EEG** to exclude complex partial seizures, and a **CT or MRI scan** of the brain are ordered. Baseline fasting blood glucose, fasting lipids, ECG, full blood count, urea, and electrolytes and liver function tests are performed and then monitored after neuroleptic medication is started.

The setting for acute treatment will depend on the risk to the patient or others, but the environment needs to be supportive because acute schizophrenia is usually frightening to the patient. The aim is to keep the patient reasonably free of psychosocial stress and conflict while maintaining as normal a daily routine as the clinical condition permits. Treatment of acute episodes in schizophrenia will take place in out-patients, the community, or in day-care unless the risks to the patients or other people are too great, in which case the patient is admitted to a mental health in-patient unit. If the risks are particularly great, a psychiatric intensive care unit, locked and with a high ratio of nursing staff to patients, may be employed. If the patient is at risk of harm to themselves or others, or is likely to reach such a risk in the near future unless treatment is initiated, then the patient is detained against their will under the Mental Health Act.

A first or second presentation of schizophrenia in a person under the age of 35 years is likely to be managed at home by a multidisciplinary team of nursing, social work, occupational therapy, clinical psychology, and psychiatric staff working in an early intervention team. Other patients in acute psychiatric episodes will be managed for 4 weeks or so at home by a similar multidisciplinary team working in a crisis resolution and home treatment team. Patients who require less urgent care will be looked after by a smaller group of multidisciplinary staff from the community mental health team.

If a patient is repeatedly in crisis resulting in admission to hospital, they will be looked after for around a year at a time by another multidisciplinary team, the assertive outreach team. In some areas, patients with acute schizophrenia episodes may be looked after in acute day hospitals open 5 to 7 days per week, supported by out of hours community mental health team staff as an alternative to admission. The number of hospital in-patient beds has been sharply reduced, so many patients will be transferred to a day hospital or one of these community teams after a few weeks.

Neuroleptic medication is given in the acute phase at sufficient doses to control the acute symptoms with the fewest side-effects. In most instances this is oral medication given in tablets, but if adherence to medication is an issue and the clinical condition requires it, liquid or intramuscular neuroleptic medication can be used. There is no reason to use intravenous neuroleptic medication.

Patients should only be **restrained** and given medication against their will *as a last resort* when the clinical situation would otherwise rapidly get out of control and there is a risk to the self or others. Restraint is a violation of the patient's consent and requires involuntarily detention under the Mental Health Act unless the situation is so urgent that there is no time to get such an order, in which case staff can use restraint under common law on one occasion only. If restraint is used it should be upright (vertical) and the patient should not be pinned down on the floor (horizontal). The use of high doses of medication and restraint (especially horizontal) has been associated with sudden death, and together with other sources of coercion, is associated with future non-adherence to treatments offered by psychiatric services.

Nursing care needs to promote self-care and in severe cases a patient will need verbal or sometimes even physical assistance with activities of daily living such as bathing, dressing, eating, drinking. A careful eye needs to be kept on the patient's self-care, hydration, nutrition (it is not unusual to see gross nutritional deficiencies such as anaemia due to poor diet), and behaviour, such as hoarding of items, including some-times perishable items (a potential hygiene issue) and items belonging to other patients (a source of conflict). Patients with schizophrenia may be unsure about what is hap-pening in their subjective world and differentiating this experience from external reality, so may need staff to help them in the acute phase of schizophrenia. While it is unrealistic to expect these approaches to change the nature of psychotic phenomena, they can help the patient to gain insight into the nature of their symptoms, for example the location of an auditory hallucination as coming from inside the mind rather than a source external to the mind. Behaviour such as social withdrawal may be a negative symptom that requires a positive motivational approach, or it could be an adaptive coping mechanism to control the intensity of the hallucinations. Some patients adopt strategies such as wearing headphones to cope with auditory hallucinations, and nursing staff should assist the patient to develop such adaptive coping mechanisms.

LONGER-TERM MANAGEMENT

The aim of longer-term treatment is to reduce distress, promote active coping with the condition, and improve function as much as possible so that the patient can have as many choices as possible in terms of the way they lead their life. Often it is not possible and not necessary for all positive and negative symptoms to disappear altogether. For instance, the goal of treatment may be to change externally located, loud, hostile and persistent auditory hallucinations to internally located, quieter, pleasant and intermittent auditory hallucinations, or to improve negative symptoms related to self-care requiring verbal assistance and social isolation to independent self-care and contact with other people through a day-centre or supported employment. The management of schizophrenia therefore requires the setting of realistic goals for treatment, and then to use the best combination of medication, psychological therapies, and social approaches to treatment.

The longer-term problems of a patient with schizophrenia can be thought of as pri-mary, secondary, and tertiary issues. Primary issues are the pre-morbid characteristics of the patient, that is, what type of person it was who got schizophrenia. The issues may be related to personality features, pre-existing medical problems, family, or social issues. Secondary issues are the features of the schizophrenia illness itself such as the severity and responsiveness to treatment of positive and negative symptoms. Tertiary issues relate to problems arising out of the treatment of schizophrenia, such as long-term hospitalization leading to loss of accommodation or inappropriate accommodation, loss of contact with friends and family, or loss of a job.

Patients with schizophrenia require the development of a long-term care plan designed to tackle these primary, secondary, and tertiary issues, including risk and incorporating the patient's and carers' wishes. The care plan needs to set out a plan of action for tackling the main issues or needs, a rationale for the plan, how and when it is to be carried out, by whom, and who will monitor its progress. The longer-term management of schizophrenia often requires a multidisciplinary team of professionals including the general practitioner, so it is normal practice to arrange a meeting of the staff, patient and carer who will implement the plan to agree its content, and then to review it at regular intervals, at least every 6 months. The person who takes lead responsibility for organizing the care plan is called the care coordinator or case manager, usually a qualified health professional who may come from any related discipline (nursing, medicine, social work, occupational therapy, or clinical psychology).

Specific pharmacological treatment

Neuroleptic drugs are dealt with in detail in Chapter 8. The specific choice of neuroleptic depends on previous response, risks, side-effects and contraindications, and choice of the patient. It is worth establishing patient concordance by explaining to the patient what they might experience in terms of effects and side-effects. For instance when prescribing a neuroleptic drug it is important to warn the patient that they may feel some sedation or get some extrapyramidal side-effects at first. The latter can be treated if they persist. Longer-term management will usually require an oral neuroleptic, but if the patient prefers and medication adherence is an issue, a depot neuroleptic, given intramuscularly every 2 to 4 weeks by a health professional such as a community mental health nurse or practice nurse taught specifically to give this medication, is an alternative.

When patients develop extrapyramidal side-effects of neuroleptic medication, such as parkinsonism, the dose of the neuroleptic is reduced or anti-parkinsonian drugs are given. Some extrapyramidal side-effects are irreversible, such as **tardive dyskinesia**. Most patients are now given **atypical antipsychotic drugs** such as olanzapine or quetiapine with fewer if any extrapyramidal side-effects, but these have brought their own problems, principally weight gain (sometimes very substantial), type 2 diabetes mellitus, and metabolic syndrome with the potential risk of premature death from cardiovascular causes.

Therefore, patients started on neuroleptic medication must have their weight (used to calculate body mass index with the patient's height) and blood sugar checked in the first month of treatment and then at 3- to 6-month intervals, with yearly checks on fasting lipids, blood pressure, ECG, abdominal circumference, full blood count, urea, and electrolytes and liver function tests. Patients with schizophrenia who have failed to improve symptomatically and functionally after two courses of different neuroleptics should be offered **clozapine** provided there are no medical contraindications. Around 30 per cent of patients respond sufficiently to this expensive drug to live independently and to justify its cost. Clozapine can cause lethal aplastic anaemia and it requires a special monitoring service to look for changes in the production of blood cells.

Specific psychological treatment

Specific psychological treatments include **cognitive behaviour therapy**, **family therapy**, **behaviour therapy** and **cognitive remediation therapy**, and early warning sign interventions. There is relatively little evidence that specific psychological treatments are more effective overall than regular contact with a support worker who is part of the community mental health team, and a psychiatrist prescribing standard medication.

However, there is a lot of evidence that any psychological treatment, including a non-specific supportive approach, is superior to just seeing a psychiatrist prescribing standard neuroleptic drug treatment. Furthermore, there is evidence that particular outcomes are improved by specific psychological therapies. In practice, obtaining these specific psychological treatments in a timely manner can be problematic and it is important that these expensive and scarce resources are targeted appropriately to make the maximum clinical impact.

Cognitive behaviour therapy seems to have benefits for positive symptoms, especially treatment-resistant symptoms such as hallucinations, when it is given by experienced therapists, and it may improve post-psychotic depression. There is also evidence that cognitive behaviour therapy may delay the onset of developing schizophrenia in those who show early signs, such as young people who display odd beliefs or behaviour, or experience some types of illusions and hallucinations.

Family therapy targeted at a single family showing high expressed emotion to the person with schizophrenia may prevent acute schizophrenia episodes and re-admission, and improve medication adherence. Early warning sign interventions can be used in some patients to identify the early stages of an acute schizophrenia episode and to prevent its onset through higher doses of neuroleptic medication or cognitive strategies taught to the patient in advance. **Social skills training** and behaviour therapy may be used to improve social interaction and shape socially unacceptable behaviour, respectively, the latter by demonstrating and then rewarding acceptable behaviour by praise or sometimes by monetary or other reward. **Cognitive remediation therapy** can be used to improve attention and concentration problems. Psychological approaches to weight gain are important given that many modern neuroleptic treatments ('atypicals') can cause substantial weight gain in a relatively short time. Often all of these interventions need to be reinforced, as there is a tendency for the benefits of psychological therapy to diminish over time.

Social approaches

The assessment of the social needs of the patient with schizophrenia along with neuroleptic treatment remain the mainstay of modern treatment for schizophrenia. A major consideration is the suitability of the accommodation and the input of carers. The patient needs to have sufficient structure and stimulation to their life to prevent negative symptoms and achieve adequate self-care, but also to live in a stress-free environment so that positive symptoms and depression are controlled. Are carers required to achieve medication adherence and prevent other problems such as substance misuse? These goals may be achieved through independent living supported by family or professional carers, or living in a group or residential environment such as a group home. Sometimes patients with schizophrenia need to go through short or more extended periods of rehabilitation in hospital and then in a sheltered environment before living successfully in their own home or a group home.

Patients with schizophrenia usually become worse in terms of negative symptoms and self-care if they do not have some structured activities in the working week. While some will be able to carry out mainstream work, many more can achieve this if they are supported at work by staff who are aware of the problems of schizophrenia and can explain and negotiate how these problems can be accommodated in the workplace. Others cannot work and are helped by day-centres, or educational or vocational placements such as horticulture. A considerable amount of information and support for the patient and carer is available from voluntary organizations.

Electrical and magnetic treatment

Electroconvulsive treatment (ECT) is only used to treat catatonic symptoms in schizophrenia. Magnetic treatment has no role in the treatment of schizophrenia at present.

Course and prognosis

Most patients show some degree of improvement in their positive symptoms and symptoms of depression with modern treatment. Overall, 20 per cent of patients with schizophrenia fully recover from their symptoms and live a normal quality of life. Thirty-five per cent have long periods of remission when they have no symptoms and function normally, but will have further acute schizophrenia episodes in their life that usually respond well to treatment. Another 35 per cent show mild, persistent positive and negative symptoms requiring continuing care in the community, in their own home or in a group setting. And 10 per cent develop chronic unremitting symptoms and need substantial care, usually in a group or residential home environment. A very small proportion of the latter group may need forensic care because their behaviour represents a danger to other people. Overall, the prognosis is much better than the public and health professionals realize.

Poor prognostic factors for outcome are:

- **Pre-morbid handicaps**: Poor work or educational achievement, poor social adjustment, schizoid personality.
- **Co-morbid psychiatric problems**: Drug and alcohol misuse.
- **Characteristics of the illness**: Long insidious onset, long delay to first treatment, obsessional symptoms, absence of affective or catatonic symptoms, pronounced negative symptoms or thought disorder, severe behaviour problems that are poorly tolerated by other people.
- **Response to treatment**: Lack of response or poor tolerance of medication and other treatment responses.
- **Current living conditions**: Lack of structure to day and lack of stimulation, exposure to high expressed emotion.

DELUSIONAL DISORDER

This diagnosis is reserved for a person who has a complex and logical system of beliefs that are based on one or more specific delusions. Sometimes there are also auditory hallucinations but there are no other features of schizophrenia. The delusions are usually persecutory or grandiose.

Some patients have single delusions, for example:

- **Dysmorphophobia** (a conviction that the body is misshapen or is releasing a disgusting smell).
- **Morbid jealousy** (the delusion is that the sexual partner has been unfaithful on the basis of flimsy and inappropriately insubstantial evidence such as the person sometimes being late).
- **Erotomania** (where someone is in love with someone else and wrongly believes they are in love with them but cannot show or reciprocate it).

Often the person with delusional disorder has a previously paranoid personality, suspicious, sensitive to criticism, and rigid in their belief system, or there is a history of sensory deprivation or temporal or parietal lobe deficits in the brain.

Treatment

The first problem is persuading the patient that he or she needs treatment at all. Treatment from the general practitioner may be more acceptable than from a mental health professional, and the patient should be tried on **pimozide** as drug of first choice, but other neuroleptics may also be successful. Full recovery may occur in about half the patients, with a further one-third showing some improvement.

14   BIPOLAR DISORDERS

There are two recognized forms of bipolar disorder, **bipolar 1 disorder**, in which there are clear-cut episodes of mania or hypomania in addition to episodes of depression, and **bipolar 2 disorder**, where the episodes of mania are either very mild, or only occur when the patient has been on antidepressant medication. A special form of bipolar disorder is rapid cycling bipolar disorder (four or more episodes of mania or depression in the same year) for which there are now specific treatment approaches.

MANIA AND HYPOMANIA

Epidemiology

Bipolar disorder has a lifetime prevalence of between 0.5 and 1.5 per cent of the population (1 per cent bipolar 1 disorder, 0.5 per cent bipolar 2 disorder). There is a slight excess of women to men with bipolar 1 disorder, but four times as many women have bipolar 2 disorder than men. The peak age of inception is 15 to 19 years, and the first onset is usually before the age of 30 years. An organic cause for the symptoms of mania or hypomania is more likely if the age of onset of the first depressive, manic, or hypomanic episode is beyond 45 years.

Clinical features

The central symptoms of mania (and hypomania) are **elated** or **irritable mood**, and **increased activity**. Elated mood is usually experienced as an infectious over-cheerfulness that may lift the mood of the observer. However, the person may experience irritable mood with displays of inappropriate anger. The mood in mania is often quite changeable, with brief periods (lasting minutes or hours) of depression interchanging with periods of elation and irritability and more normal mood. Questions to ask concerning mania are shown in *Box 14.1*. There is increased activity, with the person switching from one task to another without fully completing the first task ('**distractibility**', a form of poor attention and concentration). The person with mania often requires only **a few hours of sleep** (unlike their carers, so mania often requires hospital admission). The person may have a **grandiose** or unjustifiably heightened sense of their abilities or

---

Box 14.1 Ten-minute history and mental state examination for mania or hypomania

History

Have you felt especially happy or over-cheerful? More cheerful than you have ever felt before? Tell me more about it. Does it occur every day? How long does it last each day? How long has it lasted overall?

Have you felt more irritable or lost your temper more easily than usual? Tell me more about it. Has this occurred every day? How long has this lasted?

Have you been much more active or energetic than usual? Tell me more about it. What have you done? How long has this lasted?

If the answers to any of these questions are 'YES', ask about **reduced need for sleep**, **speed of thinking** and **speech** (increased, cannot keep up with thoughts), **agitation** and **restlessness**, **views of self-worth** (increased confidence in abilities and increased importance), **libido** (increased), **distractibility**, **buying things** that the person does not need.

Mental state examination

Appearance and behaviour. Bright, colourful appearance (clothes, make-up, hair), lack of self-care or care over appearance (cleanliness, tidiness, hydration, and nutrition), overactivity, agitation or restlessness, over-familiarity (treats doctor like a friend, may be flirtatious), disinhibited.
Speech. Fast, difficult to interrupt.
Mood. Elated, irritable, labile, or rapidly changing from elated to depressed to irritable.
Thought. Fast. Flight of ideas (sentences logical but linked by puns or clang associations, namely words sound similar, rather than sentences linked by logical argument). Increased self-confidence or grandiosity (increased ability, importance). Overvalued ideas or delusions of persecution, reference or grandiosity.
Perception. Hallucinations often congruent with elated mood.
Cognition. Poor attention or concentration because of distractibility.

---

position in life. In extreme forms they may believe they are exceptionally gifted or rich, or an important religious, political or famous person. The judgement of a person with mania is often impaired, because of grandiosity and failure to plan or consider the consequences of their actions, and their behaviour may be **reckless** and have a **high potential for harm**. Examples include excessive and unnecessary spending sprees, multiple sexual encounters, and reckless driving. They may distress other people by their tactless or inappropriate remarks or behaviour.

In mania, the person's **thoughts are speeded up** to the extent that the person cannot keep up with them. This may be observable to others as **pressure of speech**, where the person is very difficult to interrupt because the speech is relentless (pressure analogous to the steam bellowing from a kettle of boiling water). In extreme form, the person has **flight of ideas**, where words and ideas are not linked logically, but superficially by the way words sound (clang associations), double meaning, or puns (see *Box 14.1*). Subjectively, the person experiences an increased perceptual awareness so that colours are brighter and more vivid, and sounds are louder and more exciting.

Delusions and **hallucinations** are usually **mood congruent**, that is, compatible with the mood. Delusions are often grandiose if the mood is predominantly elated, but persecutory if the mood is irritable. Hallucinations also tend to fit the mood. Auditory hallucinations are usually second person, talking to the person with mania. Delusions and hallucinations can be mood incongruent, that is, unrelated to the mood, and Schneider's first rank (or positive) symptoms of schizophrenia can be experienced in mania.

Diagnosis

For a diagnosis of mania, **elated or irritable mood** has to be present with at least three of the symptoms outlined in bold (four if irritable mood only) in the same one week period. Mania lasts a week or more. It is associated with *severe loss of function and/or psychotic symptoms*. Hypomania lasts 4 days or more. It is associated with *improved function or mild impairment of function*. Psychotic symptoms never appear in hypomania. A person can have both mania and a moderate depressive episode together at the same time. If this occurs for at least a week, they have a mixed affective episode.

Different types of bipolar disorder

Episodes of mania and depression occur with a similar frequency and severity in many **bipolar 1 disorder** patients over a lifetime. In **bipolar 2 disorder** there are four or five often severe depressive episodes to one mild hypomanic episode or when hypomanic episode is precipitated by antidepressants. Both types of bipolar disorder need to be distinguished from unipolar depressive disorder because *antidepressants can precipitate mania or hypomania*, and can lead to a worse course of illness.

Differential diagnosis

Organic causes of mania ('symptomatic mania') include a **drug-induced psychosis** resulting from stimulant drugs such as cocaine, amphetamines, and high amounts of concentrated cannabis such as skunk, or hallucinogen drugs such as LSD or ecstasy. Steroids and antidepressant drugs can cause organic mania. The first month after delivery (especially the first week) is a risk for a puerperal psychosis, manic type. A number of **neurological disorders** such as multiple sclerosis, epilepsy, cerebrovascular accident, and brain tumour affecting frontal or subcortical areas of the brain, or

endocrine disorders such as thyroid disease, adrenal gland disorders, and hypopituitarism can cause symptomatic mania. An organic cause for mania should be considered when there is a known organic cause of depression and the organic cause precedes or coincides with the start of the first symptoms of depression.

Schizophrenia: The symptoms of mania with psychotic features may be very similar to those in a patient with schizophrenia who is agitated, excited, and voluble. If schizophrenia-like symptoms persist after the period of excitement has resolved, schizophrenia is the better diagnosis.

Unipolar depressive disorder: Bipolar 2 disorder can be misdiagnosed if the doctor confuses relief from not feeling depressed any more with pathological elation. The presence of the other symptoms of hypomania for sufficient duration must be established. There is especially a risk of this in people who do not come from the same cultural background. There are no features that provide a clear distinction between episodes of depression that are part of bipolar disorder, and those that are part of the more common episodes of unipolar depression – which will be dealt with in the next chapter (see p. 213). However, depression in bipolar illness is more likely to be precipitated by little evidence of the life stresses that commonly antedate the more common forms of depression, and patients may develop severe forms of depression such as melancholic depression and psychotic depression.

Borderline personality disorder: Rapid cycling bipolar disorder can be very similar to the mood instability seen in patients with borderline personality disorder. The duration and characteristic nature of the symptoms of mania and depression, and their persistence over time, should enable the episodic bipolar disorder to be distinguished from the long-standing borderline personality disorder.

Neurochemistry, neuroimaging, and neuropathology

PET scans of the brain indicate excessive post-synaptic dopamine 2 activity in mania. There is some evidence of increased central noradrenaline and serotonin turnover in mania, the opposite to depressive episodes, but the results are inconsistent. Inositol phosphatase, implicated in the metabolism of lithium, has been found to be increased in mania. Levels of lithium and valproate consistent with therapeutic levels found in the brain of patients with bipolar disorder are associated with dendronal growth in tissue culture studies. Mania has been associated with increased cortisol responsivity to stress. White matter hyper-intensities thought to be small cerebrovascular insults have been related to poor prognosis in terms of frequency of further episodes and mild cognitive impairment.

Aetiology

GENETIC FACTORS

In first-degree relatives of patients with bipolar illness, the risk of bipolar illness is substantially increased, at between 5 and 10 per cent. All twin studies have shown large differences between concordance rates for MZ and DZ twins, with one Danish study showing 62 per cent for an MZ to have a bipolar illness, and only 8 per cent for a DZ twin. If this is extended to the risk of the other twin having *either* a bipolar or a unipolar illness, the figures increase to 79 per cent for MZ co-twins, and 19 per cent for DZ co-twins. There is therefore an important genetic component in bipolar illness, but environmental factors are thought to interact with genetic factors in the production of illness in the individual. Linkage studies have implicated a number of putative sites for bipolar genes, the most notable being 12q23 to q24; and 21q22.

At least 60 per cent of patients have a genetic history of bipolar disorder, unipolar depression, and cyclothymia or hyperthymic temperament. **Cyclothymia** is a life-long tendency to experience periods of enhanced zest for life and activity followed by periods of pessimism, worry, low energy, and a sense of futility. **Hyperthymi**a is a life-long tendency to periods of enhanced zest, risk-taking and drive without contrasting periods of pessimism. This genetic history means that patients with bipolar disorder may have strong views about the illness derived from their personal experience of growing up with an affected parent, sibling, or other member of the family. Carers from the same family may also be affected with bipolar disorder or unipolar depressive disorder. There are thought to be many genes involved in either increasing or decreasing the risk of bipolar disorder, and some may code for specific features of bipolar disorder such as the COMT gene for rapid cycling bipolar disorder. In non-genetic cases of bipolar disorder, cyclothymic and hyperthymic temperaments also seem to be a predisposing factor to developing bipolar disorder.

PRECIPITATING AND MAINTAINING FACTORS

Life events leading to the disruption of sleep or the usual early morning pattern of activity such as shift work, crossing time zones, or leaving on a journey very early in the morning can precipitate mania in some vulnerable people. Positive life events can also precipitate mania. Stressful social circumstances, loss events, and criticism and hostility (expressed emotion) can all precipitate both mania and depression, mainly depression. Pregnancy, cerebrovascular accidents, and other pathology affecting frontal–subcortical structures, steroids, and stimulant or hallucinogenic drugs can all precipitate mania. Thyroid disease (including non-symptomatic elevated thyroid-stimulating hormone levels), antidepressants, steroids, high alcohol consumption, and high levels of regular cannabis use can all precipitate the onset of rapid cycling mood in patients with established bipolar disorder. All of these precipitating factors can be maintaining factors as well, and patients are likely to improve if these maintaining factors are addressed.

MANAGING RISK AND NON-SPECIFIC MANAGEMENT OF MANIA

The main risks in mania are from recklessness and aggression, but patients with mania can also neglect their self-care, nutrition, and need for sleep, leading to medical problems if they happen to suffer from co-morbid medical illness such as diabetes. In mania, they can be sexually promiscuous, leading to risks of pregnancy and both contracting and spreading sexually transmitted disease. Mania associated with little need for rest or sleep or resulting in aggressive, reckless or disinhibited behaviour can rarely be managed safely without in-patient care. Patients with mania may not accept that they are ill because they feel more healthy than normal, so they often require involuntary detention under the Mental Health Act if they are behaving in a reckless or aggressive manner posing a risk to the self or other people. Patients with mania can be easier to manage if the in-patient unit is not too small and confined, and there are activities to distract them.

PRINCIPLES OF TREATMENT IN BIPOLAR DISORDER

Acute mania

- Atypical antipsychotic. Add valproate if inadequate response. Continue or institute maintenance lithium. Women of child bearing age should not be prescribed valproate because of the high risk of fetal abnormality and polycystic ovary syndrome.

Bipolar depression

- Avoid antidepressants, especially dual-acting, since they can precipitate mania and rapid cycling.
- Use **quetiapine** or **olanzapine** first and add lamotrigine if necessary.
- If essential, use an SSRI.

Maintenance

- Avoid frequent changes and evaluate effectiveness over months not weeks before changing prescription.
- Use a compact mood diary on card, where the patient uses one letter or digit per day to indicate overall mood. Part of bedtime routine. This visualizes the pattern of mood over 12 to 18 months and whether treatment has modified it.
- Psycho-education and therapy to promote a regular diurnal activity pattern have been shown to be effective.
- Use lithium first, then add mood stabilizers until adequate control is achieved; use atypical antipsychotics or lamotrigine if depressive relapse is the main problem, and atypical antipsychotics or valproate for recurrent mania. Clozapine can be used for resistant rapid cycling.

Specific psychological treatments

Psychological treatments, like antidepressant drugs, tend to be less effective for the treatment of bipolar depression compared to unipolar depression. Patients can be taught to identify and manage **early warning signs of mania**, and prevent episodes occurring. A range of psychoeducation, family, and cognitive behaviour therapies targeted at recognizing early warning signs, coping with mild depression, stabilizing social routine, promoting adherence to medication, and avoiding substance misuse, can prevent episodes of mania and depression, and mild symptoms of depression and hypomania.

Course and prognosis

If the person has one manic episode, they will almost certainly have other manic and depressive episodes. In established bipolar disorder, there is a 50 per cent chance of another episode in the next year after a manic or depressive episode, and an 80 per cent chance of another episode in the next 4 years. Clusters of relapses interspersed with periods of fewer relapses tend to happen for the rest of the person's life.

15 INTERNALIZING DISORDERS 1: DEPRESSION, ANXIETY AND THE FEAR DISORDERS

Internalizing refers to the tendency to introspect about problems, and experience distress and dysphoria: it is seen in all disorders characterized by high anxiety and depression, as well as fear disorders such as panic disorder, post-traumatic stress disorder, and the phobic disorders. There is considerable overlap between these disorders, as their symptoms are often shared between them. Over the years, the names given to these clinical syndromes have reflected the predominant symptoms in each disorder.

These disorders frequently occur together in the general population, and they are sometimes known as *'common mental disorders'*. In this chapter each type of presentation is dealt with separately for ease of understanding, but it is important to remember that they overlap considerably, both with each other and with the limits of 'normal' experience of symptoms. In general medical settings most patients who are psychologically distressed will be found to have a combination of anxious and depressive symptoms. We describe depression, generalized anxiety, the fear disorders (panic, simple phobias, and agoraphobia), bereavement, and obsessive-compulsive disorder in this chapter.

Presentations of common mental disorders in general medical settings

Only a minority of patients with the disorders about to be described present with the symptoms that are needed for the diagnosis: most will present with somatic symptoms – either unexplained by known physical disorders, or more severe than would have been expected.

DEPRESSION

Depression can occur as a single depressive episode or a recurrent series of episodes. It is important that you recognize these symptoms, since they cause much distress to the patients, are associated with a decreased quality of life and an increased mortality, and they are eminently treatable. Depression includes terms such as 'depressive episode', 'major depression', and 'unipolar depression'.

There has been a long controversy about the best way to classify depressive illnesses, and the non-psychiatrist is well advised to ignore it. There are also more severe forms of the illness, called psychotic depression and melancholic depression. In the past, attempts were made to distinguish between 'reactive' and 'endogenous' depressions, but the distinction is no longer useful. All depressive illnesses are to at least some extent reactive to life circumstances, and there is often an unobservable component of genetic vulnerability as well. The term 'neurotic depression' is best avoided, since it implies that people who become depressed are neurotic, and this is far from being the case. It is true that people who score highly on 'neuroticism' scales are more vulnerable to develop depressive illnesses when under stress, but with sufficient adversity depressive illnesses can also develop in stable, phlegmatic people.

Epidemiology

Although *depressive symptoms* are somewhat less common than anxiety symptoms, they are nonetheless to be found in between 10 and 16 per cent of men, and between 20 and 24 per cent of women in community surveys. Once more, *depressive illnesses* – that is to say, people with more than a critical number of depressive symptoms – are very much less common, accounting for between 2.6 and 4 per cent of men, and about 7 to 8 per cent of women in surveys carried out in London, Canberra, and the United States. The annual inception rate in the community is not known, although it seems likely that it is over half the point prevalence.

The prevalence of depressive illness is very much higher in consulting populations. Depressive illnesses are the commonest diagnosis in a study of inceptions of illness in general practice, accounting for 12 per cent of all new illnesses, and 45 per cent of all psychiatric diagnoses made in this setting. It is important to emphasize that most of these depressed patients were consulting their doctors either with somatic symptoms related to their depression, or with physical illnesses that they had in addition to their depression.

Symptoms of depression

The core or essential symptoms of depression are **depressed mood** and **loss of interest and pleasure** (see *Box 15.1*).

Depressed mood may be experienced as sadness or unhappiness that lasts for at least part of the day on every day for at least 2 weeks. The person is usually more difficult to cheer up than usual (the mood is less 'reactive' to other people and the person's own interests and hobbies). More severe low mood is experienced as misery and shows no reactivity at all. In **melancholia** the patient does not experience any emotion at all (emotional numbness) (see *Box 15.2*).

Loss of interest and pleasure (sometimes known as anhedonia) is experienced as a loss of enjoyment and indifference to the person's usual pursuits and hobbies, including those involving social interaction. Often the person withdraws from social contact and keeps themselves to themselves.

A **change in sleep pattern** may be experienced as taking a long time to get off to sleep, waking up frequently in the night for no good reason, or waking up earlier than usual

> **Box 15.1** Ten-minute history and mental state examination for severe depressive episode
>
> **History**
>
> **Have you felt low or miserable?** Tell me more about it. Have you lost your emotion? (Only ask this if the person denies feeling low or miserable but looks depressed.) Does it occur every day? How long does it last each day? How long has it lasted overall? Did anything in your life seem to bring it on?
>
> **Have you lost interest and enjoyment in things you usually enjoy?** Tell me more about it. What about your hobbies? What about mixing with friends? How long has this lasted?
>
> **Are these experiences bad enough to interfere with your daily life?** In what way?
>
> If the answers to the first and/or second question plus the third are 'yes', ask about changes in **sleep pattern, weight, fatigue and energy, concentration and efficiency of thinking, views of self** (worth, guilt) and **the future**, and **suicide risk**.
>
> **Features indicating severe depression in the mental state examination:**
>
> *Appearance and behaviour.* Poor self-care (cleanliness, tidiness, hydration, and nutrition), averted eye-contact, slow movement/lack of body movement, or in contrast constant fidgeting or restlessness.
> *Speech.* In a monotone, hesitant and/or slow in speed.
> *Mood.* Observably depressed.
> *Thought.* Slow speed of thoughts. Overvalued ideas or delusions of worthlessness, inappropriate guilt. Hopelessness. Suicidal ideation or plans, or preoccupation with death or serious illness. Delusions of persecution or reference.
> *Perception.* Hallucinations often congruent with low mood.
> *Cognition.* Poor attention or concentration.

on a consistent basis. A person may sleep more than usual every day, either in one single continuous period, or as a series of naps in addition to their night-time sleep, but still feel unrefreshed.

A **change in appetite or weight** can occur, often losing their appetite for food because of loss of interest in or the taste of food, or because they feel too agitated or nauseous. The appetite can be increased ('comfort eating' to temporarily reduce distress from depression). Loss or gain of more than 5 per cent of body weight may reflect the change in appetite, although other causes for change in weight such as dieting and medical illness should disqualify this symptom from the diagnosis. There can also be change in sexual appetite, usually a loss of sexual interest or libido.

Box 15.2 Symptoms of melancholia

Distinct quality of mood – **emotional numbness**

No interest or pleasure at all

Early morning waking of 1 hour or more every day

Psychomotor retardation or **agitation**

Weight loss of more than 5 per cent over last month (not through dieting)

Diurnal mood variation (worse in the morning, improves in the afternoon and early evening)

Fatigue and **loss of energy** are common symptoms of depression, but also have many other medical, psychiatric, and social or physiological causes. Fatigue is the experience of being tired and wrung out earlier in the day than normal despite a lack of excessive activity. Loss of energy refers to the difficulty in starting tasks, primarily because of a lack of motivation and interest.

Psychomotor retardation refers to being slowed down in thoughts, speech, facial, and body movements and actions to a degree that is observable to others (see *Box 15.1*). An extremely severe depression can leave a person mute and in a stupor, unable to move any part of their body except their eyes. A person with severe depression can also be **agitated and restless**, both in mind (constantly brooding over and over the same depressive thoughts) and body (pacing up and down or getting up and then sitting or lying).

Poor concentration and **inefficient thinking** are common. A person may complain of memory problems but on formal testing of mental state (see Chapter 3), problems of attention and concentration are more obvious (so the person cannot process events sufficiently to retain or recall them).

A low opinion of the self to the degree that a person feels **worthless**, useless and a burden to other people is common in severe depression. There is also often self-blame and **inappropriate guilt** over past misdemeanours, not just for being ill and needing looking after currently. A person with depression may feel helpless and **hopeless** about the future, unable to tolerate their present mental state and unable to envisage a time or circumstances when an improvement may occur. Perhaps in such a mental state, morbid **preoccupation with death**, wishing that they were dead, believing themselves wrongly despite medical assurance to have a catastrophic medical illness, or **suicidal ideation** are understandable.

An important symptom is diurnal variation of mood, when all the symptoms of depression tend to be worse in the morning and sometimes late evening than in the afternoon and early evening. The person with severe depression can have mood-congruent delusions and hallucinations. These delusions of reference, persecution, or hypochondriasis are often seen as deserved because the person sees themselves as worthless, guilty of misdemeanours, and a burden to others. Hallucinations may be black in mood, such as funeral music or derogatory comments made in the second person such as 'you are a sinner'. Delusions, hallucinations, and Schneider's positive symptoms can also occur in severe depressive episodes. Mental state examination features are in *Box 15.1*.

Diagnosis

A diagnosis of mild, moderate, or severe depression may be made:

- In **mild depression**, a person has one of the two core symptoms (depressed mood, or loss of interest and pleasure) and three other symptoms of depression that have been outlined in bold together for at least 2 weeks (two other symptoms if both core symptoms are present).
- In **moderate depression**, they have four to seven symptoms of depression (including at least one core symptom) together for at least 2 weeks.
- In **severe depression**, seven or more symptoms of depression (including at least one core symptom) are present together for at least 2 weeks. When depression is severe, patients can develop *psychotic symptoms*, ranging from well-held ideas of worthlessness and guilt to ideas that parts of one's body are dead, and even hallucinations with an insulting or derogatory content. In *melancholic depression* there may be a distinct quality of mood with emotional numbness, no interest or pleasure at all in everyday activities, early waking, and a pronounced diurnal variation of mood – with mood being worse in the mornings

The grading of severity depends on the degree of functional impairment as well. In severe depression, the person is unable to look after themselves on a day-to-day basis, such as getting up, washing, dressing, or eating, without at least some verbal assistance from others. In moderate depression a person is usually able to look after themselves but not work, study, or look after others without some assistance. In mild depression, there is some impairment in performance at work or study, or in leisure activities. Symptoms of anxiety may be experienced to an intense degree in severe depressive episodes ('**agitated depression**') but the features of depression dominate the clinical picture.

Risks

Most completed suicides occur in people suffering from depressive episodes. Suicide is more likely if the person has a definite suicide plan (plans where, when, and how they are going to kill themselves), but any persistent suicidal ideation that is not fully formed or a suicidal act with the intent of committing suicide must be taken seriously, especially when it co-exists with the symptoms of depression. Symptoms and signs of agitation and intense hopelessness in severe depression must also be considered to indicate a risk of suicide (see *Box 4.4*, Chapter 4 to assess suicide risk).

People with severe depression may also die of neglect, usually from dehydration. Mothers with severe depression can neglect their babies, and depressed people may neglect and therefore harm other dependent people such as young children, frail elderly, people suffering from learning difficulties, and people with severe physical handicaps. A person with depression can be irritable and, especially if there are delusions of persecution directed at specific people and they are agitated, a danger to other people. A mother with severe postnatal depression may decide to kill herself and her baby as an act of humanity because the world seems such a terrible place to continue living in.

Aetiology of depression

PREDISPOSING FACTORS

Genetic factors are not as important in unipolar depression as they are in bipolar depression, but they are nonetheless present, with a **heritability** of about 37 per cent. However, at least some of these genes are likely to be concerned with the predisposition to symptoms of anxiety that so frequently co-exist with depressive symptoms. Depression is *familial* in the sense that other family members are more likely to have had similar illnesses, but there is not the clear evidence from twin studies as there is in bipolar illness. There are important interactions between the possession of particular genes and the adverse effects of stressful life events: it has been shown that people with abnormalities of their 5HT transporter gene are very much more likely to develop depression after life stress than those without this abnormality. In similar fashion, one American study showed that the increased risk for depression after a severe life event was about twice as high in subjects with a positive family history of depression. Abnormal styles of parenting – both neglectful and over-protective – have also been shown to be associated with later depression.

The personality trait '**neuroticism**' itself has an important genetic component, and people high on this trait are at increased risk for depression. Adverse experiences during infancy also put people at higher risk for depression, most notably poor **maternal attachment**, but also **maternal separation** and **maternal depression**. In early and middle childhood **emotional neglect**, and both **physical and sexual abuse** put people at greater risk of internalizing disorders – although this is not specific to depression, and involves other abnormalities such as self-harm, eating disorders, and poor sexual adjustment. Other factors with an association with later depressive illness are early bereavement, especially loss of mother by death or separation, and parental divorce. In childhood a concept of **low self-esteem** may develop. Subjects tend to regard themselves in a critical and disparaging way and have a low opinion of themselves. *Negative views about oneself, one's future, and one's surroundings* are said to constitute the '**cognitive triad**' that renders people vulnerable to mild to moderate degrees of depressive illness. It is likely that the concept of 'passive-dependent personality', which will be described next, has considerable overlap with 'low self-esteem'. The two have been kept separate in this account since it is quite possible to have the latter without the former. Recent surveys have shown early loss of mother during childhood to correlate with low self-esteem in adults, and have also identified some features in people's adult lives that relate to low self-esteem, such as women having an unemployed spouse, or more than three children living at home. Among children, those with low self-esteem have been shown to be associated with authoritarian styles of parenting, as well as with indifferent and neglectful parenting.

PROVOKING FACTORS

Loss events, physical illness, and adverse social circumstances all favour the release of depressive phenomena. **Loss events** may be bereavements, threatened future losses, such as when a near relative develops a fatal illness, the loss of a relationship, or even a failure to be promoted. These are especially likely to precipitate depression in those with low self-esteem, in those without intimate confidants, and in those with some pre-existing conflict that is exacerbated by a stressful event. The loss may precede the episode of depression by as much as 1 year. **Physical illness** commonly contributes to the genesis of depressive illnesses seen in general medical settings. The patient may have been mildly dysphoric before the onset of such illnesses, but experiences a marked exacerbation of depressive symptoms after the physical illness. Although the association between depression and infections like infectious hepatitis, influenza, and glandular fever has been recognized for many years, it should be appreciated that other infectious illnesses such as herpes zoster and urinary tract infections often seem to contribute to the development of depressive disorders. It has been shown that those with lower self-esteem are at higher risk for developing depressive illnesses after episodes of infectious illness. **Stressful social circumstances** are protean in their manifestations. Patients may have very little in the way of social support, or they may have lost what little they had. Unsatisfactory living conditions, chronic illness in close relatives, and poor interpersonal relationships are recurrent themes in individual case histories.

MAINTAINING FACTORS

The main challenge to helping patients with severe depressive episodes or other mental disorders, especially if they have been present for months or years, is to identify and then manage the physiological and psychosocial factors that are stopping the person from improving ('maintaining factors'). All the precipitating factors we identified can also be maintaining factors as well. The problem is that ways in which the person has tried to cope with their depression, the consequences of what they have neglected to do, or ways in which other people or organizations have dealt with the patient's condition, may have contributed to the lack of improvement in the patient.

Differential diagnosis

Organic causes of depression include:

- **Heavy alcohol or street drug consumption** (especially withdrawal-stimulant drugs like amphetamine and cocaine, hallucinogenic drugs such as ecstasy and LSD, or CNS depressants such as barbiturates).
- A number of **prescribed drugs** that can precipitate depression such as interferon and steroids.
- **Neurological disorders** such as disorders of the basal ganglia (e.g. Parkinson's disease, Huntington's disease), cerebrovascular accidents, head injury, dementias, space occupying lesions in the brain such as tumours, epilepsy (especially complex partial seizures or 'temporal lobe epilepsy') and encephalitis.
- **Endocrine disorders**, especially those of the thyroid, pituitary, and adrenal glands, infections such as human immunodeficiency virus (HIV), hepatitis, and glandular fever, and carcinoma (especially of the pancreas and bronchus).

An organic cause for depression should be considered when there is a known organic cause of depression and the organic cause precedes or coincides with the start of the first symptoms of depression.

Bipolar disorder: The symptoms of mania and hypomania are often missed.

Schizophrenia: Symptoms of depression occur at the same time as more florid positive symptoms of schizophrenia, or within 1 year of a florid presentation of positive symptoms.

Bereavement can present in a similar way to depressive episodes, and is dealt with on page 228.

Neurochemistry, neuroimaging, and neuropathology

According to the monoamine theory of mood disorders, depressive episodes are due to functional impairment in both noradrenaline and 5-hydroxytryptamine (5-HT or serotonin) containing neurones in the brain. In some depressed patients reduced levels of 5-hydroxyindolacetic acid (5-HIAA) are found in the cerebrospinal fluid, and there are reduced levels of 5-hydroxytryptamine in the brains of some suicide victims diagnosed with depressive episodes previously in their life. Reduced turnover of central 5-HT is the probable explanation for these findings, which are consistent with the reduced ability of drugs that are indirect 5-HT agonists (e.g. fenfluramine) to stimulate prolactin. A tryptophan-free diet can lead to both reduced 5-HT turnover in the brain on brain PET scans and also a lowering of mood in patients in remission from depressive episodes, or a worsening of symptoms of depression in patients with current depressive episodes. In severe depression, clonidine, in doses acting as an adrenoceptor agonist, has reduced effectiveness in stimulating growth hormone output, suggesting a similarly reduced noradrenaline turnover in the brain. All of these findings are consistent with a therapeutic response in depressive episodes to antidepressant drugs that increase brain turnover of 5-HT (e.g. SSRI antidepressants), noradrenaline (e.g. desipramine, reboxetine) or both (e.g. SNRI and tricyclic antidepressants). These findings do not explain why there is a therapeutic delay of 2 weeks or more, but there is growing evidence from tissue culture studies that antidepressants result in a cascade of chemical processes increasing protein production, and the sprouting of an increased density of dendrons at the ends of neurones. These effects are global in the brain.

Neuroimaging highlights that in depressive episodes there are selective reductions in blood flow to limbic and subcortical structures, including the anterior and posterior cingulated gyrus and amygdala. These areas are involved in information processing in relation to emotion and directing attention. Recovery from depression is associated with improved blood flow to these areas of the brain.

In around two-thirds of severely depressed patients, there are abnormalities of the hypothalamic–pituitary–adrenal axis (HPA), which plays a key role in controlling circadian rhythms related to sleep–wakefulness, appetite, energy, and stress responses. The adrenal glands are increased in size in moderate to severe depressive episodes, there is increased plasma cortisol and 24-hour turnover of cortisol, and cortisol production is not suppressed by the drug dexamethasone. Abnormalities of the HPA may contribute to symptoms such as diurnal variation of mood, early morning waking (the early morning surge of cortisol release occurs earlier in depression), loss of appetite and weight loss, lack of an adaptive response to and suppression of the immune system (patients with depressive episodes are more prone to upper respiratory infection).

These findings indicate that a severe depressive episode is not just a disorder of the brain or mind but affects the whole body, and that the symptoms have a real physiological and anatomical basis and that the person with depression cannot 'snap out of it' with a bit of effort on their part.

Treatment of depression

A 'stepped-care' model for the management of depression is summarized in *Figure 15.1*. This model emphasizes that many cases of depression found in general medical or primary care settings are mild in severity, and will in fact often respond to a non-medical approach, with kindly interest and general advice.

Those with **mild depression** should initially be treated by recognition, accompanied by information and general advice, and followed by 'watchful waiting'. Some patients will spontaneously improve, others may be in the process of becoming more severely depressed and then require active treatment. Many patients with milder depression respond to interventions such as taking exercise (for example through an 'exercise on prescription' scheme) or guided self-help, although many improve while being monitored without additional help. More structured therapies, such as problem-solving, brief or computer administered CBT or counselling can also be helpful. In these patients with only mild depression the risk-benefit ratio of antidepressant drugs favours a non-pharmacological approach.

Patients with a **moderate depression** should all be offered an antidepressants drug, as these are just as effective as non-pharmacological treatments, are easy to administer and cost very much less. The steps involved are summarized in *Box 15.3*. Those not wishing to take up the offer should be offered a choice of problem-solving or brief CBT (see step 3) and if there is no response these should be used in combination, with stepping up to longer-term CBT if required.

Step 5: In-patient care, crisis teams	Risk to life, severe self-neglect	Medication, combined treatments, ECT
Step 4: Mental health specialists including crisis teams	Treatment-resistant, recurrent, atypical and psychotic depression, and those at significant risk	Medication, complex psychological interventions, combined treatments
Step 3: Primary care team, primary care mental health worker	Moderate or severe depression	Medication, psychological interventions, social support
Step 2: Primary care team, primary care mental health worker	Mild depression	Watchful waiting, guided self-help, computerized CBT, exercise, brief psychological interventions
Step 1: GP, practice nurse	Recognition	Assessment

Figure 15.1 *Stepped care for depression*

Box 15.3 Negotiating treatment for depression

- Listen, empathize
- Explain diagnosis
- Explain somatic symptoms
- Address patient's **ideas**, **concerns** and **expectations (ICE)**
- Agree problem list
- Agree management plan
- Build trust
- Arrange follow-up
- Monitor progress

If prescribing antidepressant medication:
- Inform patient of efficacy and benefits
  - Mode of action
  - Not addictive
  - Side-effects
  - 10–14 days before start to work
  - When to take treatment
  - Withdraw gradually

Those with **severe depression** should all be offered antidepressants, with consideration being given to combination treatments if they are required, and in-patient admission if there is a real risk to life. In any patient with a severe depressive episode, there is evidence that recovery can be faster if the patient receives some **behavioural management** targeted at increasing their interest and confidence (these are called '**mastery and pleasure**' techniques). A task is set each day of the patient's choice, which encourages a little bit of interest and confidence. It is important to be clear what the task is and when it is to be done (bearing in mind on the one hand that the patient is often much worse in the morning and less able to do the task, and the need to get the patient out of bed and doing things). The complexity and number of tasks are increased as the patient starts to recover from their depression. Patients with depression are made worse by their tendency to brood or ruminate on all their negative, self-critical thinking if left awake in bed and on their own. They are also made worse by criticism and hostility from other people, especially from those who purport to care for them. The patient's mood is helped by distracting themselves from this thinking, solving even trivial problems effectively, and non-judgemental, empathic support from other people. It is especially important to encourage hope as long as this sounds realistic and attainable – just saying everything will be all right without explaining how tends to be ineffective. Finally patients with severe depression who are agitated and restless, or exhausted and distressed through poor sleep, can be helped with the prescription of small doses of an antipsychotic agent or other sedative agent in the short term until there is a sustained clinical response from other specific treatments for severe depression.

Electrical and magnetic treatment

Electroconvulsive treatment (ECT) is described in Chapter 8. It is especially effective for severe depressive episodes with melancholia, and depressive episodes with psychotic features. ECT should be used when a patient consents to treatment and there is urgency in obtaining a clinical response because of the risk of suicide or severe neglect, dehydration, and renal failure. ECT should also be considered when other treatments have failed. The disadvantages are frequent memory loss, and the fact that the response to ECT does not guide the clinician in the choice of antidepressant for longer-term treatment to prevent a recurrence of the depressive episode. **Magnetic treatment** (transcranial magnetic stimulation, TMS) or electrical stimulation of the vagus nerve do not provide sustained treatment responses in severe depression and should not be used.

Managing risk

The first consideration is how to keep the patient and carers safe and supported. Assessment of suicide risk and risk to others is covered in Chapter 4 pp. 51–53; and the exact questions you should use are on page 52. A common risk in severe depression is the risk of self-neglect, due principally to lack of motivation or interest, core symptoms of depression rather than laziness, indifference, or perversity on the part of the patient. In such cases, the carer will need to provide verbal assistance in a regular and assertive but also non-judgemental and encouraging manner in relation to getting up, washing, dental care, dressing, eating, drinking, and toileting. Medical and nursing staff must regularly have face-to-face contact with patients who have severe depressive episodes with evidence of self-neglect. In particular, they need to assess the patient's state of nutrition, dehydration, and general self-care, and assess the distress of the patient and carer, as managing such a patient can create frustration and therefore further distress or aggression. If there are signs that the carer is not managing the patient, then consideration will need to be given to alternative care arrangements, usually in-patient psychiatric care. If the patient normally looks after someone else, then alternative arrangements for the care of that other person need to be made on a temporary basis. Often this can be done informally through friends and family but there may be a need to contact social services to provide this.

Non-specific aspects of treatment

In drug trials of antidepressants in primary care settings many patients improve on placebo medication. It is naive to suppose that all these patients would have got better without treatment, although many would probably have done so. *The doctor's confidence that he can help his patient* – whether based on his own personal qualities or his faith in the content of his pills – *promotes hope*, and with it *an expectancy that improvement will occur*. By his offer of return visits he effectively offers to monitor the patient's return to effective social functioning, and makes the patient feel that he has a powerful ally, so that the way becomes clearer for the resolution of both hopelessness and helplessness. The doctor's power to remove both social and occupational obligations may allow the patient to *rest without a sense of failure*; and if *sleep* can be restored there is often a major improvement in how the patient feels.

Course and prognosis

Fortunately, most patients with depression will improve, and the biggest danger that the person will not make some clinical improvement is the risk of death from suicide before the treatment works. There is much variation in the outcome of depressive illnesses seen in general medical settings, and although many will become symptom free within 4 to 6 weeks, about a third are likely to follow a protracted course. Illnesses following severe loss events in those with stable pre-morbid personalities are likely to have a good outcome, while those associated with chronically adverse social and inter-personal circumstances are likely to have a poorer outcome. Depressive illnesses associated with abnormal personalities, especially those described as manipulative, unstable or highly dependent, are likely to have a poor outcome, with hostile depressive outbursts accompanied by dramatic behaviour and impulsive suicidal attempts.

Unfortunately, a minority of patients do not make a full recovery. Patients must continue to take treatment for their depression for at least 9 months otherwise there is an 80 per cent chance of recurrence, especially if the patient has not made a full recovery in terms of symptoms and function. There is a high risk of recurrence, especially if there is a history of three or more episodes in the last 5 years. The decision to continue treatment for depression beyond 9 months depends on the frequency of recurrence but is usually not necessary if the person has never had a previous episode or experiences episodes of depression infrequently.

GENERALIZED ANXIETY DISORDER

Epidemiology

Symptoms of anxiety and worry are among the commonest psychological symptoms encountered in the normal population: however, most worried people do not have enough other symptoms related to anxiety to justify a diagnosis of an anxiety state. The prevalence of anxiety states has been estimated at between 2 and 4 per cent for men, and between 3 and 4.5 per cent for women in three recent surveys of the normal population. There have been no reliable estimates of inception rate. However, one study of inceptions of illnesses seen in general practice settings showed anxiety disorders to constitute about 10 per cent of all new illness onsets, and to account for about one-third of all those with a diagnosable psychiatric disorder. There are therefore grounds for supposing that the prevalence of anxiety states is considerably higher in medical settings than in the general population. In community settings, many patients progress from anxiety states to depression, and vice versa. Many satisfy criteria for both disorders – the genes are the same, and the risk factors and the neurochemistry overlap as much as the clinical syndromes.

Most acute anxiety reactions are of relatively short duration, but phobic illnesses last longer and affect about 3 per cent of men and 6 per cent of women.

Neurochemistry

The syndrome of anxiety is characterized by increased arousal, increased sympathetic activity (mydriasis, tachycardia, perspiration), and unpleasant subjective sensations of fear and apprehension. It is believed that both ascending **noradrenaline and 5-hydroxytryptamine containing neuronal pathways**, innervating the limbic lobe and neocortex, play important roles in mediating the symptoms of anxiety. Increased activity of noradrenergic neurones appears to be involved in symptoms and signs of heightened arousal, while increased activity of 5-hydroxytryptaminergic neurones enhances responses to aversive stimuli so that blocking the effects of 5-hydroxytryptamine with antagonist drugs makes animals more likely to brave an aversive stimulus in order to gain a reward, suggesting that they are less anxious or at least less inhibited than normal. Antagonists at 5-HT2 receptors have been shown to be anxiolytic in humans, and the anxiolytic effect of antidepressant drugs may be mediated by their ability to decrease the sensitivity of 5-HT2 receptors. As is discussed elsewhere (see p. 216), changes in the functioning of noradrenergic and 5-hydroxytryptaminergic neurones are also implicated in the aetiology of depressive illness, and it is believed that different but

221

related neural pathways using different receptor subtypes are involved, which is consistent with the clinical overlap seen between the two disorders.

Neurones containing **gamma-amino butyric acid (GABA)** provide the principal inhibitory system in the brain and act to decrease the activity of other neurones, including those containing monoamines. Drugs that increase GABA function, such as barbiturates and benzodiazepines, are potent anxiolytics. Benzodiazepines act via receptors that are found in the limbic lobe and neocortex and are associated with, and modulate, post-synaptic GABA$_A$ receptors (the GABA$_A$-benziodiazepine receptor complex). Benzodiazepines increase the effect of GABA, whereas there are a group of compounds known as '**inverse agonists**' that bind to benzodiazepine receptors but have the opposite effect and act to decrease the effects of GABA. As might be predicted these compounds are anxiogenic. There are a number of candidates for endogenous compounds that bind to benzodiazepine receptors and could theoretically contribute to pathological anxiety states. Other neurotransmitters may be important in mediating anxiety. Cholecystokinin and related peptide neurotransmitters cause symptoms of panic when infused into humans.

Diagnosis of generalized anxiety disorder (GAD)

Anxious worries and ruminations often come about because the patient anxiously broods about the significance of somatic symptoms of anxiety (do the palpitations mean a heart attack, does the tiredness mean cancer?); or because he is afraid that others notice symptoms such as tremor. Such thoughts exacerbate the original anxiety, and in turn the somatic symptoms are magnified. Patients who present with a single somatic symptom of anxiety such as tachycardia or tremor may present a diagnostic problem until it is appreciated that other psychological and somatic symptoms of anxiety are present. In addition to subjective feelings of tension and worry, the symptoms of anxiety states can conveniently be thought of in three groups (see *Box 15.4*).

People with **generalized anxiety disorder** (GAD) experience **persistent anxiety** and worry that is out of proportion to actual events or circumstances and is difficult to control, leading to problems with concentration and functioning. Typically this worrying involves everyday matters such as work, relationships, money, or health.

Associated with the anxiety and worry, individuals with GAD experience **at least six of the symptoms** in *Box 15.4*, thus a wide range of symptoms that usually involve elements of:

- **Apprehension** (worries about future misfortunes, feeling 'on edge', difficulty in concentrating).
- **Motor tension** (restless fidgeting, tension headaches, trembling, inability to relax).
- **Autonomic overactivity** (light-headedness, sweating, tachycardia or tachypnoea, epigastric discomfort, dizziness, dry mouth).

Box 15.4 Symptoms of anxiety

Autonomic symptoms of anxiety include:	Symptoms relating to motor tone include:	Symptoms of hyper-vigilance include:
palpitations	shakiness	irritability
tachycardia	tremor onset	insomnia
cold, clammy hands	muscular aches	trouble staying asleep
sweating	lump in throat	easily startled
blepharospasm	distractibility	poor concentration
paraesthesiae	restlessness	feeling keyed up
dizziness	easily tired	
hot and cold spells	trouble swallowing	
frequency of micturition		
diarrhoea		
nausea		

Differential diagnosis

OTHER PSYCHIATRIC ILLNESSES

Symptoms of anxiety commonly accompany more differentiated kinds of psychiatric disorders. Easily the commonest of these is **depression**; but such symptoms also occur in any **psychotic illness** (i.e. above anxiety state in the diagnostic hierarchy). Anxiety is also an integral part of an **obsessional state** (see below), so make sure that you have elicited all the patient's symptoms, and that those you have elicited can be accounted for by morbid anxiety.

THYROTOXICOSIS

Look for symptoms suggestive of hyperthyroidism. Atrial fibrillation, exophthalmos, or a thyroid bruit make thyroid function tests mandatory.

ALCOHOL AND DRUG PROBLEMS (see p. 250 et sequ)

Patients with anxiety disorders may self-medicate with alcohol or other substances.

INTOXICATION WITH PRESCRIBED DRUGS

Think of stimulants such as caffeine and methyl phenidate; also sympathomimetic agents such as bronchodilators.

DRUG WITHDRAWAL (see pp. 104–5, 252)

Sometimes anxiety symptoms are caused by the patient running out of sedatives – whether these be benzodiazepines, alcohol, or barbiturates. Diagnostic difficulties arise when the patient wishes to conceal his drug use, but wants help for the anxiety symptoms. (If drugs are obtained illicitly, and the patient thinks the doctor may prescribe a sedative as a treatment, he may be unwilling to give an honest history.)

PHAEOCHROMOCYTOMA

Thought of by every medical student, but in fact very rare indeed! The history of flushing attacks accompanied by diarrhoea alerts one to the possibility.

Investigations

It is not necessary to carry out tests for thyrotoxicosis or phaeochromocytoma unless they are indicated by the results of the history and physical examination.

Aetiology

It is convenient to distinguish between long-term factors that predispose to symptoms of anxiety, and factors that release a particular episode.

PREDISPOSING FACTORS

The genes responsible for vulnerability to anxiety are exactly the same as those for depression. Adults with anxiety states consistently report childhoods that were more traumatic than controls, with inconsistent support from parents and higher rates of parental divorce. Sexual abuse during childhood is associated with higher levels of both depressive and anxious symptoms during adult life.

Patients who score highly on questionnaires measuring **neuroticism** or 'trait anxiety' are more vulnerable to symptoms of anxiety than those with a more phlegmatic disposition. Those with chronic social adversity are at greater risk, and this adversity may take the form of difficult interpersonal problems or unfavourable living conditions.

PRECIPITATING FACTORS

Anxiety states, like depressions, are usually in some understandable relationship to stressful life events. However, whereas the stress before a depression is more likely to be a loss, that before anxiety is more likely to be a threat of some kind. In general medical settings anxiety symptoms are often related to worries about physical health, and it is therefore essential to allow patients to express their own fears about the nature of their illness before the doctor provides information from the medical viewpoint. Anxious ruminations are especially difficult to handle if the patient has no one in whom to confide, or is unable to find reassurance from people in his immediate social field.

However, in other cases the anxiety will not be related to physical health, but will be found to be a somatic expression of some interpersonal problem. It will often be the case that the patient has not connected the psychological problem with the physical symptom for which help is sought, so that taking a proper history not only helps us to understand the aetiology of the disorder, but is also an indispensable first step in treatment.

Treatment

If anxiety co-exists with depression, it is a general rule that treatment should first focus on the treatment of depression. Many patients will not want to take medication. In general, try simple information and advice followed by either more specific psychological treatment or medication according to patient choice. If this does not work on its own, add the other.

PROVIDING INFORMATION AND ADVICE

The first step of treatment should include a clear explanation to the patient that their various symptoms make up a common syndrome with which the doctor is familiar, and that the symptoms do not indicate serious disease. Next, if appropriate, give advice on what to do at the earliest sign of a panic attack: sit down if possible, try to relax, and count to four between breathing in and breathing out, then the symptoms will pass off by themselves without developing into a full-blown attack. Finally, give advice on the advisability of going to relaxation classes, or to meditation or yoga, depending on the patient's interests. In the course of taking the history the doctor will usually have heard about other related problems, and must use judgement to decide whether the nature of these problems is such that help from others should be sought.

SPECIFIC PSYCHOLOGICAL TREATMENTS

The most effective specific psychological therapies for anxiety disorders are based on cognitive behaviour therapy (CBT). It has been demonstrated that many patients with milder disorders can benefit from being guided by a health professional through simple self-help materials based on CBT principles. If they fail to improve then they should be referred (stepped-up) to receive a course of CBT provided face-to-face by a trained therapist.

DRUG TREATMENT

In the past benzodiazepines were widely used in the treatment of anxiety – leading to problems of dependence. We would generally now advise against their use because of the risks of dependence. SSRIs are effective in anxiety, as are imipramine and clomipramine. Treatment with SSRIs needs to be continued for longer than in depression – sometimes for as long as a year.

SOCIAL INTERVENTIONS

Patients with anxiety disorders often have social or interpersonal problems that can be helped greatly by talking through their problems and directing them towards help from appropriate statutory and voluntary organizations in the community, for example a welfare rights worker or the Citizen's Advice Bureau, or if possible getting specialist advice from a social worker, although such help is less available now than in the past.

Course and prognosis

Most acute anxiety states remit, which is an excellent reason for avoiding dependence-producing drugs – however some do go on to become longer lasting, and recurrence is unfortunately quite common. Many of those put onto benzodiazepines and then thought to have developed 'chronic anxiety states' are experiencing anxiety symptoms when their drugs are withdrawn, but such symptoms often improve dramatically after a week to 10 days. Some patients with chronic anxiety will be found to have social problems, but such problems should attract social interventions. In fact, most patients with persistent anxiety symptoms will gradually develop depressive symptoms as well.

FEAR DISORDERS: PANIC, PHOBIAS AND PTSD

There is no natural dividing line between normal people and those with **fear disorders** that would enable us to lay down firm criteria for diagnosis. In this respect anxiety disorders resemble conditions like hypertension and anaemia in general medicine. There are various research criteria for the diagnosis, but they are arbitrary. In practical terms, any patient whose pronounced symptoms of anxiety are accompanied by three or more of the other symptoms given above can usefully be thought of as satisfying the requirements for diagnosis, while with increasing numbers of symptoms there is increasing certainty that such a disorder is present

Aetiology

There appear to be distinct genetic factors responsible for these disorders: rates in the general population are about 3 per cent, whereas rates in first-degree relatives are between 6 and 15 per cent. Female relatives appear at greater risk than male relatives. Where panic disorder is concerned, probands with *both depression and panic* have increased rates of panic, depression, and alcohol problems in their first-degree relatives. Rates of panic in first-degree relatives of those with *panic disorder alone* are high, whereas rates for GAD are low, just as rates for panic are low in relatives of those with GAD. In probands with depression only, rates for panic are low in first-degree relatives. All this points to overlapping but distinctive aetiologies. Twin studies of those with fear disorders show substantially higher concordance in MZ than DZ twins, with additive genetic factors accounting for about 30 to 40 per cent of the variance.

Panic disorder

Sometimes patients experience episodes of severe, uncontrollable anxiety, called **panic attacks**. These usually take the form of intense anxiety of sudden onset with both cognitive and somatic accompaniments. The patient thinks some misfortune will befall him: death by heart attack, madness, or just a nameless dread; typically accompanied by one or more symptoms such as sweating, tremor, palpitations, and paraesthesiae due to over-breathing. The attacks last for anything from a few minutes to some hours, and often present in the casualty department. When these only occur in the course of a depressive illness they resolve with treatment for the depression.

Patients whose only symptoms are panic attacks are said to suffer from **panic disorder** if they have had four or more attacks of panic in the past month. In practice, there is a strong overlap between panic attacks and other fear disorders, notably agoraphobia.

Phobias

Patients with **phobias** become anxious only in *particular situations* and have no trouble providing that they avoid the object or situation that arouses their anxiety. However, their avoidance behaviour may become extreme. Objects about which people develop specific phobias include spiders, snakes, dogs, rats, and moths; while **situations** include high places (**acrophobia**), enclosed spaces (**claustrophobia**), air-travel (**air phobia**), and social gatherings (**social phobias**). The disorder should cause the patient significant distress, and the patient should regard his fear as excessive or unreasonable. Patients with phobic illnesses should be treated with graded in vivo exposure (see p. 113).

Agoraphobia commonly develops in women between the ages of 18 and 35, and anxiety symptoms are only experienced in situations that share certain characteristics: being a long way from home, being in crowded places such as on public transport, in department stores or a cinema; shops where one must queue to pay before leaving, or any situation that is difficult to leave quickly. The anxiety may be reduced or be quite tolerable if a trusted person is with the patient: some women can manage even with a small child, others need an adult or cannot face the feared situation at all. The patient may feel quite safe in her car, but is in real trouble if the car breaks down when she is on her own. As time goes on the symptoms tend to progress and to generalize: panic attacks may occur even at the thought of going out, and eventually may occur without obvious provocation. By this time the patient is likely not to be going out at all, and is then said to be 'house-bound'. **Agoraphobia** should be diagnosed when there is marked fear in the situations described above and there is increased constriction of normal activities until fears or avoidance behaviour dominate the patient's life.

Post-traumatic stress disorder (PTSD)

This refers to a syndrome that follows exposure to unusual stress – such as a battle; or being attacked or raped; or a natural disaster like a fire or flood. The patients 're-live' the distressing experience with intrusive flashbacks or vivid memories, and may start to avoid circumstances that remind them of the original trauma. For example, a woman who has been raped in a car park may start to avoid all car parks. The symptoms begin within a few months of the original stressor, and typically occur in the setting of other symptoms of anxiety.

BEREAVEMENT AND GRIEF

Normal bereavement

Immediately following the death of a close relative, a person goes through several stages of a normal grief reaction.

Initially the person is in a state of shock, during which although he knows intellectually that the person has died, he has not yet come to terms with it. He is able to function quite well while arranging the funeral and sorting out affairs. Others may notice that the person 'is taking it so well', but the person himself feels numb and may experience depersonalization. Others will have episodes of crying even in this stage, and panic attacks may be experienced. This stage of numbness and shock usually lasts between 5 and 7 days.

This is followed by a realization of the loss, with a sharp increase in affective symptoms. This acute grief lasts for 4 to 12 weeks and resolves during the next 3 months. The phenomena during this phase are:

1. Intense **pining** for the lost person, and **preoccupation with thoughts of the deceased**, accompanied by weeping. There is a tendency to concentrate on aspects of the environment associated with the lost person. A clear visual mental picture of the deceased is often retained, and there may be dreams of the deceased. Initially the thoughts may be distressing, later they can be comforting.
2. **Illusions** are common and everyday household noises are misinterpreted as the deceased coming in or moving about. Shadows in the dark or strangers may be fleetingly misinterpreted as the deceased. **Visual or auditory pseudohallucinations** occur in which the person sees or hears the deceased. A sense of the *presence of the dead person* is common, which may be comforting. In abnormal grief reactions the sense of presence may be accompanied by talking to the dead person and preparing meals for him, and so on (see 'denial', p. 75).
3. **Depressive illness**: A triad of depressed mood, disturbed sleep, and weeping is seen in over 50 per cent of bereaved people. Other symptoms, such as anorexia, weight loss, tiredness, indecisiveness, anxiety, lack of interest and concentration, a sense of futility, and guilty feelings also occur, so that many bereaved people will satisfy the diagnostic criteria for depressive illness (see p. 213).

4. **Somatic symptoms of anxiety** may predominate, and severely distressed mourners may even express suicidal ideas because life seems hopeless without the deceased, they feel **guilty** about not having done more to prevent the death and may wish to join the dead person. The consultation rate for depressive or somatic symptoms of middle-aged widows increases three times in the 6 months following the bereavement. The somatic symptoms are sometimes similar to those experienced by the dead person.
5. The bereaved person may be **restless**, pacing the house and unable to settle. Withdrawal from social contacts occurs and consolation may be rejected. The bereaved person sometimes **searches** for the deceased, by making frequent visits to the cemetery and even calling out to him. She may constantly gaze at photographs of the dead person.
6. Feelings of **hostility** may be directed at other family members, God or the doctor 'who let my husband die'.

All these phenomena should have largely subsided by 6 months after the death. Many people will say, even years later, that they have never 'got over' their loss entirely. Loss normally becomes easier to bear with time, and less all-consuming as the weeks and months pass and an individual resumes their life. The dead person may however still be missed.

People who are grieving need an opportunity to talk about their experiences with a kind person who understands and is willing to listen. They need to talk about and remember the dead person. Often this will be done with a family member or close friend, but in the absence of a confidant, organizations in the community such as CRUSE provide support for the bereaved.

Antidepressants are indicated if there is clear evidence that a moderate to severe depressive illness has been precipitated by the bereavement in the way that depression may be precipitated by any negative life event. This may be indicated also by a pattern of *failure to improve over time* (see below – this indicates development of an atypical grief reaction) or gradual *worsening* in severity of symptoms rather than improving slowly over time (which is the norm for grief reactions although the *rate* of improvement varies enormously). Active treatment should also be instituted where the person is expressing suicidal ideas and/or experiencing definite psychotic symptoms rather than illusions or pseudohallucinations.

Atypical grief reactions

These are commoner in women than men. They can be prolonged – an initial stage of numbness lasts more than 2 weeks and the whole grief reaction lasts over 1 year or even longer. It is also more severe, with *marked social withdrawal, inability to work*, and *suicidal acts*.

Persisting difficulty accepting the loss, *guilt* feelings and *hostility* are severe. *Hypochondriacal symptoms* similar to those experienced by the deceased may occur.

Suicidal risk is raised 2.5 times during the year following bereavement, with special risk at the *anniversary* of the death. Death from physical illness is also increased in likelihood during the 6 months after bereavement, notably from cardiovascular disease.

Other forms of atypical grief include *delayed grief*, where the individual functions normally for a while, and then has a grief reaction; *denial of grief*, where the individual never appears to experience a grief reaction, but perhaps presents with otherwise inexplicable somatic symptoms much later. A psychotic form of denial was described on p. 75.

Atypical grief is more likely to occur when:

1. The death has been sudden and unexpected.
2. The person has been unable to view the body of the deceased, or to express appropriate grief at an early stage.
3. There was an ambivalent or hostile relationship with the deceased.
4. The loss involves a fully grown child.
5. The person experienced loss of their own parent as a child.
6. There are few relatives or other social supports.

ASSESSMENT AND MANAGEMENT

The aim of **assessment** is to decide whether the patient has a normal or atypical grief reaction. If it is the former, what stage has been reached and is the reaction proceeding? If the reaction is atypical, why is this so, at which stage has the reaction halted, and has the person developed a depressive illness? The presence of suicidal ideas must be assessed.

Management of those with an atypical grief reaction involves a special form of psychotherapy in which the person is guided through the remaining stages of grief. The patient brings photographs or belongings of the dead person and talks about him or her. The patient is thus confronted with the reality of the loss and the emotional expression of grief is facilitated. *Antidepressants* are prescribed if there is evidence of moderate to severe depression.

Grieving usually terminates naturally, but the patient may need encouragement to regain his former activities, or even start new ones, to combat loneliness and preoccupation with loss.

Treatment

Given that these disorders co-exist, a treatment plan may involve a variety of different measures, although there is some considerable overlap, particularly in drug treatments.

A basic principle of treatment that applies to all of these disorders is that of 'stepped care', which means that:

- Simple treatments are generally tried first as 'front-line' treatment, particularly in primary care settings.

- If a person fails to respond to simple treatment then they are 'stepped-up' to a more complex or intensive form of treatment.
- Complex or intensive treatments are reserved for those who fail to respond to first-line interventions.

OBSESSIVE-COMPULSIVE DISORDER

Epidemiology

Recent epidemiological studies report prevalence rates of 0.8 per cent in adults and 0.25 per cent in 5- to 15-year-old children. The World Health Organization rates obsessive-compulsive disorder as one of the top 20 most disabling diseases. If untreated, it generally persists.

Symptoms

In obsessive-compulsive disorder (OCD) the outstanding symptom is a sense of subjective compulsion, which the patient feels must be resisted, to carry out some action, dwell on an idea, recall an experience, or to ruminate on some abstract topic. The obsessional urge or idea is seen to be senseless but is recognized as arising from within oneself, rather than being imposed from outside. Attempts to dispel the inner thought, or to resist the compulsion to carry out some act, usually lead to anxiety (see definitions of both **obsessions** and **compulsions** in the Glossary). OCD is recognized as one of the more severe 'common' mental disorders.

Obsessional phenomena include:

- **Thoughts** of an unpleasant or obscene nature.
- **Images** in the form of disgusting but vividly imagined scenes.
- **Impulses** to perform acts of a violent or embarrassing nature.
- **Rituals** such as hand-washing or elaborate ways of dressing or cleaning oneself.
- **Ruminations** (see p. 32) about the pros and cons of everyday actions.
- **Doubts** concerning whether or not actions involving safety (locking doors, turning off gas-taps and switches) have been completed.

Diagnostic criteria

Obsessions (thoughts, images, or ideas) and compulsions share the following features, all of which must be present:

- Acknowledged as originating in the mind of the patient.
- Repetitive and unpleasant; at least one being recognized as excessive or unreasonable.

- At least one must be unsuccessfully resisted (although resistance may be minimal in some cases).
- Carrying out the obsessive thought or compulsive act is not intrinsically pleasurable.

Differential diagnosis

If obsessional symptoms occur secondary to depression, schizophrenia, or organic brain disease the treatment is usually directed at the precipitating condition.

Aetiology

Recent studies have shown obsessional illnesses to be more common in first-degree relatives of those with the disorder, and one small twin study suggests at least a partially genetic basis. Approximately two-thirds of patients who develop obsessional illness show **obsessional personality traits** (see p. 281). Indeed, those with such traits often experience some obsessional symptoms, but if they are able to function socially and occupationally they are not said to be *ill*. Such patients often experience a great increase in such symptoms if they develop a depressive illness. Conditions that commonly co-occur with OCD include **depression** (50–60 per cent), **specific phobias** (22 per cent) **social phobia** (18 per cent) **eating disorder** (17 per cent) and less commonly **alcohol dependence**, **panic disorder**, **Tourette's syndrome**, and **schizophrenia**.

Treatment

Psychological theories of obsessive-compulsive disorder suggest that ritualizing maintains the problem as it prevents habituation to the anxiety and disconfirmation of the patient's fears.

Psychological therapies aim to break this cycle by persuading patients to expose themselves to the feared situations while refraining from performing any rituals; this is known as **exposure** and **response prevention**. The patient generates a hierarchy of feared situations and then practises facing the fear (exposure), while monitoring the anxiety and experiencing that it lessens without the need to carry out a ritual (response prevention). Guided self-help, using a self-help manual, may be effective in early or mild OCD.

Drug therapies: **SSRIs** are also effective, even in the absence of depression, at slightly higher dosage than used for depression (e.g. 40 mg of fluoxetine), and **clomipramine** is also used. If either drugs or psychological therapy on their own fail, they should then be tried in combination.

FURTHER READING

Goldberg, D. and Huxley, P. (1991) *Common Mental Disorders – A Bio-social Model*. London: Routledge.

NICE (National Institute for Health and Clinical Excellence) guidelines are available on the internet at the following web addresses:

Anxiety: http://www.nice.org.uk/guidance/CG22

Depression: http://www.nice.org.uk/CG023

Obsessive-compulsive disorder (OCD): http://www.nice.org.uk/guidance/CG31/niceguidance/pdf/English

16   INTERNALIZING DISORDERS 2: SOMATIC PRESENTATIONS OF EMOTIONAL DISTRESS

Many of the patients to be described in this chapter also satisfy one or more criteria for a distress disorder given in the previous chapter. A minority do not, but neither can a satisfactory physical aetiology be demonstrated. We have already mentioned that most patients with these disorders consult their doctors for somatic symptoms.

The terminology that has been used to classify this group of disorders is confusing and complicated. Some patients have clear anxiety and/or depression of which their physical symptoms are a somatic manifestation. However there is a smaller group of patients who do not, and for these the term most commonly used in systems of classification at the present time is 'somatoform disorder'.

Some other definitions may be helpful here:

- **Somatization** is a term that is widely used and can be defined as 'a tendency to *experience* and *communicate* somatic distress and symptoms *unaccounted for by pathological findings*, to *attribute* them to physical illness and to *seek medical help* for them'. This definition has, therefore, several quite distinct components. Somatization is a term that describes a process. It is not a diagnosis.
- **Medical unexplained symptoms (MUS)** is a term that is also used a great deal at the time of writing, and is what we use here. However it has two disadvantages. Doctors often disagree among themselves on what is medically explicable, and in many cases both physical *and* psychological factors play a part in the genesis of symptoms. The majority of patients with medical unexplained symptoms (MUS) are also experiencing symptoms of depression and anxiety, but they do not present these symptoms to the doctor, or recognize their connection with current psychosocial problems. Instead, they complain of pains and other somatic symptoms, and they do not consider themselves psychiatrically unwell. They may have physical disease as well; or it may not be possible to demonstrate any physical disease.
- **Functional symptoms** is a term that is often more acceptable to patients. A range of 'functional' syndromes are recognized across medical specialities (see *Box 16.1*). However, research has demonstrated that these syndromes are rarely, in practice, distinct, and if other somatic symptoms are enquired about they will commonly be present.

Box 16.1 Functional somatic symptoms by specialty

Gastroenterology	Irritable bowel syndrome
	Non-ulcer dyspepsia
Gynaecology	Pre-menstrual syndrome
	Chronic pelvic pain
Rheumatology	Fibromyalgia
Cardiology	Atypical chest pain
Respiratory medicine	Hyperventilation syndrome
Infectious diseases	Chronic fatigue syndrome
Neurology	Tension headache
	Non-epileptic attacks or 'pseudo-seizures'
Dentistry	Temporomandibular joint dysfunction
	Atypical facial pain
Ear, nose and throat	Globus syndrome
Allergy	Multiple chemical sensitivity

NORMAL AND ABNORMAL ILLNESS BEHAVIOUR

In order to fully understand how people behave in relation to the experience of physical symptoms, it is useful to consider the concept of 'illness behaviour'.

Illness behaviour has been defined as *the ways in which given symptoms may be differentially perceived, evaluated and acted (or not acted) on*. For example, two healthy people run for a bus and both notice palpitation. One assumes that it is a normal experience, the symptom is transient and soon forgotten. The other, whose spouse recently died of a myocardial infarct, notices it more, worries that she has heart disease, and consults her general practitioner.

The definition is extremely broad and includes all aspects of thinking, emotion, and behaviour related to the symptoms of illness, whether or not these are associated with objective evidence of physical or mental disorders.

The term 'illness behaviour' does not imply that the behaviours are necessarily pathological. Illness behaviours that are appropriate are adaptive. They facilitate recovery in those with disease, for example by consultation, compliance with treatment, and rest when indicated. They also allow those with trivial symptoms to function well by recognizing them as such and avoiding unnecessary invalidism.

For individuals, illness behaviour includes both *traits* (the lifelong tendency to have a low or high threshold for being aware of and worrying about symptoms and consulting doctors) and *state* (the behaviour at a particular time). There is evidence that such traits are acquired during childhood, by learning the patterns of illness behaviour that are characteristic of the culture or family. The majority of consultations, particularly in general practice, are determined to a considerable extent by current social and psychological factors, including recent life events, the extent of social support, and distress – this is illustrated by the example of palpitation described above. Thus many of the behaviours related to illness are not directly determined by disease processes but by the psychological and social state of the patient.

'**Abnormal illness behaviour**' is used as a general term to refer to illness behaviours that are regarded as inappropriate or maladaptive, that is, they are motivated by goals other than maintaining function or recovery from disease.

There are two major aspects of abnormal illness behaviour, which have been described as *illness denial* and *illness affirmation*.

Illness denial is a term used to describe the behaviour of people with significant physical or mental disorders who use denial (see p. 75) to avoid the stigma of a physical disorder such as heart disease, or a mental disorder such as manic-depressive illness. They avoid appropriate consultations and there are also likely to be problems with treatment adherence, for example failure to follow advice about exercise, diet, or taking lithium.

Illness affirmation is a term used to describe the behaviour of those who inappropriately affirm illness although they are well or have only minor disorders. They present symptoms or are disabled to an extent that is disproportionate to any objective evidence of physical or mental disorder. All of the disorders that are described in the rest of this chapter have in common the fact that they are forms of abnormal illness affirmation.

The development of invalidism can be of benefit (whatever our state of health or disease) because it allows us to avoid unpleasant obligations or predicaments: for example, abdominal pain preventing a child from going to school when he has not done his homework or expects to be bullied; or headaches preventing a man who has recently been made redundant from seeking work, despite his limited skills.

If successful this leads to *primary gain*, that is, relief from stress, because of avoidance of the underlying predicament. (An example is described in the section on dissociative disorders.) Following the onset of invalidism, there may be other tangible benefits (referred to as *secondary gain*), such as increased care and concern from family, friends and medical services, as well as financial gains such as disability benefits, pensions, and compensation payments. If successful, such mechanisms are more likely to be used in the future. Invalidism can benefit others too – this process has been referred to as *tertiary gain*:

> A man who has been made redundant develops 'tension headaches'. His wife has devoted her life to bringing up their children, who have left home, and her life is now empty. She responds to his headaches with increasing care, so that she satisfies her own thwarted need to care for others, and consequently he does less for himself, worries about the significance of his headaches, and becomes disabled.

Similarly, some doctors are able to resolve uncomfortable feelings of uncertainty by diagnosing non-existent illnesses or offering inappropriate treatments. This also illustrates the way in which abnormal illness behaviour is commonly facilitated by doctors – that is, it is partly *iatrogenic*.

Usually, patients and others who are involved do not consciously plan to benefit from invalidism, that is, these are **unconscious defence mechanisms** (the exception is 'malingering' – see below).

MEDICALLY UNEXPLAINED SYMPTOMS (MUS)

Epidemiology

Community-based surveys indicate that the most severe and chronic MUS are found in about 0.5 per cent of the general adult population, and that about 10 per cent are suffering from less severe disorders. In primary care almost 20 per cent of patients presenting to their doctors with new episodes of illness can be shown to satisfy criteria for acute or subacute MUS because, in addition to the features described above, a research diagnosis of a depressive illness or an anxiety state can be made, treatment of which would ameliorate the patient's presenting somatic symptoms. A physical disease will also be demonstrable in about 70 per cent of such patients, but it will not by itself account for all of the patient's symptoms.

Symptoms

Acute MUS tend to be associated with sudden brief fear or panic, such as when someone develops palpitations before an examination, worries about having a 'heart attack', but then probably recognizes the true nature of the experience as soon as their anxiety, and its cause, subside. The psychological disorders will probably be viewed as '**adjustment reactions**'.

However **persistent MUS** may last for weeks or several months, and are more commonly related to anxiety states and depressive disorders. *Chronic MUS* is best regarded as lasting for 6 months or more, and is particularly associated with somatoform disorder diagnoses.

In most settings the majority of people with MUS have **depressive or anxiety disorders** (often with mixed symptoms), and others have **adjustment reactions**. An important minority have **alcohol and drug related disorders**. In addition there is a smaller group of psychiatric disorders that are particularly characterized by abnormal illness behaviour and the presentation of medical unexplained symptoms, that is, these constitute the core of the symptoms and signs. They include the **somatoform disorders – somatization disorder, somatoform pain disorder**, and **hypochondriacal disorder** (see below).

Aetiology

We must now understand why these patients choose to focus on somatic symptoms to the relative neglect of their affective symptoms and psychosocial problems:

- The patient does not connect his affective symptoms with his physical symptom, for example pain, and concentrates on the pain **because it hurts**.

- The patient is afraid that the pain may indicate some **serious physical disease**, so he gives it increasing attention, leading to further exacerbation of the pain.
- The patient may feel that his emotional problems are his own affair, but excluding physical causes for pains is very much his doctor's job. Some doctors share this view, feel unfamiliar with or intolerant of their patients' emotional problems, and may respond with greater interest to physical symptoms than they do to psychological symptoms. This is '**differential reinforcement**' by the doctor. Doctors may investigate physical symptoms repeatedly despite negative findings, give misleading and conflicting diagnoses, and give physical treatments for non-existent disorders. This encourages their patients' inappropriate worry about a physical disorder. So the problem is often at least partly *iatrogenic*, that is, caused by doctors.
- Focusing on somatic symptoms tends to run in families. One reason is that the patterns of behaviour are copied (or 'modelled'). Another is that key people in the patient's family may be more sympathetic to physical symptoms than they are to psychological problems: this is **differential reinforcement** by relatives.
- The patient may feel that there is some **social stigma** attached to emotional illness: societies vary in the extent to which they stigmatize such illnesses, but even in our own it is more acceptable to be thought to have a physical illness.
- The last reason is a development of the same point and employs the concept of the process of somatization, which is defined above: a patient who fails to recognize that he is emotionally unwell does not have to ask himself awkward questions about his own personal contribution to the life predicament that he is in, particularly if it can be blamed on physical illness. To have a physical illness is a misfortune, but in most cases one does not need to feel responsible for it. A patient who somatizes his distress by converting it into a physical symptom **need not blame himself**, examine the life problem in which he is enmeshed, or accept some responsibility for resolving it. Thus **somatization acts as a defence mechanism**.

Research into MUS in primary care settings has indicated that adults who present with MUS are more likely to have experienced lack of care from physical illness in a parent during their childhood, serious illness before the age of 17, and serious physical illness in one or both parents. The more of these experiences, the more likely are they to develop chronic MUS. It has also been shown that, when compared with patients in primary care who present psychological complaints, somatizers are less depressed, report lower levels of social dissatisfaction and stress, have a less sympathetic attitude towards mental illness, are less likely to consult doctors about psychological symptoms, and have received more medical in-patient care for previous complaints.

CHRONIC MEDICALLY UNEXPLAINED SYMPTOMS

A variety of different terms are used by psychiatrists to describe this group of disorders, and classification systems regularly undergo changes and revision.

Presentation is characterized by repeated physical complaints and concern about health, requests for medical examinations, investigations and treatments, often from many different doctors, and failure to be reassured by negative findings and explanations. Although there may be some evidence of a physical disorder, this cannot account for either the complaints or the associated disability, which is sometimes so severe that the patient may become chair- or bed-bound. Anxiety and depressed mood may be present (and there may be an associated diagnosis of an affective disorder – see above), but this may be denied or there may be no clear evidence of it. Precipitation and maintenance of the physical complaints are often closely related to distressing life events, but the patient tends to resist any exploration of possible psychological causes. Although the following disorders are described, in practice there is often some overlap and it is uncertain to what extent they are separate conditions.

Somatization disorder is a term used for a disorder in which the patient has many different symptoms that fluctuate and recur over many years. Very few complaints will have adequate physical explanation. It is much more common in women than men, starts in early adult life or even childhood, and tends to run in families. Symptoms may be referred to any system of the body, and are particularly likely to include various aches and pains, and other gastrointestinal, sexual, and menstrual complaints.

Patients are likely to have visited numerous hospital departments (for example, the neurology department for headaches, cardiology for palpitation and breathlessness, gastroenterology for abdominal distension and flatulence, gynaecology for dysmenorrhoea and menorrhagia), where they receive multiple inappropriate diagnoses and accumulate thick medical records. Doctors feel frustrated by these patients, as attempts to relieve their symptoms are unsuccessful. Often they claim that their symptoms have been caused by treatments, particularly surgery, given by previous doctors.

Diagnosis

The following are all required:

1. At least **2 years of multiple and variable physical symptoms** for which no adequate physical explanation has been found.
2. **Persistent refusal to accept reassurance** from doctors that there is no physical explanation.
3. **Impairment in social function** associated with the symptoms.

In **persistent somatoform pain disorder** the essential feature is pain that persists for at least some months and often for many years, and cannot be adequately explained by any identifiable organic pathology or physiological process, despite appropriate examination and investigation. The disorder is diagnosed more often in women than in men and can start at any age. The pain may be felt at a single site, multiple sites, or may be diffuse (chronic widespread pain), and may affect different sites at different times. Its distribution is usually incompatible with any recognizable pain representation of the central or peripheral nervous systems, such as a dermatome or peripheral nerve distribution. On examination, clinical signs are either absent or inconsistent with any known organic syndrome. Patients with this disorder often have additional physical complaints, and preoccupation with ill health and 'missed' diagnoses, so that they tend to see many different doctors in their search for a 'cure' and cannot be reassured by negative findings.

Although there is often evidence of current or past organic disorders that have contributed to the symptoms, this is never sufficient to account for the severity or distribution of the pain, or for the associated disability, which may be profound. In some cases the pain is initiated by trauma, for example following a road traffic accident, but fails to improve as expected, and this pattern is seen particularly in those seeking compensation.

Often there is evidence of social and psychological predisposing factors (such as childhood physical or psychological neglect or abuse), precipitating factors (such as negative life-events), and gain resulting from the symptoms. These are not always obvious from the history because the patient tends to present an idealized picture of a 'perfect' life.

The essential characteristic of **hypochondriasis** is persistent preoccupation with the possibility of having a serious physical disorder (e.g. heart disease or cancer), or an abnormality in physical appearance (e.g. nose or breasts too small or too large), despite appropriate medical examination, explanation and reassurance about the lack of physical abnormality. The beliefs take the form of **overvalued ideas** (see p. 33) – they are not delusions – and their content and strength are liable to vary from time to time. The physical symptoms that the patient presents to support his case can often be recognized as elaborations of normal bodily sensations (e.g. heart beat or gut peristalsis) to which the patient pays excessive attention and attributes inappropriate significance. The patient may present specific diagnoses, but often will be quite vague, saying 'I'm not the doctor but I know something has been missed.' The prevalence is similar in men and women, usually starts before the age of 50, and tends to run a chronic course.

The term **dysmorphophobia** is used to describe the idea that the body is deformed in some way; particularly the nose, but sometimes other parts of the body such as the face, hair, breasts, or genitalia. Patients with such beliefs commonly and repeatedly consult plastic surgeons but are unlikely to be helped by surgery. These ideas are included in the syndrome of hypochondriacal disorder if they take the form of overvalued ideas but not if they are delusions, in which case they indicate the presence of a psychosis (usually schizophrenia).

DISSOCIATIVE AND CONVERSION DISORDERS

Epidemiology

The prevalence of these disorders in the community is uncertain as the nature of the disorder may go unrecognized. However, they are thought to have become less common in recent years, although they remain a common presentation in developing countries. Hospital surveys show that between 1 and 5 per cent of all referrals have this disorder, which is more common in women than in men. The onset may be at any age but the majority start before age 30, and it is likely that transient symptoms may be quite common in children. Of patients who have been referred to hospital, about 70 per cent recover during the first year, 80 per cent in 5 years, and few of the remainder recover subsequently.

Conversion and dissociative symptoms are liable to show **epidemic spread** (referred to as '**mass hysteria**'), particularly among adolescents and young adults who are in close proximity. There are generally several accounts of outbreaks that can affect hundreds of people, for example in schools or at 'pop' concerts, reported in the national press each year, sometimes masquerading as some new or mysterious disease. One interesting facet is the widespread vulnerability of the general population to the development of conversion symptoms by suggestion, given 'favourable' conditions; they are by no means limited to a few 'weak' or abnormal personalities.

Symptoms

These disorders are a form of abnormal illness behaviour in which the patient develops an often dramatic symptom of physical or mental illness, usually with an acute onset. Thus the patients may present with **paralysis, pseudo-seizures, anaesthesia, amnesia, dysphonia** or **blindness** – but there are many others. These symptoms all involve unconscious simulation of the symptoms of illness. In addition, the physical symptoms, such as paralysis and blindness, involve somatization.

However, all these symptoms are thought to share an additional underlying psychological mechanism – the defence mechanisms of **dissociation** and/or **conversion**. Our normal function is based on our ability to exert some degree of conscious control over our memories, sensations selected for attention, and choice of movements. It is thought that in the conversion disorders this ability is partly or completely lost and this can result in impairment of many different functions.

The word '**conversion**' is conventionally applied to somatic symptoms produced in the above fashion. If the symptom is psychological (e.g. loss of memory rather than loss of function of a limb) it is regarded as **dissociative**.

Symptoms have two distinguishing characteristics:

1. First, they mimic the phenomena of neurological and psychiatric disorders, but *reflect the patient's concept of how such disorders present*. Thus a dissociative paralysis will not show the range of features of a typical upper or lower motor neurone lesion. A dissociative anaesthesia will fail to show the distribution of either a central or a peripheral sensory loss: for example, it may be of 'glove' or 'stocking' distribution on perhaps a single limb, rather than conforming to the distribution of a dermatome, a peripheral nerve, or the symmetrical distribution of a peripheral neuropathy.
2. Second, the function that appears to be lost *can often be demonstrated to be intact* in conditions that the patient does not associate with the symptom. For example, a leg that is 'paralysed' when the patient attempts to walk may show normal tone and reflexes in the relevant muscle groups and may be raised against gravity from the examination couch. Similarly a patient with hysterical dysphonia may phonate normally if coughing or laughing, and the vocal cords are seen to be normal on laryngoscopy. It is often possible to remove dissociative symptoms by hypnotic suggestion and this may be helpful diagnostically.

241

An important difference between hypochondriacal disorder and dissociative symptoms is that patients with the former show excessive concern about their health, but the latter present with clinical signs. Because of their value, dissociative symptoms often result in a surprising lack of distress, and the patient may pay little more than lip service to the wish to overcome his disorder. French physicians have referred to this bland lack of concern as '**la belle indifférence**'.

Generally, dissociative/conversion symptoms tend to have a sudden onset, following a major stress, a seemingly insoluble predicament, or an interpersonal problem. This may not be evident from the history provided by the patient, and information from other informants is essential. The patient clearly believes that the symptoms are organic and will usually reject any suggestion that they are psychological in origin.

A complicating factor is that symptoms which are themselves dissociative/conversion may be released by other mental disorders – particularly organic brain disorders, functional psychoses, and affective disorders. For this reason, in the presence of symptoms suggestive of one of these other disorders, the dissociative/conversion symptoms have no diagnostic value and are ignored.

Dissociative and conversion symptoms can also occur in the setting of somatization disorder. The latter diagnosis is made rather than dissociative or conversion disorder if there have been many different symptoms over a number of years.

Aetiology

The predisposing factors and unconscious mechanisms involved are those described for abnormal illness behaviour and somatization (see above). Primary gain is thought to play a particularly important role, but secondary and tertiary gain may also contribute. It should be possible to demonstrate that the symptoms have some adaptive value for the patient. For example, anxiety is at least partly relieved when the development of a symptom removes the patient from conflict.

> A student who feared he might fail his exams developed a paralysis of his arm which prevented him from completing his course and sitting the exams.

Diagnosis

1. The main requirement is a symptom or impairment of sensory or motor function suggestive of disease of the central nervous system, which is inconsistent in form with the characteristics of such disease, and occurs in the absence of any objective evidence of organic pathology that can account for it. It follows that dissociative symptoms cannot be identified correctly unless you are thoroughly familiar with the symptoms of organic disorders.
2. There should be no evidence of other major psychiatric disorders – this point is explained above.
3. There should be some evidence of psychological causes, based on the onset following stress, and of gain, although this may not be evident from the patient's history.

242

A note on 'hysteria'

The terms 'hysteria' and 'hysterical' originated in ancient Greek medicine and, like many other long-established concepts, have acquired a wide range of different and ambiguous meanings. In order to avoid confusion, we have abandoned the use of these terms (but not the concepts), in line with the major classifications of mental disorder. We advise you to do the same. Because these terms are likely to continue in medical usage for some time to come, we include a summary of the commonest ways in which they have recently been used.

1. 'Hysterical' has been used by lay people as a pejorative term to describe dramatic or **histrionic behaviour**: these latter terms are more appropriate.
2. 'Hysterical personality' is an old-fashioned term for **histrionic personality** (see p. 280).
3. 'Hysterical symptoms' are now referred to as **dissociative symptoms** (or conversion symptoms).
4 'Hysteria' and 'hysterical neurosis' have now been replaced by **dissociative (or conversion) disorder**.

These usages have nothing to commend them and they should be avoided. We are left with 'mass hysteria' (see p. 241), for which the only synonym is epidemic hysteria. Fortunately, it is rare.

SIMULATED DISORDERS

Finally, there are three forms of abnormal illness behaviour in which organic disorders are simulated by the patient: **factitious disorder**, **malingering**, and **dissociative disorder**.

In **factitious disorder** the patient is aware of the simulation but not the gain; the **malingerer** is aware of both simulation and gain. In **dissociative disorders** it is thought that the patient lacks insight into the fact that symptoms are simulated and also into the gain derived from them; the simulation is at an unconscious level. However, it is possible for them to overlap, as in the case of a patient with a dissociative disorder who gradually acquires insight and then consciously maintains his symptoms in order to 'save face'. It can therefore sometimes be extremely difficult to differentiate between them.

Factitious disorder

Some patients consciously feign the symptoms and signs of disease, by self-injury or other subterfuge, in order to deceive doctors ('factitious' means artificial). They may present with many different signs, including rashes – **'dermatitis artefacta'**; infections, for example of the urinary tract, or septic arthritis, as a result of the introduction of infected material; 'pyrexia of unknown origin', which results, for example, from putting the thermometer in a cup of tea; or lapses of consciousness caused by the injection of insulin. Usually the patients are well aware of the deception, but they may have little or no insight into the motives for their behaviour. In this respect they differ from malingerers. Their motives in general are to maintain themselves in the role of invalidism, from which they derive comfort and care: they either fail to receive these normal human requirements from the more usual sources, or they are dependent personalities with excessive needs. Formal psychiatric assessment rarely leads to any diagnosis other than personality disorder.

Munchausen syndrome

This is a form of factitious disorder. Baron Munchausen was an eighteenth-century Hanoverian cavalry officer who was famous for his inventive story-telling. His name has therefore been given to this form of factitious illness, sometimes referred to as 'hospital addiction'. Patients may present to any department but particularly to surgical units, usually as an emergency, for example with signs of an 'acute abdomen', or with haematemesis, complete with blood-stained vomitus. The patient may give a polished but totally invented history, which can include a false name and past medical history, and this often has the desired result of major surgery. Characteristically, the patient bears the scars of many previous episodes. If the suspicions of staff are raised and the patient's history is checked by contacting other hospitals, he is often found to have mysteriously left the ward and is never seen again. Such patients tend to roam the country, from one hospital to the next, using different names at each admission. They rarely wait to be seen by psychiatrists but if assessed appear to have grossly disturbed personalities, or may be seeking narcotic analgaesics.

Munchausen syndrome by proxy

'Munchausen syndrome by proxy' consists of factitious disorder presenting in children, caused by a parent, almost always the mother. Apart from demonstrating the abnormal needs of the mother, it often results in serious physical and psychological abuse of the child. It is thought to be relatively common and sometimes leads to the child's death, for example as a result of hypoxia caused by smothering, hypoglycaemia resulting from insulin, or poisoning with other medication. These are either caused directly by the mother, or by doctors who are induced by the mother to give inappropriate treatments. The range of presentations is as broad as those resulting from factitious disorder in adults. It is important to be aware of this if you work on a paediatric unit, but it is also important to be aware that this is, because of recent legal cases in the United Kingdom, a controversial diagnosis – as it is often made by mistake.

Malingering

Malingering is a form of feigned illness in which the subject is conscious both that he is simulating the symptoms of disease, and also of the purpose (the nature of the gain): for example this may be to get time off work, to avoid responsibility for some criminal action, or to obtain financial compensation for an alleged injury. The presentations are similar to those of dissociative and factitious disorders. In practice it can be extremely difficult to differentiate between them.

Differential diagnosis of abnormal illness behaviour

The following must be considered:

1. **Physical disorders**: Patients suffering from medically unexplained symptoms have the same risk of developing a new physical disorder as others, but it is unusual to discover an organic cause for long-standing multiple symptoms that have previously been adequately investigated with negative results. Organic disorders are particularly likely to be missed in patients who present their symptoms in dramatic ways. Also, dissociative or conversion symptoms are liable to be misidentified as resulting from physical disease.
2. **Affective disorders**: If the presentation satisfies the criteria for a somatoform disorder then it should be diagnosed as such, but there may also be grounds for an additional diagnosis of a mood disorder. Because patients with these disorders tend to confirm that they have symptoms that are suggested to them, it is important to base diagnoses of the affective disorders on objective changes (e.g. observed sleep disturbance and measured weight loss) rather than rely entirely on the patient's own account.

    Some patients focus on symptoms that are limited to the autonomic nervous system and appear to represent physiological responses to anxiety, such as sweating, palpitation, hyperventilation, and 'tension' headaches. The diagnosis will depend on the other clinical features: they may justify an anxiety disorder diagnosis, or that of a somatoform disorder.
3. **Other somatoform disorders**, dissociative disorder, factitious disorder and malingering: In practice, patients may satisfy criteria for more than one of these diagnoses. The preferred diagnosis should be the one that fits the syndrome best.
4. **Dementias**, particularly in the elderly, who sometimes have multiple complaints related to a combination of physical and mental disorders. Also remember that dissociative symptoms may be released by organic brain disorders.
5. **Substance misuse**: Alcohol misuse may cause multiple physical complaints as a result of physical pathology, as well as an associated mood disorder. There is also some evidence that alcohol abuse may predate the onset of somatoform disorders. Alcohol and drug misuse may result from the patient's or doctor's attempts to achieve symptomatic relief. Substance misuse must therefore be considered as part of the differential diagnosis and also as an additional diagnosis.
6. **Schizophrenia and depressive psychosis** must both be considered in the differential diagnosis of hypochondriacal disorder, because in these disorders there may be **delusions with hypochondriacal content** or of **distorted body image** – in these the beliefs take the form of absolute conviction and the patient cannot be argued out of them. These can occur in any of the **organic and functional psychoses**. In **schizophrenia**, delusions about disease or changes in the shape of one's body may be

grotesque, for example a young man who thought his face was changing into that of a pig, developing a snout and bristles. In depressive psychosis, delusions tend to be 'mood congruent', that is, in keeping with depressive cognitions of hopelessness, and may take the form of impending and certain death due to cancer. In extreme cases the patient may believe that he is already dead: this would be an example of a nihilistic delusion.

7. **Personality disorders** are commonly found in patients who develop somatoform disorders, dissociative disorders, and factitious disorder. They should therefore be diagnosed in addition.

Treatment of medically unexplained symptoms

Management can be divided into prevention; general measures, which can be applied in any medical setting; and specialized psychological approaches, particularly for the more severe and persistent disorders – these will be considered briefly.

PREVENTION

Doctors make a major contribution to the development and chronicity of abnormal illness behaviour by responding inappropriately. It is important to avoid this by recognizing these problems and learning more appropriate ways of responding. We have already described how to avoid differential reinforcement of somatic complaints by acknowledging mood disorders and psychosocial problems. In addition:

1. Always provide clear information about negative clinical findings when you examine patients, and about negative investigations, otherwise they may assume the worst.
2. Avoid giving patients speculative or spurious diagnoses – medical records are full of these – the patient always remembers these diagnoses rather than the subsequent retractions.
3. Avoid treating disorders that the patient does not have – it is not unusual to find that patients who are told 'there's nothing wrong with your heart' have been offered medication commonly used for heart disease, without adequate explanation. Obviously, the patient will believe he is seriously ill.
4. Avoid carrying out and repeating investigations unless you think they are indicated, based on objective clinical findings. If you think they are indicated it is important to inform the patient both of the purpose and of the result.
5. Avoid arranging consultations and referrals unless you think they are indicated. Always explain why.

THE MANAGEMENT OF SOMATIC PRESENTATIONS OF ANXIETY OR DEPRESSION

In cases where either no physical disease is demonstrable, or the physical disease that is present does not account for the patient's symptoms, it is essential to help the patient to

246

see his symptoms in a different way. The **worst thing you can do** is to indicate by your words or actions that:

Our investigations are normal, so there's nothing wrong with you.

The patient knows that isn't correct since his pain is real enough. The patient will usually be complaining of numerous other psychiatric symptoms, but he will not have connected them with the pain. You will have to help him.

Let us suppose that a patient with severe epigastric pain has reported numerous symptoms of a depressive illness, and you have been asked to tell him that the results of all investigations, including a gastroscopy, are quite normal. You should now go through the following steps:

1. **Provide clear information about negative physical findings, while acknowledging the reality of the physical symptoms:**

   I'm glad to be able to tell you that you haven't got an ulcer or a tumour causing this pain, and all our investigations have been completely normal. Nevertheless, you have had a lot of pain, haven't you, and it has gone well beyond your usual indigestion pain? . . . (Having acknowledged the reality of the pain, pause for agreement)

2. **Specify the relevant mood state and associated symptoms and refer to the psychosocial factors that were previously noticed:**

   When you came into hospital you told me how depressed you have been feeling since you didn't manage to get promoted at work. You mentioned that you have lost over a stone in weight and tended to wake early in the morning brooding about the things that you feel you've made a mess of in your life . . . (Mention about three of the more striking symptoms, always including the mood disorder. Be prepared to remind your patient about the others if necessary. This is called 'broadening the agenda' – moving on from the somatic complaints only to include the possible psychosocial causes)

3. **Explain about the relationship of mood and pain:**

   We think that you are undoubtedly depressed, and that your depression has made your pain very much worse than it would have been otherwise. It's one of the things that depression does, I'm afraid . . . (Pause for the patient's response; be prepared to repeat that you know that the pain is real, but depression can cause real pain)

4. **Emphasize the positive aspects of treatment and provide reassurance, based on a realistic idea of outcome:**

   We think that it is very important to give you some treatment for your depression. Most people get over this sort of illness completely but it is likely to take some time. I would now like to discuss some of the ways we might help you . . . (If you have got this far, you have done well. From now on the management is as described earlier in this chapter, but with one advantage. The patient's pain will act as a key symptom to indicate your success – or lack of it! – in dealing with the problem)

THE MANAGEMENT OF MORE PERSISTENT DISORDERS

All the points covered in the preceding sections on treatment are relevant. If the problems continue, this is how to proceed.

1. Remember that anyone may have a physical disease, however obviously they show features of abnormal illness behaviour or an abnormal mental state. Frequently both physical and mental disorders occur in the same patient, so always look for evidence of both. All patients must be physically examined and investigated if they have a new episode of illness or new symptoms.
2. Few physical diagnoses are made as a result of further investigations more than 6 months after the initial presentation. Apart from the iatrogenic effects, repeated and inappropriate investigations also result in delay in initiating the appropriate psychiatric management.
3. At this stage it is essential to have a full psychiatric assessment, and the purpose should be explained to the patient and his cooperation sought. The first step is to look for evidence of affective disorder (described above) or other treatable mental disorders, and to treat them.
4. Review the past medical records, particularly if they are voluminous, because it may become evident that far from being a new disorder the present symptoms are part of a chronic or recurrent pattern.
5. Arrange to see a key relative yourself in order to find out more about the psychological and social background of the disorder, to assess their knowledge and beliefs about the patient's symptoms (usually they have not been seen previously by a doctor and will probably share the patient's views that he has an undiagnosed physical illness), and to explain the nature of the disorder.
6. Ask the medical social worker to help by carrying out a home visit, by seeing other relatives on your behalf, or by providing some tangible social help for the family.
7. It is essential for all doctors involved to work closely together and to take a consistent approach towards psychiatric management.
8. The cause of these disorders is primarily psychological and therefore the management should be psychological. However the specific causes of a patient's illness will rarely be evident from the initial history: usually the patient is unaware of underlying problems and relates all his difficulties to physical disease. Other factors will usually only come to light after taking detailed histories from the patient and others.
9. Insight-orientated psychotherapy can help the patient to face underlying problems and find more constructive ways to adjust to them. Behavioural psychotherapy can help the patient to give up inappropriate disability, by using a structured rehabilitation programme. Cognitive therapy is used to reduce inappropriate focus on and

beliefs about symptoms, and to encourage positive attitudes and approaches to coping.

10. Often inappropriate attitudes and behaviours are reinforced by family members who are over-solicitous. They must therefore be included in the treatment plan to modify the effect they have on the patient. Sometimes they have a particular need to care for an invalid and are unable to tolerate the patient's recovery. They may then need help to find new ways of adjusting to their own problems.

11 Somatoform and dissociative disorders are often resistant to treatment, perhaps because they are rarely seen by psychiatrists in the early stages, and because of poor compliance by patients and/or their families. Those that fail to improve within the first year or two often run a chronic course subsequently.

FURTHER READING

Bass, C. and Benjamin, S. (1993) The management of chronic somatization. *British Journal of Psychiatry*, *162*, 472–480.

Creed, F. and Guthrie, E. (1993) Techniques for interviewing the somatizing patient. *British Journal of Psychiatry*, *162*, 467–471.

17 EXTERNALIZING DISORDERS: MISUSE OF ALCOHOL AND DRUGS, AND EATING DISORDERS

Externalizing refers to the tendency to act out one's problems, and includes conduct disorders (see Chapter 20, p. 297) and anti-social personality (see Chapter 18, p. 276). This chapter is concerned with disorders that are common in adults attending general hospitals: namely, alcohol dependence, drug dependence, and eating disorders.

ALCOHOL MISUSE AND DEPENDENCE

Epidemiology of alcohol problems

General population surveys of alcohol problems are notoriously difficult, but also demonstrate that many problem drinkers are not known to any form of helping agency. However, recent evidence from England suggests that:

- Thirty-eight per cent of men and 16 per cent of women (age 16–64) have an alcohol problem (26 per cent overall), which is equivalent to approximately 8.2 million people in England.
- Twenty-one per cent of men and 9 per cent of women are binge drinkers. There is a considerable overlap between drinking above 'sensible' daily benchmarks and 'sensible' weekly benchmarks for both men and women.
- The prevalence of alcohol dependence is 3.6 per cent, with 6 per cent of men and 2 per cent of women meeting these criteria nationally. This equates to 1.1 million people with alcohol dependence nationally.
- There is a decline in all alcohol-related problems with age.
- Black and minority ethnic groups have a considerably lower prevalence of hazardous/harmful alcohol use but a similar prevalence of alcohol dependence compared with the white population.

Problem drinkers are greatly over-represented among medical in-patients. Eight per cent of women and 29 per cent of men in general medical and orthopaedic wards have been found to be problem drinkers. Higher figures will be found in casualty departments because accidents often involve those with a high blood alcohol, and in gastrointestinal clinics, since these deal with many of the physical complications of alcohol. Yet most

250

alcohol abusers in the general hospital go undetected. Twenty per cent of psychiatric admissions are associated with alcohol dependence.

Although problems of drug and alcohol misuse have traditionally been considered separately, they increasingly co-exist, and that is reflected in this chapter. 'Misuse' of substances (alcohol and drugs) can occur without the development of 'dependence'. Services for people with drug and alcohol problems are now generally known as 'substance misuse' services and offer advice and support to many people who would not technically meet the criteria for 'dependence' (see below).

What are 'safe limits' for alcohol?

- It is recommended that **men** should drink no more than 21 units of alcohol per week (and no more than four units in any one day).
- **Women** should drink no more than 14 units of alcohol per week (and no more than three units in any one day).

Limits are higher for males than for females, because when they both consume the same amount of alcohol the female will achieve a higher level in the bloodstream. The higher proportion of body fat in women is an important contributing factor. Details of units of alcohol are shown in *Box 17.1*.

Problem drinking occurs when a person is not dependent on alcohol, but drinks enough to cause actual physical, psychological, or social harm. Many people misuse drugs without becoming dependent, but may still experience a variety of drug-related harms.

Box 17.1 Units of alcohol

One unit of alcohol is 10 ml (1 cl) by volume, or 8 g by weight, of pure alcohol. For example:

1. **One unit of alcohol** is about equal to:

   - Half a pint of ordinary strength beer, lager, or cider (3–4 per cent alcohol by volume), or
   - A **small** pub measure (25 ml) of spirits (40 per cent alcohol by volume), or
   - A standard pub measure (50 ml) of fortified wine such as sherry or port (20 per cent alcohol by volume).

2. There are **one and a half units of alcohol** in:

   - A small glass (125 ml) of ordinary strength wine (12 per cent alcohol by volume), or
   - A standard pub measure (35 ml) of spirits (40 per cent alcohol by volume).

Any drug becomes a drug of **dependence** when there is a compulsion to take it on a continuous or a periodic basis. The concept of dependence has several components (see *Box 17.2*). By 'addiction' or 'dependence syndrome' we mean a state in which the drug takes up an overriding importance in life.

Awareness of a **compulsion to use the substance** is reported by the person so that, for example, the first drink of alcohol after a period of abstinence inevitably leads to a return to the previous level of consumption. The desire for a further drink is seen as irrational, the desire is resisted, yet the further drink is taken. If the person tries to abstain, he may experience cravings for alcohol.

Box 17.2 Features of the dependence syndrome

- Strong desire (compulsion) to take the substance
- Difficulty controlling its use
- Withdrawal state
- Tolerance
- Persistence despite knowing there will be harmful consequences
- Neglecting other interests and pleasures

Increased tolerance develops so that large amounts can be consumed without inebriation. The patient may have derived confidence from this, when in fact it indicates that dependence is beginning.

Withdrawal symptoms occur when there is an abrupt drop in the level of the substance in someone who has maintained a high intake over a prolonged period of time. With **alcohol** these typically occur in the morning, since this is the time when blood alcohol is at its lowest. They consist of shaking of the hands ('morning shakes'), nausea, sweating, and agitation. They are relieved by taking an alcoholic drink. More severe withdrawal symptoms include illusions, a sense of dread, and jumbled auditory hallucinations. *Generalized epileptic* seizures may occur; and after some 48 hours **delirium tremens** (see pp. 165–166). After a while, drinking begins to take priority over everything else: work, family life, social life, and even health. The drinking repertoire is restricted to a stereotyped pattern each day and drinking acquires salience over other activities. The concept of dependence leads to the discussion of whether someone is 'an alcoholic' or not. This is seldom a useful discussion. *It is better to ask whether a dependent individual has developed any related disabilities.*

Taking a history of drinking

Establish with the patient what their consumption has been over the previous week, taking each day at a time back over the previous 7 days, so that you can estimate the **total number of units consumed per week**. It may be helpful to obtain a simple guide to

252

the alcohol content of various types of beer, wine and spirits as an *aide-memoire* (easily found on the internet, see Further reading) and carry this with you.

Ask if this has been a typical week – some people have a pattern of *binge drinking* for several days at a time followed by a period of abstinence. Because some people may be at very high risk of alcohol-related harm as a result of bingeing on one or two nights of the week, it is important to check out not just a 'typical day' but also consumption over the week.

Then focus on the following:

1. Establish if the **first drink of the day** is taken to combat withdrawal symptoms.
2. Does the patient **drink throughout the day** without getting drunk, or in **bouts** – usually at lunchtime and the evening?
3. How much is drunk at each session?
4. Does a single drink always leads to many more, and the person generally becomes drunk? If so, has this led to **blackouts** or falls?
5. Establish whether drinking takes place alone, and whether the person drinks only in response to certain moods or situations.

Having established the current drinking pattern, try to ascertain the **development of heavy drinking** over the years. There are often key points in the patient's life, such as working in the armed forces or in the wine trade, where a great increase in drinking occurred. The patient may recall his daily drinking pattern at times when he lost a particular job or when his marriage broke up. What has been the longest period of abstinence? Contacts with the police may also be dated. In this way the doctor establishes the duration of heavy drinking, which of the related disabilities have developed, and the pattern of their development over time.

Where possible, and where it is indicated, you should also get a history from a family member or other informant.

Taking a drug history

This is similar to a drinking history but focuses *for each substance* that the person takes on establishing: **quantity, frequency, typical pattern of use, age of starting, time of most recent use, method of administration**.

Try to find out how much money is spent on drugs each day and week.

Ask about **risky behaviours**: frequency of intoxication, bingeing, overdosing, driving habits, unsafe sex, sharing needles.

Enquire about development of **tolerance**: does the patient need more of the substance now, compared with before, to achieve same effect?

Establish, as with alcohol, whether there is evidence of **physical, psychological**, or **social harm** related to the drug misuse, for example the development of HIV or hepatitis C, episodes of depression or psychosis, or problems with the police.

Establish what help has been received in the past and the person's response to that help. What is the best that they have achieved? What problems have they faced in staying off drugs?

Clinical features

PHYSICAL EXAMINATION

Is there evidence of intoxication? *Alcohol*: alcohol on the breath, sedated, slurred speech, or ataxic gait? *Opiates*: pinpoint pupils, low blood pressure, or venepuncture marks? *Benzodiazepines:* disinhibited or intoxicated but not drunk? *Psychostimulants*: rapid speech, large pupils, agitation, restlessness, or high blood pressure?

Is there evidence of withdrawal? *Alcohol*: tremulous, or high blood pressure? *Opiates:* dilated pupils, high blood pressure, sweaty, rhinorrhoea, or cramps? *Benzodiazepines:* tremulous, hyper-reflexia, depersonalization, hypersensitivity? *Psychostimulants*: agitation or restlessness?

ALCOHOL-RELATED PHYSICAL DAMAGE

Cirrhosis of the liver is the best-recognized complication. Deaths from cirrhosis have risen in the UK recently because of the marked increase in alcohol consumption. For men the risk of cirrhosis increases as a result of drinking four pints of beer a day (or a quarter of a bottle of spirits or one bottle of wine), for women two pints of beer or equivalent is sufficient. Persistent heavy drinking is most likely to lead to cirrhosis, which will occur in 80 per cent of those who drink 10 or more pints a day for 15 years. **Hepatitis** is also common among heavy drinkers and may lead on to cirrhosis. **Hepatic encephalopathy** occurs in liver failure.

Half the cases of **chronic pancreatitis** occur in heavy drinkers, especially chronic calcifying pancreatitis. **Acute gastritis** is common among heavy drinkers, and peptic ulcers are three times more common than in non-drinkers. These illnesses together with **oesophageal varices** and **oesophagitis** mean that a problem drinker may present with abdominal pain, with a haematemesis, or with an iron-deficient anaemia. **Macrocytosis without anaemia** occurs as a result of folate deficiency. **Megaloblastic anaemia** may result from folate or vitamin B_{12} deficiency, or a direct toxic effect of alcohol. **Haemolytic anaemia** or **thrombocytopenia** may arise from cirrhosis.

The risk of **ischaemic heart disease** and **cerebrovascular accidents** is increased with alcohol abuse. **Cardiomyopathy** is more specifically linked to alcohol, which is associated with 50 per cent of cases of primary degeneration of the heart muscle.

Peripheral neuropathy occurs in 10 per cent of dependent drinkers and affects both sensory and motor systems, especially in the lower limbs. It is due to thiamine deficiency but rarely responds to treatment. **Cerebellar degeneration**, **myopathy**, and **Wernicke's encephalopathy** (see p. 179) occur. The alcoholic is at greater risk of **subdural haematoma** and **traumatic neuropathy**, as well as injuries of all kinds resulting from accidents at home and at work, road traffic accidents, and episodes of violence.

Many of these physical disabilities are a result of, or are made worse by, dietary deficiencies and general poor health which predispose the alcohol-dependent patient to develop infection.

PSYCHOLOGICAL DISABILITIES

Depression is common among alcohol abusers. Three patterns may be discerned:

1. Alcohol has a **direct depressant effect** and the alcohol abuser may have a persistently depressed mood that responds to abstinence.
2. Alcohol abuse leads to **social problems**, such as unemployment, divorce, and debts, and these lead to the person becoming depressed.
3. Depression, occurring for some other reason, may be **relieved temporarily** by drinking. This is one way in which heavy drinking starts, with an eventual worsening of the depression.

The depression may lead to deliberate self-harm. Nearly half of the males who take overdoses are dependent on alcohol. The risk of **suicide** is increased many times among the population of alcohol abusers admitted for treatment.

Anxiety is related to alcohol abuse in a similar way to depression. In addition, anxiety is marked during alcohol withdrawal.

Alcoholic hallucinosis is a rare condition separate from the acute effects of withdrawal. In the setting of clear consciousness, auditory hallucinations occur that are generally in the second person and may be derogatory. They are often in the form of a conversation about the patient. The phenomenon usually occurs when prolonged heavy drinking ceases or is considerably reduced. It generally clears within a few days. If not, a state similar to schizophrenia develops. In this case it is likely that latent schizophrenia is released by the heavy alcohol intake.

Dis-social personality disorder (see p. 278) may lead to alcoholism, but a normal personality may be evident before persistent heavy drinking leads to mood changes, inability to hold a job, and disruption of personal relationships.

MEMORY IMPAIRMENT

1. This occurs during acute intoxication with alcohol. Although the person may function quite normally during an evening of heavy drinking, on waking the next day there will be a dense amnesia for those hours (**alcoholic amnesia**, or 'palimpsest', or alcoholic 'blackout').
2. A specific memory impairment occurs, **Korsakoff's syndrome** (see pp. 174, 179).
3. **Alcoholic dementia**, which may resolve if the person stops drinking.

SOCIAL DISABILITIES

Marital problems occur because the alcohol abuser is late coming home, and may be abusive or violent while drunk, incur debts, lose his job, and become impotent. The spouse may be disgusted by her drunk husband and embarrassed by his social behaviour. She may therefore become depressed and anxious herself, or even take an overdose, and the astute general practitioner may detect alcohol abuse in this indirect way. Effects on the children may predominate if it is the wife who is abusing alcohol.

Work problems develop if the person attends late, is drunk and argumentative at work, and fails to perform at his former standard. Alcoholics miss much time from work and lose their jobs more frequently than their sober colleagues.

Heavy drinkers often come into contact with the police because of anti-social behaviour while intoxicated, either being disorderly or committing a petty crime.

Vagrancy has many causes but alcohol abuse often combines with other factors to lead to this state. Such people may present very considerable problems to the health services because of their multiple physical illnesses, their poor living conditions, and their insistence on continued drinking.

WHEN TO SUSPECT A PROBLEM MAY BE PRESENT

The detection of alcohol-related disabilities

Doctors do not detect alcohol abuse in general medical practice because they fail to ask the appropriate questions.

1. When any of the physical problems mentioned on page 254 present (do not be satisfied with diagnosing a peptic ulcer, ask yourself whether alcohol could be responsible).
2. When the patient seems evasive or unclear while describing his complaint (this might represent concealment of heavy drinking or indicate a memory impairment).
3. When the patient is in a high-risk occupation (barman, publican, wine merchant or brewer carries a high risk; well above average are company directors, commercial travellers, the armed forces, journalists, entertainers, and doctors).
4. When another family member has alcohol-related problems.
5. When investigations provide evidence of pathology that may be a result of alcohol (for example, an unexpected elevation of the γ-GT).

USEFUL QUESTIONNAIRES

In any of these circumstances, you may find that the CAGE questions are useful (see *Box 17.3*), but the AUDIT questionnaire, which can be easily downloaded from the internet (see Further reading), is more sensitive in picking up early problem drinking.

Aetiology

GENETIC FACTORS

The prevalence of alcohol dependence among parents and siblings of people with alcohol dependence is two and a half times that of the general population. This is not solely an environmental effect as sons of alcoholic fathers adopted away are just as likely

---

Box 17.3 The CAGE questions

C.   Have you ever felt you ought to CUT down on your drinking?
A.   Have people ANNOYED you by criticizing your drinking?
G.   Have you ever felt bad or GUILTY about your drinking?
E.   Have you ever had a drink first thing in the morning to steady your nerves or get rid of a hangover (EYE OPENER)?

If you get positive replies to any *two* of these questions, it is worth taking a proper 'drinking history'. (Probability of being a case if score is 2 or > 2 = 45 per cent; probability of being a non-case if score is 0 or 1 = 97 per cent.)

---

to become alcoholics as those who remain in the original parental home. Twin studies suggest a small genetic component, and adoption studies show that alcohol dependence in the biological parent produces significantly higher rates of alcoholism in their adopted-away children.

PSYCHOLOGICAL FACTORS

Prospective studies have shown that although neurotic traits in childhood do not relate to the later development of alcohol problems, children who were **impulsive**, **aggressive** and **hyperactive** are more likely to develop alcohol problems as adults.

However, alcohol is a potent anxiolytic, so agoraphobics, social phobics, and other neurotic personalities are likely to use alcohol in this way. In some this will lead on to clear dependence on alcohol. The relief of tension or distress by alcohol can be viewed as a reward in behavioural terms. If this happens repeatedly the consumption of alcohol becomes a self-perpetuating habit. Any difficulties that arise from heavy drinking, including withdrawal symptoms, increase anxiety that can once again be relieved by the ingestion of alcohol. Thus a vicious circle with increasing consumption is set up.

SOCIAL FACTORS

Several *occupations* have more people with alcohol problems than would be expected, and these have been listed above. Predisposing effects of these occupations include availability of cheap or free alcohol, strong peer pressure to drink, lack of supervision at work, and estrangement from the stabilizing influences of home life.

Cultural factors are important as the taboos against drinking among Muslims and Mormons, and against drunkenness among Jews, lead to very low rates of alcohol problems compared to cultures where drinking is equated with masculinity.

Availability of alcohol is being increasingly recognized as a factor. There is evidence for a direct relationship between per capita consumption in a population and the number of people with alcohol-related problems. The former is determined by the real price of alcoholic beverages and as this is reduced the mortality rate from cirrhosis increases.

Investigations

TO ESTABLISH THE DIAGNOSIS

Physical

Test blood or urinary alcohol to detect alcohol in the patient's bloodstream when he denies having drunk; or abnormal liver function in someone who denies drinking very much.

Social

Interview an informant to establish the patient's true drinking pattern and extent of related disabilities when these are not clear from the patient. Assessment of family relationships, financial position, and job situation will reveal the true extent of social disabilities, which are often more serious than the patient has led the doctor to believe.

A knowledge of these social factors may allow the doctor to understand the aetiology of the person's heavy drinking (this may be years previously) but also allow him to assess the factors that reinforce his current consumption.

TO ESTABLISH THE EXTENT OF ALCOHOL-RELATED DAMAGE

Physical

Test liver function, especially γ-glutamyl transpeptidase (γ-GT), which is raised (> 40 iu/l) in 75 per cent of dependent drinkers. Test blood film for **macrocytosis** in the absence of anaemia, and thereafter test to detect the physical sequelae of heavy drinking listed above.

Psychological

Test for memory impairment (see p. 255).

Treatment – alcohol dependence

It is essential to clarify and agree with the patient what the **aims and goals of treatment** are – abstinence or a reduction in intake.

People who have not yet become physically dependent on alcohol, and do not have serious alcohol-related physical or psychological harm *may* be able to learn how to cut down their drinking successfully. This process is called **controlled drinking**, and community alcohol agencies specialize in providing self-help materials (which usually involve keeping a drinking diary to record daily consumption) and offering counselling in order to help people reduce the amount that they are consuming. However, this is highly unlikely to be successful in someone who has developed the symptoms of alcohol dependence, and if the patient is suffering from problems that will be exacerbated by continuing ingestion, for example liver disease, depression, then the doctor should advise that **abstinence** really ought to be the goal. However some people will find this a very difficult goal to aim for initially.

PHYSICAL

Many patients who are physically dependent on alcohol undergo detoxification at home under the care of their GP, and close daily supervision from community alcohol teams. This is only suitable for those who have no history of alcohol withdrawal fits or delirium tremens, who have good social support, and who are not otherwise at risk from physical (e.g. liver disease) or psychological complications (e.g. depression, suicide, psychosis) of their drinking.

Chlordiazepoxide is the drug of choice for alcohol withdrawal regimes in a reducing daily dose over 7 days, starting at 80 mg per day. Chlormethiazole is no longer used because of the risk of development of dependence and lethality in overdose, but diazepam is an alternative.

Treatment for delirium tremens is described on page 166.

High dose oral thiamine (200 mg per day) together with vitamin B strong tablets (30 mg per day) will be sufficient to prevent the complications of vitamin deficiency in most patients undergoing detoxification, but patients at high risk of developing Wernicke's encephalopathy should be given intravenous therapy (*Pabrinex*).

Serious depression or anxiety occasionally requires drug treatment, but usually depression improves as the person is detoxified.

Any accompanying physical illnesses must be treated.

Disulfiram (Antabuse) causes an accumulation of acetaldehyde, which results in flushing, nausea and vomiting, palpitations, and difficulty in breathing. It can be given daily and will help the impulsive drinker who knows that he will become acutely ill if he drinks during the subsequent 24 hours. The patient must be motivated to take the tablet each day for this to be a useful adjunct to other treatment, and it is considerably less popular than it was in the past.

Acamprosate (Campril) has been shown in research to produce a small increase in abstinence and reduced levels of drinking and relapse compared with placebo, but it is still unclear which patients are most likely to benefit.

PSYCHOLOGICAL

Motivational interviewing strategies (see p. 118) will be essential to help the patient to make a decision about their goals, and about when, how, or if they wish to try to change their behaviour.

Supportive psychotherapy is essential (see p. 120). Developing an empathic but *honest* relationship with the doctor will help the patient to achieve their goals.

SOCIAL

Where possible, involve the family so they can understand the nature of the problem, provide support for the patient, and help them cope.

Activities other than going to the pub or mixing with drinking friends should be encouraged. The patient has to adopt a new lifestyle that does not revolve around drinking, and this can be a challenge.

With more serious cases *admission to a psychiatric ward or alcohol treatment unit* is recommended so that the commencement of psychological treatments occurs together with the detoxification.

Group therapy is useful to help the person to be honest about the nature of the problem and find ways of coping without alcohol.

Alcoholics Anonymous is very helpful for many patients. It advocates a strict abstinence policy, and provides a social structure to replace drinking. Support is available at all times and often from ex-alcoholics with whom the patient can identify.

DRUG MISUSE AND DEPENDENCE

Much of what has been written about alcohol-related problems applies to drug-related problems. There are high levels of health and social problems associated with drug misuse and dependence, and many who misuse drugs use several different types of substance (polysubstance misuse/dependence). A person may move through the use of several different substances throughout their lives. In the past there was much less overlap between people who were misusers of alcohol and those who used drugs, but this is no longer the case, and many people misuse a wide range of substances including both drugs and alcohol. They may only become dependent on *some* of the substances that they misuse, but still experience (and cause) a variety of types of drug-related harm.

Harm to the drug user

The drug user is at risk from **blood-borne viruses** (if injecting), **overdose and death** (both a high risk of suicide and of homicide), **mental illness, infection, cardiovascular disease and thrombo-embolism, injury and general ill health, social exclusion**, and **poverty**.

Harm to the community

Drug use is associated with **crime** (for example burglary to fund the habit, or drug-related gang crime) and **violence** and has a long-term and deeply negative effect on communities where it becomes prevalent.

General principles of treatment

Treatment is aimed at:

- Helping to stop or reduce drug use, or to ensure that drug use is safer (harm minimization).
- Reducing the amount and frequency of polysubstance use.
- Improving physical and mental health.
- Improving social functioning.
- Reducing the impact on the community.

The next sections examine specific substances in detail.

Opiate dependence

These drugs in the UK come from three sources: legal prescriptions, theft from chemists, and smuggled oriental heroin. The addict takes the drug by mouth ('dropping'), inhales the fumes of burning heroin ('chasing the dragon'), nasally inhales it ('snorting'), or injects it intramuscularly (a 'fix'), subcutaneously ('skin pop'), or intravenously ('mainlining'). Initially the drug taker experiences a 'rush, thrill, buzz or flash' following intravenous heroin. This is described like a rather superior sexual orgasm and is the reason for taking heroin at first. Appetite and sexual desire are decreased, and constipation is common.

As tolerance develops larger doses are required, dysphoria and somatic side-effects are experienced, and the person takes the drug increasingly to avoid withdrawal symptoms.

WITHDRAWAL SYMPTOMS

These start 8–10 hours after the last dose, with **rhinorrhoea, lacrimation, yawning, sweating**, and **craving. Nausea, vomiting, diarrhoea, abdominal cramps** and **muscle pains** develop.

Central nervous system rebound excitability is shown by **mydriasis, tachycardia, hypertension, flushing**, and **involuntary movements**.

These symptoms ('cold turkey') are much feared by addicts because they are so unpleasant, but in fact they recede after 72 hours and do not carry the same risk to life as delirium tremens.

MORTALITY AND MORBIDITY

Mortality among opiate addicts is almost 15 times that of the non-drug-taking population. This is accounted for by the **morbidity** associated with opiate dependence, itself mainly related to:

1. **Dirty injection technique** leading to **sepsis, hepatitis, endocarditis, tuberculosis,** and **nephrotic syndrome**. There is an increased risk of infection at all sites,

superficial, deep and systemic. Abcesses can lead to general septicaemia, and thrombo-embolism is also a risk, particularly among groin injectors.

Infection with HIV from sharing injecting equipment is a risk, but there are also an increasing number of drug users with hepatitis B and hepatitis C who may go on to develop cirrhosis and liver cancer.

2. **Drug overdosage** (accidental poisoning and self-harm – which may be hard to distinguish) may cause **respiratory failure**.
3. Feelings of **desperation and depression** often lead to **suicide**.

CLINICAL FEATURES

During withdrawal, the patient will have widely dilated pupils, tachycardia and pilo-erection as well as the symptoms listed above. Look for thrombosed veins, and other complications of dirty injections.

TREATMENT

As with alcohol-related problems this is largely concerned with helping the individual in the longer term to develop a new lifestyle free of the drug. This may involve changing the social group in which the person mixes if this includes other drug misusers. Financial and family problems and involvement with the law will all require social help. Treatment may include:

- **Detoxification**. This may be done by a GP with close support from the community drug team and involves prescription of a reducing regime of oral methadone (usually in 1 mg/ml solution). For serious cases of dependence, admission to a *specialist treatment unit* is advisable so that rapid detoxification may take place with minimal withdrawal symptoms, and a long-term treatment plan commenced.
- **Urine testing** for the presence of substances, especially if replacement drugs are being prescribed.
- Longer term **methadone replacement therapy** may be arranged by the community drug services. This option enables the drug user to stabilize their lifestyle, and helps to minimize drug-related harm. Specialist services supply injectable as well as oral methadone. The aim is generally that the person will eventually undergo withdrawal, but some patients do stay on maintenance treatment for long periods while trying to achieve stability in other aspects of their lives and generally improve their health.
- 'Harm minimization' strategies with the use of a **needle exchange** to prevent HIV. Some community pharmacies also provide this service.
- A range of **psychotherapeutic interventions** as specifically indicated by the nature of the underlying problems. This will involve individual and/or group therapy.
- Health promotion and **general health care** including testing and **immunization** against hepatitis.
- **Social interventions**. Working with the probation service, further education, employment.

It is often the general practitioner, casualty officer, or general physician who is initially faced with an addict claiming to be in withdrawal.

When deciding whether to prescribe **methadone** (this drug is used because it can be given orally, it prevents withdrawal symptoms, but does not produce the pleasurable 'buzz' of heroin) it is best to err on the side of caution – there are some heroin users who only take the drug occasionally and are not dependent.

In the GP surgery and casualty department it is always better not to prescribe in the absence of clear withdrawal symptoms or without the patient agreeing specific goals of treatment. A *treatment contract* defines a withdrawal regime of reducing doses over a 2 to 3 week period, and states conditions the patient must fulfil (for example, abstinence from additional drug-taking checked by urine samples each visit) if the doctor is to continue prescribing. Without such precautions the doctor may find himself becoming obliged to continue prescribing, and it is in such circumstances that most problems occur.

A small minority of patients have developed dependence on opiates as a result of prescriptions from a doctor ('iatrogenic drug dependence'). In the case of terminally ill patients this does not matter. For the remainder opiates have usually been prescribed for a painful condition, so alternative methods of controlling the pain must be sought before the opiate can be withdrawn gradually.

Benzodiazepine dependence

These widely prescribed drugs are a major cause of dependence in the community. They cease to be effective anxiolytics once the user is habituated to them, yet severe symptoms of anxiety will be experienced if withdrawal is attempted. The withdrawal *symptoms* also include **giddiness, trembling, faintness, insomnia, and hypersensitivity** and abrupt withdrawal may result in confusion and fits. Withdrawal symptoms can be minimized by using a long-acting drug, such as diazepam, and withdrawing it very slowly. Benzodiazepines can be withdrawn in steps of about one-eighth of the daily dose per fortnight. Irritability and insomnia are severe in the first 2 weeks after withdrawal, but have virtually disappeared 3 months later. Large numbers of people have become dependent on these drugs as a result of their widespread therapeutic use. In addition, young polydrug abusers often use them (especially Temazepam) in extremely high doses in combination with other drugs.

Barbiturate dependence

These drugs are now very little used, but there are still some young multiple drug-abusers who manage to obtain these drugs through medical channels.

Barbiturate abusers may develop *tolerance* but the risk of **respiratory depression** increases with large doses and these may be fatal. Drug-dependent individuals are particularly likely to take an overdose of barbiturates. A **withdrawal syndrome** similar to that of alcohol is recognized, **epileptic fits** and **delirium** are common.

Clinical features

The younger barbiturate addict may have injected these highly irritant drugs in aqueous solution, and so produced phlebitis, indolent abscesses, and sloughing ulcers. He may be unkempt, dirty, and malnourished. He may appear drunk, with slurred speech and incoherence, or be sleepy. Nystagmus is usually present, and depression is a common complication.

Treatment

Replacement with a short-acting barbiturate (for example pentobarbitone) is recommended for those dependent on high doses, with 10 per cent reduction of dosage per day and possible concurrent cover with an anticonvulsant. Subsequently prolonged difficulty with sleep occurs and **nightmares** result from REM rebound.

Drugs causing abnormal mental states, but not dependence

They are often used alongside other drugs, and they may precipitate psychotic illness.

CANNABIS

Cannabis is widely abused in the population. 'Grass' refers to the dried plant, *Cannabis sativa*, while 'resin' is secreted by the female parts of the flowering plant. The effects largely depend on the circumstances in which the drug is taken, and it is generally used as a social drug. There is no withdrawal syndrome, nor is there evidence of tolerance. Feelings of well-being, relaxation and tranquillity are induced within minutes of inhalation, but prevailing moods of anger or depression may be aggravated. Perceptual disturbances of time, sight, and sound may occur but the person generally retains insight throughout.

Although relatively harmless for most adults when taken in small or moderate doses, those carrying the (recessive!) genes for schizophrenia are at risk of developing **schizophrenia**. Those with a positive family history are at much greater risk than those without such a history. The higher the dose, the more likely is an episode of schizophrenia. The longer exposure occurs in those who have had an episode, the greater the likelihood of developing the illness.

AMPHETAMINES

There are three basic types of amphetamine: laevoamphetamine, dextroamphetamine, and methylamphetamine. Most street usage is of a very impure powdered preparation containing the first two of these in equal proportions ('amp', 'speed', 'whizz' or 'sulph').

They are taken to produce a state of increased awareness, energy and concentration, together with reduced hunger and fatigue. Taken intravenously they may produce a

264

short-lived 'flush' and are used in this way by opiate addicts. These effects are followed by depression, anxiety, irritability, and anergia.

Clinical features

The patient will be talkative and over-active if intoxicated; sleepy or depressed if withdrawn. He may be malnourished because of the anorexia, and lick his lips because of the dry mouth. The pupils are dilated, there may be sweating, tachycardia, high blood pressure, or arrhythmias, and there is usually a generalized hyper-reflexia.

Amphetamines may produce **organic psychosis** with schizophrenic symptoms (see p. 191) in otherwise normal people, with persecutory delusions, accompanied by visual, tactile, and auditory hallucinations in a state of clear consciousness. They will also exacerbate schizophrenic symptoms in those vulnerable to the disorder. In other patients a **symptomatic mania** can be precipitated. The mental state usually returns to normal over 5–7 days as the drug is excreted, but occasionally a persistent psychosis requires treatment with phenothiazines.

COCAINE

Cocaine may be 'snorted' into the nostril and absorbed through the nasal mucosa, injected, or smoked (the 'crack' preparation of the drug is used in this way). It is a central nervous stimulant with effects similar to amphetamine, but said to be less sharp and more subtle. It may produce disorientation and depression. It resembles amphetamine in its ability to produce a symptomatic psychosis.

Clinical features

The intoxicated patient may be excited, with dilated pupils and tremulousness. He may report a feeling of insects crawling under his skin ('formication'). At later stages, dizziness, convulsions, and cardiac arrhythmias occur. Death may be from cardiac arrest.

HALLUCINOGENS

Mescalin, lysergic acid diethylamide (LSD, or 'acid'), dimethyltryptamine ('angel dust') and psilocybin ('the magic mushroom') are hallucinogens. LSD and psilocybin are most commonly used in this country.

Clinical features

Taken orally LSD causes perceptual changes within 40 minutes. Sensation in all modalities is heightened and distorted and may be translated from one modality to another so sounds may be seen and colour smelled: 'synaesthesia'. The **body image** may be terrifyingly distorted; the patient may regard himself as able to fly or to walk on water. Numerous deaths have occurred in this way. **Extreme emotional changes** may occur,

265

which result in anxiety and terror of imminent insanity: these are described as a 'bad trip'. Such states are best managed by someone 'talking down' the patient, emphasizing that the alarming experiences are caused by the drug.

The acute effects die down over 24 hours, but perceptual changes may last longer. A more prolonged psychosis may result as with amphetamines, although it may be that the drug has merely released the psychosis in a vulnerable personality. Sometimes **flash-back experiences** occur some months later when, under stress or the effect of another drug, the person re-lives part of the perceptual distortion that occurred during an LSD trip.

ECSTASY

Ecstasy is a stimulant drug that also has mild hallucinogenic effects and has been popular in the club and dance culture in the last two decades. It has been described as being like a mixture of amphetamine and a weak form of LSD. The effects of taking a moderate dose start after 20–60 minutes (longer if on a full stomach) and can last for up to several hours.

Clinical features

The pupils become dilated, the jaw tightens and there is often brief nausea, sweating, dry mouth and throat. The blood pressure rises, the heart rate increases, and loss of appetite is common. Many users experience an initial rushing feeling followed by a combination of feeling energetic and yet calm. Loss of anger, empathy with other people, and an enhanced sense of communication are commonly reported. Some users also report a heightened sense of their surroundings, greater appreciation of music, and increased sexual and sensual experience. Some users have bad experiences. This may include feeling anxious and panicky for days or even weeks.

SOLVENT SNIFFING

Psychological dependence occurs and this causes concern because it involves children, especially those from a deprived background. The mortality is considerable; about 50 per cent as a result of direct toxic effects of the solvent, the remainder mainly as a result of asphyxia from the plastic bag from which the solvent was inhaled, or from inhalation of gastric contents.

Clinical features

Euphoria may result from the sniffing of solvents that contain toluene and acetone, but continued inhalation leads to stupor and loss of consciousness as these toxic substances are powerful CNS depressants and may cause neuronal destruction. Look for glue on the hands, face or clothes, and the glue sniffer's rash over the mouth and nasal area. The patient is usually a child or adolescent, and males outnumber females by 13 to 1. The glue may be smelled. There are rapid variations in the level of consciousness, disorientation, sometimes slurred speech, and an ataxic gait.

NON-OPIATE ANALGESICS

Those who regularly take large doses of aspirin, phenacetin, and paracetamol may do so secretively, against medical advice and with serious physical consequences.

Psychological dependence occurs, and women with chronic depressive illness or personality disturbance are particularly prone to use these drugs in this way. The principal physical related problem is **analgesic nephropathy**.

Multiple drug abuse seems to be the norm rather than the exception, especially if alcohol is included as a drug. Therefore a drug-dependent person who has taken an overdose may have done so with several drugs. An opiate-dependent person denied his normal dose will turn to other drugs.

'Dual diagnosis'

This term applies to those people who have a diagnosed mental illness, usually a psychotic illness, and who also experience problems with drugs and/or alcohol. The relationship between the two is often quite complex and it can be difficult to work out which came first, the drug use or the mental illness. However some people may use drugs as a form of continued 'self-medication' for their symptoms in the belief that there is little difference between street drugs and those prescribed by doctors, and treatment can be difficult.

About half of those who experience serious mental illness will have a positive history of substance use. This will include not only those with schizophrenia who use drugs, but also people with a diagnosis of bipolar disorder, depression, or anxiety who use drugs and/or alcohol.

Doctors, drugs and alcohol

Health professionals are susceptible to developing dependence on alcohol and drugs, and medical students are increasingly known to use substances during their period at university when they are not (yet) subject to the professional regulation of the General Medical Council. Services exist in most countries in order specifically to engage doctors and dentists in therapy, and even Alcoholics Anonymous has groups for doctors in the UK. Doctors have a duty to protect patients from risk of harm by another colleague's conduct, performance, or health. You should discuss your concerns with an impartial colleague, consult your defence body, professional organization or the General Medical Council for advice.

EATING DISORDERS

Eating disorders comprise anorexia nervosa, bulimia nervosa, and their variants. These disorders typically develop in adolescence or early adulthood, predominantly in females.

They share much the same psychopathology and many patients migrate between the two disorders over time.

Anorexia nervosa

EPIDEMIOLOGY

Anorexia nervosa is relatively rare. Most estimates of the point prevalence come from studies of adolescent girls or young adult women and give a figure within this group of around 0.3 per cent. The prevalence is probably higher in boarding schools and ballet schools. The ratio of females to males is about 10 to 1 in adults, but somewhat lower in adolescents. Anorexia nervosa appears to have become more common over recent decades, but the apparent increase could well be due to greater help-seeking, better detection, and changes in diagnostic practice rather than any true increase in the incidence of the disorder. It is more commonly recognized in developed countries.

CLINICAL FEATURES

This condition presents with self-induced weight loss, so that body weight is maintained at least 15 per cent below expected weight and is accompanied by an intense wish to be thin. In adults, the body mass index (weight in kg/height in metres^2) is 17.5 or less. The patient has an intense fear of fatness, and this takes the form of an *over-valued idea* (see p. 33) that she is fat, although aware that others regard her as thin – this feature distinguishes anorexia nervosa from all other causes of either weight loss or anorexia. There is a widespread endocrine disorder involving the hypothalamic–pituitary–gonadal axis, manifested in females by amenorrhea, and in males by loss of sexual interest and potency. If the onset is pre-pubertal, the sequence of pubertal events is delayed or arrested.

The patient may successfully conceal abnormal eating habits, and sometimes be under medical investigation for somatic complaints such as diarrhoea, metabolic disorder, or amenorrhoea before the diagnosis is recognized.

The core features of anorexia nervosa are the **over-evaluation of shape** and **weight**. This results in dieting behaviour and intense fear of weight gain and fatness. Most of the other features are secondary to this psychopathology and its consequences (for example **severe weight loss** and **endocrine dysfunction**). Thus weight loss tends to be viewed as an accomplishment and, as a consequence, patients have a limited desire to change. The core belief leads many patients to mislabel adverse physical and emotional states as 'feeling fat' and equate these with actually being fat. The commonest presentations are **emaciation** and complications of starvation or weight loss. The patient may present with fainting, oedema, or menstrual irregularity. She may wear heavy clothes to mask her thinness.

Weight loss is primarily the result of a severe and selective restriction of food intake, with foods viewed as fattening being excluded. There is generally no loss of appetite. The dieting may also be an expression of other motives including asceticism and competitiveness with others. Some people engage in a driven type of exercising that also contributes to their weight loss. Self-induced vomiting and other forms of weight-control behaviour (such as the misuse of laxatives or diuretics) are practised by a subgroup. These patients may also sometimes engage in binge eating. **Abuse of diuretics** leads to dehydration and **laxative abuse** may result in diarrhoea and hypokalaemia.

Depressive and anxiety features, irritability, lability of mood, impaired concentration, loss of sexual appetite, and obsessional symptoms are frequently present. Interest in the outside world also declines as patients lose weight and most become socially withdrawn and isolated. These psychosocial features tend to get worse with weight loss and improve with weight regain.

DIFFERENTIAL DIAGNOSIS

Careful history-taking usually elicits the attitudes to weight, shape, and fattening foods characteristic of anorexia and the diagnosis is not made by exclusion of other disorders. Anorexia nervosa can be distinguished from *normal dieting* by the degree of emaciation and over-valued ideas about fatness.

Weight loss may result from other psychological or physical illnesses: **hyperthyroidism** and **diabetes** are examples that occur at this age. Organic causes of diarrhoea, such as **idiopathic steatorrhea** or **inflammatory bowel disease**, may need to be considered. Amenorrhoea may result from **ovarian** or **pituitary disease**, following use of the **contraceptive pill**, or from **psychological stress**.

Depressive and obsessional features may suggest these disorders, and occasionally **psychotic illnesses** can present with avoidance of food, but the central fear of weight gain and distorted body image generally indicate the true diagnosis.

AETIOLOGY

The cause of anorexia nervosa is thought to be multi-determined, a genetic predisposition acted on by a range of environmental risk factors. Eating disorders and certain associated traits run in families, with cross-transmission between anorexia nervosa and bulimia nervosa. There is also a raised prevalence of depression in these families and an increase in rates of substance abuse. Twin studies suggest a significant heritability.

Some risk factors comprise non-specific adverse experiences of the type associated with many psychiatric disorders (e.g. **childhood sexual abuse**). Others are more specific (e.g. parental concerns about shape and weight; a family history of eating disorder, childhood and parental obesity, early menarche, parental alcoholism). Certain of these factors are likely to operate by **sensitizing the person** to their shape, thereby encouraging dieting, an effect that is most likely to be seen in women in western societies in view of the **social pressure on them to be slim**. Others are character traits, the two most prominent being low self-esteem and perfectionism.

Brain imaging studies have identified altered activity in the cortex in both anorexia nervosa and bulimia nervosa, and there is some evidence that these alterations persist after recovery. Whether they are a consequence of the eating disorder or have somehow contributed to it is not known.

Specific psychological theories such as the cognitive-behavioural theory have been proposed to account for the development and maintenance of eating disorders. In brief, this proposes that the restriction of food intake has two main origins. The first is a need to feel 'in control' of life that gets displaced onto controlling eating. The second is an over-evaluation of shape and weight in those who have been sensitized to their appearance. In both instances, the resulting dietary restriction and weight loss are highly reinforcing. Subsequently, other processes begin to operate and serve to maintain the eating disorder. These might include a crisis within the family, such as parental marital breakdown, or psychiatric illness in a family member, or the condition may be reinforced through renewed commitment to school work.

INVESTIGATIONS

Physical investigations

These may be indicated to exclude other medical conditions. More important is the need to assess the extent of malnutrition and electrolyte disturbance resulting from vomiting or purging. Weight, height, and BMI should be calculated and for adolescents compared with norms from BMI centile charts. Temperature, pulse and blood pressure should be recorded and an ECG carried out if the patient is emaciated. Muscle weakness can be gauged by asking the patient to sit up from lying down and stand from a sitting position without using her hands.

Assessment of body image in a standardized way may be useful for evaluating body image disturbance, and self-report questionnaires may provide a useful baseline of eating, weight, shape, and other concerns.

Luteinizing hormone levels have been shown to be low, and to show an impaired response to LH-releasing factor. Even when weight is restored, cyclical LH activity may not resume for some time. Ovarian ultrasonography may be useful in such cases to assess ovarian maturity. There may be raised levels of growth hormone and cortisol, and abnormalities of insulin secretion.

Social investigations

Family, social, or educational stressors that may be acting as maintaining factors should be explored. In younger patients a member of the multi-disciplinary team should assess the capacity of parents to assume responsibility for eating, activity, and exercise planning.

TREATMENT

This aims at restoration of normal body weight, correction of distorted cognitions, and to provide support with developmental challenges appropriate to the patient's age.

Restoration of body weight

Most patients can be treated on an out-patient basis. A weight-restoring diet plan should be implemented, supported by parents or other family members, with the aim of achieving a weight gain of 0.5–1 kg per week. A dietician can provide useful education and advice. In-patient treatment may be required from the outset if the patient's weight is very low or there are significant physical complications. Rarely the emaciation is extreme and the patient refuses voluntary treatment so admission under section 3 of the Mental Health Act (see p. 365) has to be considered.

Drug treatment

There is no evidence to support the use of drugs in the treatment of anorexia nervosa. Although one initial report suggested that *fluoxetine* reduced the rate of relapse following in-patient treatment, a subsequent study failed to replicate the finding. *Olanzepine* is occasionally used to manage extreme anxiety around eating and *antidepressants* (chiefly fluoxetine) are sometimes used for concurrent depressive illness. Correction of *hypokalaemia* may be urgent if vomiting has been a pronounced feature, and severe dehydration if diuretics have been abused. A multivitamin, multimineral preparation should be prescribed to address and prevent other nutritional deficiencies that may be unmasked during weight regain.

Psychotherapies

There is currently a lack of evidence to support any specific psychological treatment, though it is clear that weight restoration alone does not lead to recovery in the absence of psychological change. Cognitive-behaviour therapy has theoretical appeal, based on the proposed psychological model and the characteristic distorted cognitions. There is preliminary evidence to suggest a role for family therapy to treat adolescents with the disorder, but uncertainties exist over the merits of conjoint therapy over parental counselling. Pure behaviour therapy is contra-indicated. A trusting relationship with a therapist who empathizes with the patient is beneficial, and motivational approaches are often helpful in increasing the patient's commitment to treatment. In the longer term the psychotherapeutic relationship may help the patient address maturational issues such as their developing sexuality and leaving home.

COURSE AND PROGNOSIS

An episode of anorexia nervosa usually lasts for at least 2 years, with about 50 per cent recovering by 5 years. Weight gain can generally be achieved in the short term but is only maintained in about 50 per cent. There is significant progression to other eating disorders, with a proportion going on to develop bulimia nervosa and some becoming obese. Other psychiatric disorders occur in approximately one third; the main ones being anxiety, depressive disorders, and personality disorders. The condition carries a **mortality rate** of up to 10 per cent; death occurring through emaciation or suicide.

Factors that indicate a *good prognosis* are an adolescent onset, a brief illness with rapid response to treatment, and satisfactory family relationships. A poor prognosis is indicated by the presence of vomiting, purgative abuse, attainment of a very low weight, and chronicity.

Bulimia nervosa

EPIDEMIOLOGY

Unlike anorexia nervosa, epidemiological data indicate that bulimia nervosa is more a disorder of early adulthood than adolescence, with most cases being in their twenties It is about three times more common than anorexia nervosa and partial syndromes are more common still. There are no reliable data on the prevalence of bulimia nervosa in boys or men. Clinical experience suggests that bulimia nervosa became considerably more common in the 1970s and 1980s, and limited epidemiological data support this, although there is evidence that the rise has now ceased. The explanation for these changes is not clear.

CLINICAL FEATURES

The central psychological disturbance in bulimia nervosa is similar to that of anorexia nervosa; hence patients commonly move between the two diagnoses. In bulimia nervosa attempts to restrict food intake are punctuated by repeated episodes of binge eating, with the result that patients may describe themselves as 'failed anorexics'. Uncontrolled and excessive binges are followed either by **self-induced vomiting**, by the use of **laxatives**, or by **rigorous dieting** to counteract the effects of the binge. The patient typically eats high-calorie foods and reports a relief from tension during the binge. The great majority of these patients are distressed by their loss of control over eating, which makes them easier to engage in treatment, but because of the associated shame and secrecy there is typically a delay of many years before they seek help.

The diagnosis is based on the following features:

1. Recurrent episodes of **binge-eating**.
2. A feeling of **lack of control** during binges.
3. **Self-induced vomiting, purgation**, or **severe dieting** afterwards.
4. At least **two binges per week** for at least 3 months.

Patients presenting with bulimia tend to be older than those with anorexia nervosa, but often report a previous episode of anorexia that may have gone undetected. Body weight is within the normal range (a diagnosis of anorexia nervosa taking precedence in those who are underweight). Menstrual disorders occur in about half of the cases. Mood disturbances are common. The eating disorder tends often to mask other psychological problems, and binges may be a repeated way of relieving distress.

Physical complications are either mechanical, the result of acid erosion (particularly of the teeth), or biochemical. Vomiting and purgation result in potassium deficiency, with weakness, cardiac arrhythmias, and occasionally renal damage.

The maintenance factors underlying bulimia differ from those in anorexia. For example, rigid dietary restraint increases the likelihood of binge eating, which in turn encourages further dietary restraint. Self-induced vomiting, while used to compensate for binge eating, results in the binges becoming larger and more frequent. External processes are important too. In those prone to binge eat, adverse events and negative moods may trigger episodes of binge eating, with the binges tending to modulate the negative mood and distract the person from the problem at hand.

TREATMENT

The evidence base for the treatment of bulimia nervosa is much stronger than that for anorexia, and several psychological approaches have been shown to be effective. The aim is to normalize eating, break the abstinence–bingeing–purging cycle, and challenge the underlying cognitive assumptions. The most effective treatment to date is a form of cognitive-behaviour therapy specifically developed for bulimia. Interpersonal therapy (IPT) is also effective, but appears to achieve its outcomes more slowly.

For patients who do not have access to these therapies or are unable to take them up, self-help in which patients follow cognitive and behavioural tasks in a book, can be effective. This is especially so when delivered in a 'guided' form, in which a supportive counsellor encourages adherence to the programme.

Selective serotonin re-uptake inhibitor (SSRI) antidepressants (particularly fluoxetine at a high dose of 60 mg/day) have a specific antibulimic effect that reduces binge eating and therefore disrupts the bulimic cycle. It is unclear whether any positive effects continue after the drug is discontinued.

OBESITY

Obesity is not a mental disorder or classified within existing eating disorder classification systems. It refers to an abnormally high proportion of body fat, but is usually estimated by comparing body weight with height. The *body mass index* (weight in kilograms divided by height in metres^2) is greater than 30. About one-third of adults in Britain and the USA are obese by this definition. A proportion of these will have *binge eating disorder* in which binges similar to those occurring in bulimia nervosa are not followed by compensatory behaviours.

Aetiology

The aetiology is partly constitutional, partly social – a combination of over-eating and under-exercise. In some obese people an additional contribution comes from *abnormal eating patterns* such as eating to deal with stress, comfort eating, night-eating, continuous snacking, and binge eating. Those who have been overweight since childhood have a greater rate of abnormal eating patterns, and higher rates of psychosocial difficulties. Many of these are similar to those seen in anorexia and bulimia and include low self-esteem, guilt, feelings of ineffectiveness, and social relationship problems.

Obese patients seen in medical clinics may be an unrepresentative sample, and have higher rates of mental health problems such as anxiety and depression. Their excessive weight may enable the patient to avoid problems in interpersonal and intimate relationships. If weight loss is successfully achieved these problems may become prominent and disrupt relationships whose precarious stability seems to have depended on the patient being obese. Some of these may give a history of an earlier eating disorder.

Treatment

All obese patients should be given advice on *diet and exercise*, and many benefit from self-help groups, although relapse is frequent.

Those who have binge eating disorder, low self-esteem, and a negative attitude towards their body image have been shown to benefit from cognitive-behaviour therapy. *Appetite suppressant drugs* have no place in the treatment of obesity: they produce dependence and any effect that they may have on body weight is likely to be shortlasting.

Good results have been reported by surgical procedures in the treatment of morbid obesity (where body mass index > 40). Both *gastric resection* and *jejuno-ileal bypass* are followed by weight reduction as a result of decreased food intake, and there may be psychological benefits including increased self-confidence, elevation of mood, and decrease in negative self-image.

FURTHER READING

Alcohol and Drugs

Gerarda, C. (2005) *The RCGP Guide to the Management of Substance Misuse in Primary Care*. London: Royal College of General Practitioners.

USEFUL WEBSITES:

AUDIT questionnaire, available at http://whqlibdoc.who.int/hq/2001/WHO_MSD_MSB_01.6a.pdf
Drugscope is useful for information, at http://www.drugscope.org.uk/home.asp
Alcohol Concern (large UK charity), see http://www.alcoholconcern.org.uk/servlets/home
British doctors and dentists group (have 16 groups in the UK and also help students), see http://www.medicouncilalcol.demon.co.uk/bddg.htm

SERVICES IN THE UK FOR BMA MEMBERS

BMA Counselling Service and Doctors Advisory Service: For help, counselling, and personal support just call 08459 200 169, and you will be offered the choice of speaking to a counsellor or being given the details of a doctor-adviser whom you can call directly.

Eating disorders

Jaffa, A. and McDermott, B. (Eds) (2007) *Eating Disorders in Children and Adolescents*. Cambridge: Cambridge University Press.

Treasure, J. and Schmidt, U. (Eds) (2003) *Handbook of Eating Disorders*, 2nd edition. Chichester: Wiley.

18 PERSONALITY DISORDERS

Personality is a term used to describe enduring traits and behaviours that differentiate individuals from each other. Personality traits are usually present since adolescence, are stable over time, and are evident in a range of different environments. Personality disorders, on the other hand, are mental disorders characterized by enduring patterns of inner experience and behaviour that deviate from the individual's culture and are pervasive and inflexible. A core defining feature of personality disorders is that the traits and associated behaviour are associated with significant personal, social, or occupational impairment.

CATEGORIES OR DIMENSIONS?

Doctors tend to prefer the use of categories when describing abnormal states. However, the categorical model of personality disturbance has its limitations. Criteria for categories of personality disorder frequently overlap, and clinicians often disagree on whether categories are present or not. In fact, personality is probably more accurately conceptualized in terms of variation along the 'Big 5' dimensions of neuroticism, extroversion, openness to experience, agreeableness, and conscientiousness. However, although the research evidence favours dimensions, categories lead more readily to treatment decisions and convey more vividly the disturbance demonstrated by the highly abnormal people that psychiatrists are called on to assess.

Personality disorders refer to characteristics of individuals that cause them to suffer or that cause others in society to suffer: they have been described as deeply ingrained maladaptive patterns of behaviour generally recognizable by the time of adolescence or earlier and continuing throughout most of adult life, although often becoming less obvious in middle or old age.

We are concerned here with those aspects of personality that are of particular importance to doctors: either because they **increase an individual's vulnerability** to a particular disease, or because they help us to understand **how an individual is likely to behave when he is ill**.

Possession of some of the traits can be quite adaptive: for example, mildly obsessional people make good doctors, accountants, or lawyers; mildly histrionic people are good public speakers and fun to be with; schizoid people may run a good computer system;

and dependent personalities may play supportive roles in human organizations. People with cyclothymia can be very creative during upswings of mood.

Two points must be emphasized from the outset. First, a personality disorder is not an illness, so concepts of 'treatment' and 'recovery' are simply irrelevant. It is sometimes possible to modify habitual patterns of behaviour to some extent, although typically such modification takes a great deal of time and effort if it succeeds at all. Second, by their very nature, personality disorders are dimensional rather than categorical. That is to say, there are infinitely graded steps between normality and any of the 'disorders' described below. The distinction between having and not having such a disorder is arbitrary: individuals present such traits to a greater or lesser extent, and it is possible to have some traits but not others under each heading.

SOME ABNORMAL PERSONALITY TYPES OF MEDICAL IMPORTANCE

Paranoid personality (also known as 'sensitive personality')

DESCRIPTION

The patient has displayed excessive sensitiveness to humiliations and rebuffs, a tendency to misconstrue neutral or friendly actions of others as hostile and contemptuous, and a combative and tenacious sense of personal rights. There may be proneness to jealousy or excessive self-importance. Such people feel easily humiliated and put-upon, and there is excessive self-reference. They bear grudges, and are unforgiving.

AETIOLOGY

Unknown. There is a high incidence of this disorder in first-degree relatives of patients with paranoid psychoses.

MEDICAL RELEVANCE

Those with pronounced sensitive traits are especially likely to develop ideas of reference when depressed; some will even progress to frank persecutory symptoms during illnesses that respond to treatment with antidepressants. In the general wards of the hospital such patients readily misinterpret medical advice, and may be hostile and critical about treatment given to themselves or to their relatives.

Schizoid personality

DESCRIPTION

A withdrawal from social and interpersonal contacts, with emotional coldness and a preference for fantasy and introspection. The patient will have had few friends outside his immediate family and is often indifferent to praise or criticism from others. Prefers solitary activities – such as computing. He tends to be aloof and cold, and has little enjoyment in close personal relationships and no desire for sexual experience. Rarely experiences strong emotions such as anger or joy.

AETIOLOGY

Uncertain; probably genetically related to schizophrenia. Increased incidence of schizoid personalities in the first-degree relatives of schizophrenic probands.

MEDICAL RELEVANCE

Schizoid personalities are at somewhat greater risk for developing an episode of schizophrenia, and, having developed such an illness, the prognosis will be worse. However, it must be emphasized that only a minority of schizoid personalities develop schizophrenia; and many schizophrenics have normal personalities before they become ill.

Dis-social personality (originally called 'psychopathic personality' or 'anti-social personality')

DESCRIPTION

A life-long tendency to disregard social obligations, and a lack of real feeling for other people that may show itself either in impetuous violence or in callous unconcern. The patient may be abnormally aggressive, and tends to be affectively cold and irresponsible. They tolerate frustration poorly and tend to be impulsive. They tend to blame others or offer plausible rationalizations for the behaviour that brings them into conflict with society. The assessment is made from the personal history, which will show at least four of the following features:

1. An **inability to sustain enduring relationships** with others: most easily indicated by an **unstable work record**, with significant periods of unemployment at times when work was available, repeated episodes of absence from work, or repeated episodes of walking out of jobs without good cause; and a failure to sustain a monogamous **sexual relationship** for a prolonged period of time.
2. **Failure to conform to social norms** indicated by admitting to offences that have not been detected, a repeated failure to honour financial obligations, or a *forensic history* showing episodes of larceny, destroying property, assault and so on.
3. **Low tolerance for frustration**, with irritability and aggressiveness indicated by fights, assaults, wife-beating or child abuse.
4. **A callous unconcern for the feelings of others**, and a marked tendency to blame others for behaviour that brings the patient into conflict with society. Lacks remorse.
5. **Failure to plan ahead, and impulsive behaviour**: travels without clear destination; long periods with no fixed address.
6. **No regard for truth**: repeated lying, use of aliases, or 'conning' others.

278

7, **Disregard for own personal safety and the safety of others**: drives while drunk or disqualified; recurrent speeding offences.
8 If a parent or guardian, **neglects the child**, squanders money that should be spent on the child.
9. **Recklessness, impulsiveness**, disregard for truth and lack of remorse for offences.

AETIOLOGY

Perhaps because of its enormous social importance, much work has been done on the aetiology of what has been called 'sociopathic personality'. Both genetic and environmental factors are undoubtedly important. There is a very much higher concordance for criminality in monozygotic than in dizygotic twins. Adoption studies show that adopted offspring of criminal parents have a much higher expectancy of sociopathic personality than adopted children whose biological parents were not offenders. In one Danish study the expectancy of criminality in adopted children whose biological parents were not known to the police was not affected by criminality in the father of the adopting family. However since the MZ concordance rate for criminality in twins is only about 50 per cent, it is evident that environmental factors must also be important. Criminality and social deviance in parents have repeatedly been shown in surveys of anti-social behaviour; as have conflict-ridden and 'broken' homes, lack of early training, and lack of caring supervision. Parents have repeatedly been shown to use poor disciplinary techniques: thus mothers have little control over their (delinquent) children and don't enforce obedience; while fathers are either too lax or too strict.

MEDICAL RELEVANCE

Many of the injured patients you see in an accident room on a Saturday night will either have been injured by dis-social personalities, or be dis-social personalities who have managed to injure themselves in fights. Dis-social personalities are at higher risk than others for alcoholism and drug dependence.

Emotionally unstable personality disorder (includes explosive personality; borderline personality)

DESCRIPTION

A marked tendency to act impulsively without considering the consequences, combined with easily aroused symptoms of anxiety and depression. In the **'explosive'** type, outbursts of intense anger often lead to violence with minimal provocation. The individual has outbursts of violence or threatening behaviour, often accompanied by feelings of tension. In the **'borderline'** type the same tendency for emotional instability is accompanied by chronic feelings of emptiness and a lack of clarity about emotional preferences and long-term aims. The patient's anger is often directed against the self. Intense and unstable relationships are associated with attempts to avoid abandonment, with suicidal threats and self-harm.

AETIOLOGY

Little is known.

MEDICAL RELEVANCE

'Explosive' patients often injure others, and may themselves ask for medical help in controlling their temper. They are best dealt with by teaching them **'anger management'** in which they learn to recognize early signs of becoming angry, and either remove themselves from the encounter or learn to engage in displacement activities. They sometimes derive benefit from beta blockers like **propanolol**. 'Borderline' patients most often come to medical notice in A&E departments after they have taken overdoses, or tried to harm themselves after a crisis in some interpersonal relationship. They respond poorly to most forms of medical treatment.

Histrionic personality (originally, and confusingly, called 'hysterical personality')

DESCRIPTION

The patient – who is usually female – behaves in a histrionic way, tending to exaggerate and dramatize her descriptions of both symptoms and circumstances. Aspects of her own behaviour that are inconsistent with the romanticized version she relates are either ignored or denied. Displays of emotion (both weeping and angry tantrums) commonly accompany the history – but they strike the observer as being too easily aroused, and they disappear as quickly. She tends to be egocentric in personal relationships, showing too little attention to other people's feelings to form any very deep relationships. Indeed, although she tends to be sexually provocative, her own sexual relationships tend to be unsatisfactory, and she tends to be both frigid and sexually naive. She is often an attractive girl, who has learned to be flirtatious as a way of gaining her own ends rather than as a way of initiating a sexual relationship.

DIAGNOSTIC CRITERIA

The label tends to be fixed onto any female patient who succeeds in irritating the (male) medical staff, by giving an exaggerated account of her symptoms, or who behaves in a manipulative way. This is a pity, since if the term is used in this way it becomes meaningless. In this one case we will therefore give some simplified diagnostic criteria. **All three of the following** should be present:

1. **Attention-seeking** or histrionic behaviour.
2. **Demanding interpersonal behaviour**.
3. **Displays of emotion** that are easily aroused, or more intense than the circumstances require.

AETIOLOGY

Unknown. When measured as a personality trait there appears to be no genetic component, although the disorder does tend to run in families. It can probably best be thought of as a set of behaviours that are learned by some immature girls who have been starved of parental affection. It is difficult to escape the impression that these patients use their behaviour to gain attention and admiration from older men, but there have been no systematic studies on this point.

MEDICAL RELEVANCE

The concept came about as a way of describing those thought to be at high risk for hysteria: thus the original name. Although these girls are at higher risk for conversion phenomena than those without such traits, it is now recognized that the majority of those with hysterical illnesses do not have such personalities. You are far more likely to meet these patients in the accident room than in the neurological wards. They are certainly at very high risk for manipulative and attention-seeking interpersonal behaviours, and they will arrive in hospital having poisoned themselves with drugs, or having made superficial cuts on their forearms. You should be on your guard when someone begins to behave in this way for the first time in adult life: the diagnosis is much more likely to be an affective illness than a personality disorder!

Obsessional personality (also called 'anankastic personality')

DESCRIPTION

Feelings of personal insecurity, doubt, and incompleteness lead to excessive conscientiousness, checking, stubbornness, and caution. There is perfectionism and meticulous accuracy and the need to check repeatedly in an attempt to secure this. Patients may become indecisive. They may also show unreasonable insistence that others do things their way; excessive devotion to work to the exclusion of leisure and friendships; restricted expressions of affection and a lack of generosity. Rigidity and excessive doubt may be conspicuous, and there may be insistent and unwelcome thoughts. They may be unable to discard worthless or worn-out items.

AETIOLOGY

Twin studies have shown that genetic factors are important in determining obsessional traits, and that there is an association between such traits and 'neuroticism' – which together may manifest as obsessional symptoms. Ritualistic behaviour and excessive orderliness appear to be a normal developmental stage in childhood. There is no association between such traits and coercive toilet training, although there is some association between such traits in mothers and children. One study showed that parenting practices characterized as 'restrictive warmth' were associated with children who were submissive, dependent, polite, neat, and obedient: but that is about as near as the various studies of child development seem to get to 'obsessional personality'.

MEDICAL RELEVANCE

People with obsessional traits are especially likely to develop obsessional symptoms during episodes of depressive illness: in such patients special treatment for the obsessional symptoms is not required since they will respond to antidepressants. Obsessional personalities are commonly observed in the pre-morbid personalities of those with obsessional illness (see p. 231).

Dependent personality (includes asthenic personality; passive-dependent personality)

DESCRIPTION

The patient has always let others make decisions for him, and has few resources of his own. He has difficulty initiating projects or doing things on his own. He will agree with people with whom he really disagrees to avoid disturbing a relationship, and will remain in a relationship in which he is mistreated for fear of being left alone. When a close relationship ends he is devastated and helpless, as he is often preoccupied with a fear of being abandoned. He constantly seeks reassurance and approval from others, and is easily hurt by disapproval.

AETIOLOGY

No systematic studies have been reported. Authoritarian parents, who enforce rules and edicts without discussion, have been shown to produce children who are miserable, socially withdrawn, and have low self-esteem. It is possible that this might form the basis of the adult disorder, marked as it is by resourcelessness and a desire to please dominant people.

MEDICAL RELEVANCE

These people are at high risk for depressive illness when they lose the dominant person by death or separation. Left to themselves, they may drift down the social scale and become unemployed or homeless.

HOW TO EVALUATE PERSONALITY

It is usual to divide personality types into three broad groups, each of which has several members:

- **Cluster A** (the 'odd or eccentric' types): paranoid, schizoid and schizotypal personality disorder.

- **Cluster B** (the 'dramatic, emotional or erratic' types): histrionic, narcissistic, antisocial and borderline personality disorders.
- **Cluster C** (the 'anxious and fearful' types): obsessive-compulsive, avoidant, and dependent.

It is important to be sure that the informant or patient (as their own informant) understands that this interview concerns a time of life when the patient was well. Agree on that time (e.g. 5 years ago, or before the marriage broke down) and focus the interview on that period.

Start your discussion of personality with a general screening question, like *'How does he/she get on with other people?'* Replies to this question may take you directly to the right cluster. Go on to the following, asking clarifying questions only if you have a positive reply to a screen question:

A. Odd, eccentric cluster

Does he/she trust other people?   (*Paranoid*)

- Is he/she a suspicious person who misinterprets the actions of others as threatening?
- Does he/she consistently bear grudges?

Would you describe him/her as a loner?   (*Schizoid*)

- Does he/she almost always prefer to do solitary things?
- Is he/she a detached, aloof, or cold person?

Does he/she have difficulty controlling his/her temper?   (*Dissocial*)

- Is he/she consistently irresponsible?
- Does he/she lack remorse when he/she has done something wrong?

B. 'Dramatic, emotional or erratic' cluster

Is he/she impulsive?   (*Emotionally unstable*)

- Does he/she have an unstable mood?
- Does he/she make frantic efforts to avoid abandonment?

Does he/she dislike situations where he/she is not the centre of attention? (*Histrionic*)

- Is he/she a dramatic or theatrical person?
- Do his/her emotions change rapidly (over the course of minutes or hours – not days)?

Are his/her relationships with people he/she really cares about characterized by lots of extreme ups and downs? (*Borderline*)

- Does his/her sense of who he/she is often change dramatically?
- When he/she is under stress, does he/she get suspicious of other people, or feel especially spaced out?

C. 'Anxious and fearful' cluster

Is he/she a worrier or a shy person? (*Anxious*)

- Does he/she view him/herself as inferior compared to others?
- Is he/she unwilling to get involved with people unless he/she is certain of being liked?

Does he/she depend on others a lot? (*Dependent*)

- Does he/she allow others to make most of his/her important decisions?
- Does he/she have difficulty expressing disagreement with others for fear of rejection?

Does he/she have unusually high standards at work or home? (*Anankastic*)

- Is he/she so preoccupied with details and rules that the main point of an activity gets lost?
- Does he/she insist that others do things the way he/she wants them to be done?

PART 3

DISORDERS RELATED TO STAGES OF THE LIFE CYCLE

19 DISORDERS OF EARLY LIFE: LEARNING DISABILITY

EPIDEMIOLOGY

Intellectual ability and social competence are continuously distributed variables, so there is no clear cut-off between normality and disability, or between the various degrees of disability. It became possible to examine the distribution of intelligence in a population when psychologists developed methods for measuring cognitive performance in the first half of the twentieth century. Performance on intelligence tests approximates to a Gaussian ('normal') distribution. The frequency distribution of a Gaussian curve may be described completely by the mean and standard deviation: about 95 per cent of the population falls within two standard deviations either side of the mean. IQ ('intelligence quotient') scores are adjusted so that the population mean is 100 and the standard deviation is 15. An IQ of less than 70 (i.e. two standard deviations below the mean) is generally considered subnormal. About 2.5 per cent of the population might be expected to have an IQ below 70, but in practice the figure depends on factors such as education and welfare provision.

The prevalence of IQ less than 50 is between 0.3 per cent and 0.4 per cent, and is similar wherever it has been measured. Minor changes occur from time to time because of changes in incidence and survival. For example, there has been a reduction in the proportion of pregnancies occurring in the second half of the childbearing age; this has led to a fall in the rate of **Down's syndrome** (trisomy 21) births. On the other hand, factors such as cardiac surgery, treatment of childhood infections, and improvements in social care have led to increased survival in Down's syndrome. Demographic factors are responsible for some of the minor variation in prevalence from place to place. For example, families with disabled members have different patterns of migration compared to the rest of the population, and tend not to move from inner cities that are otherwise becoming depopulated, so in the UK the prevalence in cities is higher than in rural areas.

Most studies show a male preponderance among people with a learning disability. Mild and moderate disability are well known to be associated with low socioeconomic status. Early studies of severe disability showed no association with socioeconomic status; a weak association is evident in more recent studies.

TERMINOLOGY

A distinction has always been made between disorders of mental functioning that are developmental and those that are acquired. By definition, developmental disorders are first evident in infancy, childhood, or adolescence, and lead to permanent impairment of function. This chapter concerns developmental disorders of intellectual ability and adaptive behaviour.

Historically many terms have been used to describe individuals with learning disabilities: natural fool, idiot, imbecile, and moron to name but a few. The nineteenth and early twentieth century use of the term 'mongol' for someone with Down's syndrome (suggesting that sufferers had 'retrogressed' to share features with the supposedly less advanced Mongolian race) serves as a salutary reminder that the medical profession is as capable of prejudice as any other. Other defunct and obsolescent terms have been introduced by educationalists and by legislators (e.g. educational subnormality, mental subnormality, and mental impairment).

The term **mental retardation** is widely used (including in ICD-10) for developmental disorders including combinations of cognitive, linguistic, motor, and social skills. This term is understood internationally, but even this has a connotation of stigma in some cultures. As a result the United Kingdom Department of Health introduced the term **learning disability** to replace the term mental retardation in the 1990s, and this is the term we use in the remainder of this chapter. Such terminological variation is problematic (1) because it is necessary to discuss patients' difficulties with colleagues, patients and their families with stable meaning, and (2) because the relevant terminology varies across national boundaries, so there is a possibility of misunderstanding. In the UK the term 'learning disability' remains current and appears likely to be in use for some time.

CLINICAL FEATURES

There are three main features, all of which must be present for a diagnosis of learning disability (mental retardation in ICD-10):

1. Impairment of intelligence.
2. Impairment of adaptive behaviour.
3. Onset before adulthood.

Intelligence is not easy to define, and there is some truth in the old adage 'intelligence is whatever intelligence tests measure'. Nevertheless, it is obviously concerned with speed of understanding and the ability to learn from experience. Other aspects include focusing attention (concentrating), registering, retaining and recalling information, and thinking. In a clinical setting, impairment of intelligence is often detected by attending to the complexity of language that a patient uses and understands, and how the patient compares to their similar-aged peers in adaptive or academic performance.

By definition, a person with a learning disability will have a significant impairment of adaptive and social functioning that may affect their ability to act or live independently. It is helpful to remember five areas of skills required for various degrees of independence: *self-care, domestic activity, communication, social skills,* and *coping with stress.* Deficits may be found in some or all of these, and the diagnosis of a learning disability depends as much on their quantification as it does on quantification of IQ. Specific rating scales exist for this purpose.

It should be noted that some developmental disorders affect aspects of cognitive development without necessarily giving rise to a learning disability (in the sense of an ICD-10 diagnosis of mental retardation), in particular autism spectrum and hyperkinetic disorders (attention deficit hyperactivity disorder). Moreover, several forms of *specific* developmental disorders of scholastic skills (e.g. *specific* disorders of reading, spelling, or arithmetical skills) may cause a person without a learning disability to require special education or social support.

DIAGNOSTIC CRITERIA

The classification of learning disability is not without problems. IQ measurements have limited reliability, and an incomplete correlation with practical and social competence. The IQ should be determined from standardized, individually administered intelligence tests for which local and cultural norms have been determined, and the test should be appropriate to the individual's level of functioning and additional deficits (e.g. expressive language problems and hearing impairment, if present). The criteria below are best thought of as clinical guidelines, not absolute rules. The age at which mental development is regarded as stable is arbitrary; international classifications use the age of 18, but in clinical practice, leaving school is the dividing line.

Mild learning disability is defined by IQ measurements in the range of 50 to 69. It accounts for 2–3 per cent of the population, and 75 per cent of all people with learning disability. In general, affected individuals acquire language with some delay, but can generally use speech for everyday purposes. Individuals in this category are able to cope with self-care and domestic activity independently most of the time, but may have problems when faced with new or complex situations, as executive speech problems interfere with independence. They are most likely to present to services such as GPs if they are faced with stress (e.g. minor illness) and are unable to cope, but they may not necessarily come to the attention of specialist services. Such people are usually able to learn simple occupational skills, but may have problems with the social skills required for employment. Common problems include budgeting, planning a healthy menu, and using the health service to best effect.

Moderate learning disability is defined by IQ measurements in the range of 35 to 49. In general, people with moderate learning disability need supervision or assistance with complex activities, such as cooking, but the level of support needed is usually within the resources and abilities of families with no special training. They can usually participate

289

in simple conversations and can communicate their basic needs, although some never learn to use language. An organic aetiology can be identified in a majority, and the majority will have been considered to have special educational needs. These people are likely to require specialist services if there is not a high degree of family support.

Severe learning disability is defined by IQ measurements in the range of 20 to 34. People with severe learning disability are unable to cope independently because they need supervision or assistance with skills required for independence (self-care, domestic, social, communication, and coping with stress). Most will require supervision by a responsible person on a daily basis; they are overwhelmingly likely to be detected at school as having special educational needs. The great majority come to the attention of specialist services at some time, as they usually have a marked degree of motor impairment or other deficits indicating maldevelopment of the CNS.

Profound learning disability accounts for less than 0.1 per cent of the population, and 5 per cent of all people with learning disabilities. IQ testing is unreliable at this level of ability, where the person's development of language and other skills is equivalent to a normal child of 2 years or less, but it is estimated to be under 20. Comprehension of language is limited, at best, to understanding simple commands. An organic aetiology can be identified in the majority of cases; severe neurological and physical disability is common. Such people require assistance with all areas of life, including some skills required for basic survival (e.g. feeding, clothing).

AETIOLOGY

There are more than two thousand disorders recognized that can lead to learning disability, and it is hopeless to try to remember them all. Instead, it is better to think in terms of an aetiological framework that will enable you to conduct a rational investigation in any particular patient. One such considers the onset of the cause of disability to be prenatal, perinatal, postnatal, or unknown (see *Table 19.1*).

Figures are not available for developing countries, but it is known that **maternal malnutrition, dietary insufficiency of iodine**, and **inadequate perinatal care** are major causes of disability. In Western Europe 'birth trauma' is an uncommon cause. Despite recent controversy there is no significant evidence that childhood vaccinations are implicated in the aetiology of learning disability or childhood autism.

Down's syndrome

The commonest single cause of learning disability, which accounts for the overwhelming majority of chromosomal causes of severe and profound disability, is **Down's syndrome**. This is a result of trisomy 21, and demonstrates the classical increase in incidence with increasing maternal age. Diagnostic characteristics include oblique eye fissures with epicanthic folds, hypotonia, a flat nasal bridge, a single palmar crease, a protruding tongue, and Brushfield spots (white spots on the iris). There has been a sharp increase in

Table 19.1 *The relative frequencies of causes of learning disability in Western Europe (adapted from various sources)*

Aetiology	Severe and profound mental retardation (%)	Mild and moderate mental retardation (%)
Prenatal	60	35
Chromosomal	35	15
Single gene	5	1
Alcohol	0	8
Infection	7	0
Other	13	9
Perinatal	15	18
Postnatal	10	2
Unknown	15	55

the number of cases of Down's syndrome detected prenatally since the 1980s. The diagnosis may be confirmed by examining the chromosomes of cultured leucocytes.

Fragile-X syndrome

Fragile-X syndrome is now known to be the second commonest cause of learning disability. It accounts for 10 per cent of mild learning disability and 6 per cent of more severe learning disability in boys, and a small proportion in girls. It is a familial condition associated with a gene whose length increases with successive generations, and with a 'fragile' site on the X chromosome, detectable by examining chromosomes in leucocytes cultured under special conditions. The length of the gene is correlated with the degree of intellectual impairment. Dysmorphic features include macro-orchidism, large ears, a long face, and a high-arched palate.

Less common causes

Further details of the many conditions associated with learning disability should be obtained from a paediatric text. Conditions that are important because they are treatable if detected early include **hypothyroidism, phenylketonuria**, some **metabolic disorders** (e.g. hypernatraemia resulting from incorrectly formulated feeds), and some **infections**. Doctors treating pregnant women should be aware of the risks caused by **alcohol, drugs** (especially anticonvulsants), and **radiation** (including diagnostic radiography).

Most people with more severe learning disability are disabled as a result of a biological impairment, but no biological impairment can be detected in about half of people with mild learning disability in whom there is likely to be a relatively greater aetiological contribution from **social deprivation** and **poverty**.

It is important to remember that where the distribution of a variable is Gaussian, by definition approximately 2.5 per cent of the values lie at more than two standard deviations below the mean. Therefore, if a statistical approach is taken, approximately 2.5 per cent of the population will always have 'subnormal' intelligence, whatever their absolute intelligence.

DIFFERENTIAL DIAGNOSIS

1. Developmental Disorders without impaired intelligence
   - **Communication problems**: Any disorder that impairs communication may lead to an underestimation of the person's intelligence; these include sensory impairments (deafness, blindness), motor impairments (cerebral palsy), other speech impairments (deformities of the mouth such as cleft palate), and other disorders that affect cognitive function (autism, hyperkinetic disorder, and specific learning disabilities).
   - **Emotional dependency**: People who are more dependent than expected for their chronological age may have the skills they require, yet fail to use them for some reason.
2. Acquired impairment of intelligence
   - **Dementia** may occur at any age, and dementia before the age of 18 leads to learning disability. There are a wide range of metabolic and infective causes of childhood dementia. Non-progressive loss of cognitive function may be caused by brain injury that may be traumatic, toxic (e.g. heavy metals, alcohol), infective (e.g. herpes encephalitis), anoxic, and so on.
3. Acquired disorders without impairment of intelligence
   Severe psychiatric illness may cause impairment of social functioning, and in some cases the person may have slowing or inhibition of cognitive function, or appear to have intellectual impairment, because of poor concentration or lack of cooperation with testing. This non-specific phenomenon most notably occurs with schizophrenia and depression.
4. Impaired social functioning, but no intellectual disorder
   - **Lack of education** may mean that a person has not acquired the skills required for independence, especially if their intelligence is at the lower end of the normal range.
   - **Lack of opportunity** resulting from living in a very restricted environment (such as a prison or an institution) may have the same effect.
   - **'Functional behaviour'**, in other words, behaviour that serves a purpose (whether or not the person is aware of it), may sometimes convey the impression of learning disability. This is uncommon, and occurs mainly when a person is strongly motivated to avoid unwelcome responsibilities or demands; for example, a person charged with murder who wishes the charge to be reduced to manslaughter.

INVESTIGATIONS

Assessment of social and practical competence

In ordinary clinical practice, the method of assessing competence is to ask the patient about their 'typical day', and to seek confirmation and elaboration from an informant. Details should be obtained concerning rising, washing, choosing clothes, dressing, preparing breakfast, eating, clearing up, going out, using transport and roads, attending a place of occupation or education, shopping and using money, eating away from home, returning home, cooking, leisure, and recreation. For each activity, the degree of independence may be:

- Unsupervised.
- Checked after the event.
- Prompted and checked.
- Physically prompted or helped.
- Done for the person by another.

It is important to distinguish between activities that the person cannot do despite having the opportunity, and those that they never have the opportunity to try.

Specialist services use standardized assessments that yield a profile of the person's abilities, and indicate the areas to focus on for further training.

Developmental history

The patient's parents (often but not always the mother) can provide most detail about their child's cognitive and motor histories. Unfortunately, memory is unreliable, and it is vital to obtain and record this information at the earliest opportunity. Paediatric and community child health records are invaluable, and developmental records of disabled children should be preserved. Problems during pregnancy, delivery and the neonatal period should be elicited, as should the ages at which developmental milestones are reached. It is important to memorize some basic cognitive, social and motor milestones for 'internal' reference. We suggest the ones shown in *Table 19.2*.

Psychometric assessments (measurement of cognitive ability)

Where cognitive delay is unequivocal and associated with obvious deficits in adaptive function, it may not be necessary to perform IQ testing in order to establish a diagnosis of learning disability. Nevertheless, such testing is advisable as it may provide a baseline against which to measure possible future change. Where the disability is mild or equivocal an IQ test using a standardized instrument should always be performed (usually by a clinical psychologist trained in administration). More detailed testing of component psychological functions (e.g. of memory, executive function) should be performed if:

1. There appears to be a substantial variation between one aspect of a person's ability and another.
2. There is a history of disturbed/challenging behaviour (e.g. executive deficits may underlie impulsive or disinhibited behaviour).
3. There is a suspicion of cognitive decline and such testing is being used to explore the hypothesis that the patient is dementing.

Table 19.2 *Developmental milestones (adapted from the Denver Developmental Screening Test)*

	6 months	12 months	24 months
Posture and large movements	Pulls to sit with no head lag	Walks to the side holding furniture	Kicks ball forwards
Vision and fine movements	Watches adult move, reaches for toy	Grasps with thumb and finger	Scribbles spontaneously
Hearing and language	Vocalizes with two syllables	Imitates speech sounds	Points to one named body part
Social behaviour and play	Smiles spontaneously	Initially shy with strangers	Uses spoon, spilling little

In addition, data relating to diverse cognitive functions may be particularly useful in planning rehabilitative strategies.

Special investigations

An attempt should always be made to diagnose the cause of the disability. In childhood, the cause may be remediable, and in adulthood may have significance for the onset of physical or mental illness (e.g. Down's syndrome is associated with early onset Alzheimer's disease). It is also very likely to be important in determining how to advise family members planning to have children.

Most 'diagnosable' disorders are identified in childhood by neonatologists, paediatricians, clinical geneticists, psychiatrists, or biochemists. A strategy for planning investigations should be based on available clinical signs. Where these do not exist, the search strategy should be based on relative aetiological frequency (see *Table 19.2*, above). As a minimum, investigation should include chromosomal analysis, urine and blood screens for the more common inborn errors of metabolism (these days using tandem mass spectrometry), and investigations for infective intrauterine causes of learning disability (including toxoplasmosis, rubella, cytomegalovirus, herpes simplex virus, and syphilis; remember the acronym TORCHES).

TREATMENT

When developmental delay is first detected, it is important that the news is broken to parents in a sensitive way. This means telling them the facts at a speed and in a language that they can understand. As a rule, parents should be told jointly, in private, at the earliest opportunity after a problem is suspected. This will usually be done by a paediatrician, although it might be done by a GP. Non-technical language should be used, and it is important to realize that people retain only a very small amount of information when they first hear unwelcome news. There must be a follow-up interview soon, and preferably a written report for the parents. If a heritable condition is detected, families should be offered referral to a clinical genetics service.

Some conditions leading to learning disability are susceptible to medical treatment during childhood (e.g. phenylketonuria). In later life, people with learning disabilities are entitled to the same standard of medical care as the rest of the population. While they have higher rates of some illnesses, they use medical services proportionally less than the rest of the population. People with learning disabilities therefore require additional support in accessing health surveillance and screening.

Associated health problems may be considered under three headings:

1. **Specific associations**: For example, **Down's syndrome** (trisomy 21) is associated with cardiac defects, obesity, respiratory tract infections, conductive deafness, skin problems (acne), chronic lymphatic leukaemia, Alzheimer's disease (leading to dementia, epilepsy, and early death), and hypothyroidism.

    Other examples (among many) include congenital **rubella syndrome**, which is associated with deafness, blindness, and cardiac defects, and congenital **hypothyroidism**, which is associated with deafness.
2. **Shared aetiologies**: The presence of learning disability should make the physician alert to the possibility of associated neurological abnormality that may be manifest in epilepsy, sensory impairment, motor impairment (cerebral palsy), autism, or hyperkinetic disorder. People with learning disabilities have a significantly increased risk of mental illness, partly because of impaired brain function.
3. **Increased susceptibility**: People with learning disability are more likely than the rest of the population to live in social circumstances that carry risks to health. They are more likely to live in poverty, subject to crime, exploitation and cruelty, and are likely to be unemployed and unmarried. Some still live in large institutions, with associated risks of TB, hepatitis, and malnutrition. Even where they receive good general care, inappropriate demands may be made of people without sufficient intellectual resources, leading to stress-related illness. Alternatively, there may be a paucity of appropriate activity, resulting in institutionalization and social impoverishment.

The majority of people with learning disabilities are likely to require support with:

1. Housing. A person with a disability needs supported housing, such as a substitute family or a staffed house, or a house with support from a neighbour or a warden.
2. Education. People with learning disabilities have special educational needs and should be able to receive appropriate primary, secondary, and continuing education.
3. Occupation. There are various ways of supporting disabled workers in the workplace, or in sheltered sections of the workplace, or in wholly sheltered workshops.
4. Leisure and recreation. Sports and social activities also offer opportunities for personal and social development.

Other support needs may include:

1. Prevention of primary and secondary disability.
2. Specialized interventions to address sensory, motor, communication, and behavioural problems.

3.   Advocacy.
4.   Family support, respite care, holidays, and family advocacy.

Services are provided by social service and education departments of local authorities, and by community support teams for people with learning disabilities (sometimes called community learning disability teams). General practitioners are responsible for a person's primary health care, and may refer to consultants in psychiatry of learning disability, or to child psychiatrists or neurologists as appropriate.

COURSE AND PROGNOSIS

The course of a learning disability depends on the interaction between the pathology causing the disability, and the treatment, education, training, and support the person receives. Most developmental disorders are stable in adult life, with a tendency to progressive improvement. Behavioural problems coming to medical or social agency attention are much less common after the age of 25 to 30. People who receive suitable education, training, and care, and who receive treatment for intercurrent illness, often do well, with gradually increasing independence. Nevertheless, morbidity and mortality remain substantially above baseline rates.

FURTHER READING

Gelder, M., Lopez-Ibor, J. and Andreasen, N. (2003) *The New Oxford Textbook of Psychiatry*. Oxford: Oxford University Press.
(This book provides further information on psychiatry for learning disability.)

Jones, K.L. (1997) *Smith's Recognizable Patterns of Human Malformation*. Philadelphia: W.B. Saunders.
(This is the standard reference text in human dysmorphology.)

The reader will be aware of the pace of genetic and biochemical research into single gene disorders. Some of these disorders are responsible for inherited learning disability. All physicians these days should be familiar with the superb web resource *Online Mendelian Inheritance in Man* (www.ncbi.nlm.nih.gov/omim) for its utility in this as well as in many other fields of medicine.

20   CHILDHOOD AND ADOLESCENCE

Understanding psychiatric presentations in children requires an understanding of normal development and the range of normal emotions and behaviours present at each age. Some disorders represent abnormalities in terms of degree, or presentations that are outside the norm for a child's age, whereas others are qualitatively abnormal; that is to say they involve features that are abnormal at any stage of development. Emotional and behavioural problems are very common during childhood and adolescence. They are considered disorders when they cause suffering, affect education or relationships, or seriously interfere with development; that is, when they pass a threshold of impairment.

ASSESSMENT

Assessment in child and adolescent mental health is a complex task requiring the ability to synthesize verbal and non-verbal information obtained from several sources.
The aims of assessment are:

- To engage the young person and family.
- To gather information on the nature and extent of the child's difficulties.
- To assess the young person's mental health and evaluate risk arising from it.
- To plan further steps in assessment and management.
- To agree a formulation and treatment plan with the family, including obtaining their consent.
- To communicate one's findings with other professionals.

Preparation

Consideration should be given to the setting of the assessment, its age appropriateness, and the importance of privacy. Arrangements for the use of interpreters or translators should be made in advance.

Engagement

Use of leaflets and other written material can provide information for parents and young people, prior to the appointment. The introductions should explain the basic premise for the assessment, how long you will be meeting for, how the time will be structured, and the use of cameras or one-way screens, if applicable. For younger children, permission or encouragement to use toys should be given. Explanation should be given around the boundaries of confidentiality. A neutral non-judgemental approach to the referral problem should be used, especially when adolescents are being assessed, or when the child's behaviour is being complained about.

Gathering information

Assessment information is usually gathered through meetings with the child alone, and with parents and/or other family members. An interview with the parents is often conducted and other sources of information consulted. The stages involved are these:

1. The joint (family) **interview**.
2. The **parental interview**.
3. The **interview with the child**.
4. Obtaining **other sources of information**.

THE JOINT INTERVIEW

It is often helpful to see all of the family together at the start of the assessment. Conjoint interviews provide a way of setting the scene, engaging family members, and observing interactions between them. The extent of agreement between family members about the nature of difficulties can be gauged. The interviewer can assess how the parents respond to the child's communications (e.g. sympathetically, critically), and form a view of relationships within the family. The interviewer should avoid exclusive questioning of individuals, but should set up opportunities for interactions between family members. This can be achieved by setting the family a task, such as drawing the family tree, or by asking questions that encourage such interactions. This is also a good time to establish the background to the referral and to identify who is concerned about the child and in what way.

THE PARENTAL INTERVIEW

It is invariably important to gain a background history and understanding of the presenting complaint from a parent or carer. With an older child or adolescent this will usually be carried out in their presence, but parents of younger children may be seen alone. The interview with the parents should start with open questions to obtain the history of the presenting complaint. Try to clarify precisely what the parent means, and distinguish observation from inference. Is the situation getting better or worse? What effects have the child's problems had on schoolwork, peer relationships, and the family? How long has there been a problem?

Next it is necessary to cover systematically the child's recent health and behaviour (but bear in mind that parents do not have direct knowledge of the child's mental state, and may be unaware of important symptoms such as suicidal ideation). Direct enquiry should be made about each of the following areas: *emotional symptoms* (anxiety, fears, depression, suicidality); *behavioural problems* (stealing, aggression, disobedience, fighting, truancy, running away); *attention and concentration*; *motor skills* (activity level, clumsiness); *fits or faints*; *abnormal movements*; *school performance* (attendance, bullying, relationships with teachers); *peer and sibling relationships*; *bladder and bowel control*; *physical health* (appetite, weight, sleep, major illnesses); *recent adversity* (e.g. bereavement or separations).

The family history should then be obtained. It is especially important to know about mental illness or personality problems in the parents. Find out about the parents' relationship, including marital problems. If the parents have separated, obtain details. Does the child have continuing contact with the non-custodial parent? How have family members adjusted to the introduction of step-parents or siblings? To whom is the child closest?

The child's family life and relationships should be enquired about next. Key areas here include disciplinary practices, family activities that involve the child, and the child's role in the family.

Ask next about the child's personal history. Where was he or she born? Were there any problems during the pregnancy or delivery? Enquire about birth weight, neonatal problems, and immunizations. Have there been any early separations or attachment difficulties? Ask about motor and language milestones, major illnesses, and schools attended.

Finally, ask about the child's temperamental characteristics. Has the child always been a regular sleeper and eater? How well does the child adapt to new situations? Does he or she show strong emotions? Is the child habitually sociable, or inhibited and slow to warm up?

THE INTERVIEW WITH THE CHILD OR ADOLESCENT

There are two main aims in this part of the assessment; to achieve a sympathetic understanding of the young person's point of view, and to make a full assessment of their mental state. A good rapport and communication are essential both to complete the assessment and also as a prelude to future therapeutic work. An understanding of normal developmental milestones (especially with young children) is important in order that speech, coordination, motor skills and social functioning can be evaluated. Very young children might best be assessed in their parents' company throughout.

An explanation should be given to the child that this is a 'private' interview in which they have an opportunity to describe what they think and feel, however one should not give a false impression of complete confidentiality. It should be clear that the detail of the interview is confidential, but that the clinician may need to discuss certain issues that arise from the assessment with parents, but that you will tell them what these are. Occasionally a clear conflict arises, for example if a young person discloses serious abuse, suicidal plans, or high-risk behaviours.

For younger children, it is helpful to explain that you would like to spend some time on your own with them and to describe what you will be doing, for example, 'playing with these toys together' or 'talking and doing some drawing'. Older children from middle childhood onwards can be asked gently about the problem at hand, after putting them at ease, or maybe starting the conversation on other more general topics. It is important to use simple age-appropriate language and clear questions (closed questions are used more often than with adults).

It may be possible with older children to follow a similar procedure as used to examine an adult's mental state, but in young children formal examination of the mental state is often difficult. Every opportunity should be taken to observe the child's behaviour, and this should be recorded systematically and objectively. Do not forget to obtain the child's view of the situation, including their likes, dislikes, and hopes for the future. Establishing a useful conversation with the child requires you to show warmth, interest, and respect for the child. Approach emotive topics gradually and carefully and use language that is appropriate.

THE MENTAL STATE

General behaviour

Dress and appearance.
(*Is the child appropriately and cleanly dressed?*)

Parent–child interaction and separation.
(*What is the parents' manner with the child; is there any evidence of separation difficulty?*)

Emotional responsiveness and relationship with the interviewer.
(*Describe your own feelings about the quality of your interaction with the child*)

Habitual mannerisms.
(*Does the child have tics, or stereotypic movements or mannerisms?*)

Description of the course of the interview.
(*What went on: drawing, play, tears, temper?*)

Anxiety and mood

Signs of tension and sadness.
(*Include facial expression, apprehension, tearfulness*)

Whether preoccupied by fears, worries, depressive thoughts.
Whether restless, disinhibited, assertive, aggressive.
Whether apathetic, withdrawn, or shy.

Talk (form)

Spontaneity, flow.
(Is speech painfully difficult to elicit, is the child overly talkative; or is the flow and exchange of talk normal?)

Defects of prosody, articulation, or sentence structure.

Coherence.
(Can you follow what is being said, or does it lose its point?)

Talk (content)

Attention or persistence.
(Whether easily distracted; whether interrupted by preoccupying thoughts or by hallucinatory experience)

Degree and duration of interests in topics, activities or objects.
(Does the child flit quickly from one topic to another?)

Spontaneous interruptions of attention.
(Is speech suddenly arrested, the point lost?)

Activity Level

Gross activity.
(In particular, whether 'over-active' or 'hyperkinetic')

Intellectual Function

Obtain a rough assessment of reading level, spelling, arithmetic, writing, general knowledge.
The child can be asked to write their name and address, draw a man, copy a triangle, a diamond, a cross, and a circle.
If there are concerns, testing by a clinical or educational psychologist should be arranged, including assessment of basic intellectual ability, educational attainments, and specific learning problems.

Other sources of information

Obtain (with parental consent) a school report or, for younger children, an account from nursery school or play group. School can provide results of standardized assessment tests (SATS), and information on behaviour and peer relations. Any other agencies who are involved with the child or the family (such as medical and social services) should be contacted (again with consent).

THE FORMULATION

Aetiology

PREDISPOSING FACTORS

A child's vulnerability to psychiatric disorders is increased by several factors. Genetic influences can be *direct*, as in the parent–child transmission of schizophrenia, or *indirect*, as when a child's temperamental characteristics lead to parental rejection, which in turn leads to disorder. The *goodness of fit* between a child's characteristics and the environment seems to be especially important. For instance, difficult children who are brought up in stable, warm families are at lower risk of behavioural disorders than difficult children who are brought up in unstable, discordant families. Children with generalized learning difficulties or specific delays in development such as reading retardation are at increased risk of psychiatric disturbance.

The child's early attachment relationships to the parents are also of importance. Brief disruptions of this relationship during infancy do not usually carry serious long-term consequences. Indeed, as long as alternative care is adequate, many children can survive even severe disruptions of attachment without psychological damage. However, separations that are followed by chronic lack of care, or were preceded by severe family disruption, can lead to insecure attachment, which may in turn predispose the infant to problems later in childhood. Other causes of abnormalities of attachment include parental mental illness, parental personality disorder, and being brought up in care.

PRECIPITANTS AND MAINTAINING FACTORS

Psychiatric disorders in children are commonly precipitated by adversities. Factors within the family may include marital difficulties or separations. Parental mental illness is also strongly associated with disturbance in children, mainly because it leads to impaired quality of parental care. For example, depressed mothers are less able to respond to their child's needs and provide less consistent discipline. Emotional and sexual abuse are also important precipitants.

Factors outside the family may include educational failure or bullying. Sometimes physical injury can trigger an emotional or behavioural disorder. For instance, severe head injuries may have a direct effect on brain function, while injuries that prevent a child taking part in sports may have an effect on self-esteem.

STRENGTHS AND PROTECTIVE FACTORS

The strengths and assets within the child and family should be recorded so these can be worked with.

Diagnosis

Different components of the child's problems are recorded separately using a **multi-axial framework**:

302

1. **Psychiatric syndromes.**
2. **Specific developmental disorders.**
3. **Intellectual level.**
4. **Medical conditions.**
5. **Abnormal psychosocial situations.**

The use of this framework makes it much easier to devise a precise formulation of the child's difficulties. Thus, a child with conduct disorder (axis 1), specific reading disorder (axis 2) and epilepsy (axis 4) from a home in which there is parental conflict (axis 5), would receive a coding in four areas.

PSYCHIATRIC SYNDROMES

Disorders in children and adolescents can be broadly classified into three groups: **emotional disorders**, **disruptive behaviour disorders**, and **developmental disorders**. Comorbidity is common particularly with conditions in the same group. Thus depressed children commonly have other emotional symptoms such as anxiety, and children with hyperkinetic disorder often have conduct problems. In adolescence young people may present with adult mental illnesses such as schizophrenia and bipolar disorder as well as abnormalities of personality development.

Emotional disorders

Emotional disorders comprise anxiety disorders, phobias, mood disorders, obsessive compulsive disorder, and somatization disorders. Most anxiety and phobic disorders of childhood are exaggerations of normal developmental trends. For example, it is normal for pre-school children to show a degree of anxiety over separation from people to whom they are attached. When this anxiety becomes severe, or persists beyond the usual age period, *separation anxiety disorder* may be diagnosed. Similarly, when stranger anxiety (which is also normal in toddlers) persists beyond the pre-school years and/or is associated with impairment, the diagnosis of *social anxiety disorder* is justified. In adolescence generalized anxiety becomes less common, but when it does occur it usually takes the form of school refusal, social phobia, or agoraphobia.

EPIDEMIOLOGY

Anxiety disorders are among the most common psychiatric problems in childhood, occurring in about 3 per cent of 10 year olds.

AETIOLOGY

Genetic and temperamental factors are of some importance, with children who are constitutionally 'slow to warm up' and inhibited being at greatest risk. The parents are often anxious, and communicate their anxiety by behaviours such as over-protectiveness. Some anxiety disorders, especially specific fears, may be precipitated by stressful life events.

TREATMENT

Treatment consists of the reduction of stress, behavioural treatment of specific symptoms (e.g. graded exposure to the feared situation), and general treatments for anxiety such as relaxation. Anxiolytics may occasionally be helpful for severe cases, but should not be prescribed for long periods. The prognosis of anxiety disorder is usually good, but about one third will subsequently have another episode. Adult type anxiety disorders arising in adolescence (such as agoraphobia) have a worse prognosis.

Mood disorders

Depressive disorders occur relatively rarely in pre-pubertal children, but by mid-adolescence the prevalence rises to about 4 per cent in boys and 8 per cent in girls. The main clinical features are similar to those found in adult depression, but pre-pubertal children have more somatic complaints and anxiety than their adolescent or adult counterparts. Biological symptoms such as weight loss are uncommon. Mania is extremely uncommon in pre-pubertal children, but about 10 per cent of adults with bipolar disorder have had their first episode in adolescence.

Children and adolescents with depressive disorders commonly have parents who are depressed, but these links are a reflection of environmental factors (such as parenting problems) as well as genetic predisposition. Depression in young people is often precipitated by adversity.

Suicide is very rare before puberty, amounting to only 1 in 200 deaths in this age group. By late adolescence it is the second commonest cause of mortality, accounting for 14 per cent of deaths. **Self-harm** is much more common, overdosage often being an impulsive act that draws attention to an unsatisfactory situation rather than the result of depressive disorder. Cutting rarely has suicidal intent, but any presentation with self-harm should result in a careful risk assessment.

TREATMENT

Treatment consists of reducing this adversity, individual psychological interventions such as cognitive-behaviour therapy (which can be administered to children of 10 years and older), and/or family therapy. Antidepressants may be useful for severe adolescent depression, but should be used with caution because of the dangers of overdose and the unpredictable nature of unwanted effects. Most depressed children will recover in a few months, but relapse is common.

Obsessive compulsive disorder

The presentation of OCD in childhood is remarkably similar to the disorder in adults, with typical rituals and ruminations, chiefly around contamination, cleaning, checking, touching, and pursuit of symmetry. Depression and anxiety are common associated features. Family members may be drawn into complying with rituals and demands for reassurance.

Individual cognitive-behavioural approaches are the mainstay of **treatment**, supported by family therapy/parental counselling.

Somatization disorders

Unexplained physical symptoms, such as abdominal pain and headaches, are present in a substantial proportion of children attending medical services. Emotional disorders are found in excess in such children, but most of them are not otherwise psychiatrically disturbed. They tend to come from families in which there are health problems and high academic expectations. In many cases the child is in some kind of *predicament* in which other avenues have been blocked. For instance, the child may feel unable to perform academically according to family expectations. Pre-existing physical problems in the child or in a relative may determine the kind of symptomatology that is shown.

Treatment involves close liaison between the psychiatrist and the paediatrician, changing the family focus from physical to psychological issues, and an emphasis on leading as normal a life as possible (such as returning to school).

Disruptive behaviour disorders

CONDUCT DISORDER

Conduct disorder is characterized by **persistent anti-social behaviour**, generally lasting at least 12 months. In the majority of epidemiological studies it is the most common child psychiatric syndrome, though whether it should be seen as a health problem is controversial. Defiance and aggression are common features. In older age groups behaviours such as stealing, truancy, fighting, lying, and running away are seen. In the most severe cases there may be fire-setting or cruelty to animals or other children. Conduct disorder is usually associated with poor peer relationships, but sometimes occurs in children who are generally well integrated into their peer group.

Epidemiology

Conduct disorders occur in about 5 per cent of 10-year-olds living in cities, with lower rates in rural areas. They are twice as common in boys as in girls.

Aetiology

There is a strong link between conduct disorder and family factors, especially discordant intrafamilial relationships and personality disorder in one of the parents. Parents are often inconsistent in applying rules, and are frequently very critical and rejecting of the child. The role of genetic factors is unclear, though temperamentally 'difficult' babies

305

seem to be at greater risk of behavioural problems later in life. About one-third of children with conduct disorder have specific reading disorder, and educational failure is common.

Treatment

The kind of treatment that is offered will depend very much on the presenting problem and on the commitment of the parent/s. Behavioural modification techniques may be effective, especially in younger children with few symptoms. Parent management training has promising results when focusing on desired behaviour and improving parent–child relationships. Medication is of little value. Children with conduct disorder commonly cause substantial disruption in the community, and it is often necessary to work closely with other agencies such as the school, social services, and the courts. The outcome of conduct disorder is variable. Children with few symptoms and good peer relationships often do well. Children with an early onset, poor peer relationships, and a large number of symptoms are at risk of personality disorder and delinquency. Almost all adults with anti-social personality disorder or delinquency have had conduct disorder as children.

OPPOSITIONAL DEFIANT DISORDER

In young children, conduct problems tend to be dominated by markedly oppositional behaviour such as defiance, hostility, and disruptiveness that is clearly outside the normal range. Children often lose their temper, argue with adults, and deliberately annoy others. They are often spiteful and vindictive and shift the blame onto others when challenged.

Treatment

Similar family risk factors to other conduct disorders apply, and parent management training is the treatment of choice.

HYPERACTIVITY

Hyperkinetic disorders are characterized by the early onset of *over-active behaviour* and *marked inattention*, often accompanied by *impulsiveness*. To diagnose the disorder these features should be evident in more than one situation (e.g. home, clinic, classroom) and persist over time. The diagnosis is difficult to make in children under the age of 5 as there is wide normal variation in activity levels in this age group. Hyperkinetic disorders are associated with an increased risk of conduct disorder and learning difficulties.

Epidemiology

Prevalence estimates have varied widely over time and between countries, as a result of differences in diagnostic practice, but current estimates give a rate of around 2 per cent. Boys are three times as likely to have the disorder as girls.

Aetiology

Family and twin studies suggest genetic factors are important in the aetiology. Brain dysfunction as evidenced for example by epilepsy is common, but most children with hyperactivity have no evidence of brain damage. Additives in the diet have also been implicated, but attempts to prove an association have not generally been successful. Hyperkinesis may sometimes be the result of early social deprivation and institutional rearing.

Treatment

The first step in treatment is to counsel the parents on the probable importance of biological factors. Behaviour modification programmes that aim to encourage the child to concentrate for increasingly lengthy periods can be effective, especially when they are carried out at school as well as at home. Stimulant medication, such as methylphenidate, is very effective in moderate to severe cases without emotional symptoms, though side-effects such as sleep disturbance and reduced appetite may occur. Many parents will have tried diets of one kind or another, and if these are not too restrictive and the parents feel they have helped then it is sensible to continue them.

DEVELOPMENTAL DISORDERS

These comprise delays or abnormalities in maturational development most of which are not psychiatric disorders in themselves, but are conveniently considered here as they pose a risk for psychiatric syndromes.

Pervasive disorders

Mental retardation (learning disability) – see Chapter 19.

Autistic disorders

This group of disorders is characterized by:

1. An onset **before the age of 3** years.
2. Grossly **abnormal social interactions** (such as social withdrawal and lack of responses to other people).
3. Abnormalities in **verbal and non-verbal communication** (such as lack of social usage and, in severe cases, absence of useful speech).
4. A **restricted, repetitive repertoire of interests** (such as preoccupation with unusual activities).

EPIDEMIOLOGY

Autism has a prevalence of about 5 per 10,000 and is three times more common in boys than in girls. Two-thirds of children with autism have mental retardation. Autistic-like syndromes are sometimes associated with medical conditions such as congenital rubella or the fragile-X chromosome condition, but in the majority of cases no diagnosable physical disorder can be found.

AETIOLOGY

Twin studies suggest that genetic factors are important. The prognosis of autism is poor, with most cases unable to live independently in adulthood. **Asperger's syndrome** is sometimes considered to be a mild variety of autism, in which there is no mental retardation and the language disorder may be limited to a stilted or pedantic style of speech. Social relationships are characterized by a lack of responsiveness or empathy. Autism should be differentiated from the **disintegrative disorders**, in which there is loss of acquired skills.

TREATMENT

There is no specific treatment for autism, though children and their families can be greatly assisted by provision of appropriate educational facilities and other forms of practical help. Children do best in a well-structured educational environment with experience of the condition, while home-based behavioural treatments may reduce tantrums and aggressive outbursts.

Specific developmental delays

These disorders have an onset in infancy or childhood and involve impairment or delay in a *specific* psychological function such as speech, language, or reading, not accounted for by general intellectual retardation. The impairments often lessen as the child grows older, though some forms, such as specific reading disorder, show strong continuity into adult life. From a psychiatric point of view, the most important specific developmental disorders are language disorders and reading disorders, both of which have a strong association with behavioural and emotional difficulties. Special educational provision is crucial in minimizing the effects.

Specific developmental disorders of language may be sensory or expressive in nature. Both varieties present with slowness in speaking. There should be concern about children who show no interest in sounds by 6 months, who fail to develop repetitive babble by 1 year, or who do not understand simple commands by 18 months. Developmental language disorders should be distinguished from mental retardation, the most common cause of speech delay, by the fact that the delay is out of keeping with the general level of cognitive functioning. Other causes of delayed speech include deafness, autism, and selective **mutism** (which is characterized by a lack of speech outside the home but normal speech at home).

AETIOLOGY

In developmental language disorders there is commonly a family history of similar or related disorders, and it is likely that many cases have a genetic basis. However, in some cases environmental factors, such as deprivation or lack of stimulation, may be important. Such children are often helped by advice to parents on the ways to further communication, such as devoting special time to play with the child. Speech therapy and educational assessment are also helpful.

Specific reading disorder (SRD)

SRD is a *specific* and significant impairment of reading skills. It should be distinguished from *general reading backwardness*, in which reading problems are part of a general delay.

EPIDEMIOLOGY

SRD is three times more common in boys than in girls, and occurs in about 5 per cent of children. It is commonly accompanied by perceptual deficits, such as difficulty telling left from right.

AETIOLOGY

Social factors, such as large family size and a lack of books in the home seem to be important, but in some varieties there is probably a genetic component. There are increased rates of behavioural problems.

TREATMENT

Treatment is mainly educational, but some children are also helped by the treatment of associated psychiatric problems. Early intervention is very important so that the child does not fall behind their contemporaries, which leads to frustration and behavioural problems, and may explain why SRD is over-represented in the prisons and in the special hospitals. Many children with SRD continue to show reading problems in adulthood.

Enuresis and encopresis

ENURESIS

Enuresis is inappropriate emptying of the bladder in the absence of organic disease in a child over the age of 5 years, and it may be nocturnal, diurnal, or both. By the age of 5 years about 10 per cent of children will still be wet at night, and about 3 per cent will be wet by day. The most common cause is an inherited delay in maturation of the nervous pathways that control micturition. However, referrals to child psychiatrists commonly have increased rates of behavioural problems, especially in girls and in association with day-time wetting. Enuresis can also be maintained by inconsistent or negative approaches to toilet training.

Treatment

The first step in management is a careful history and physical examination. Symptoms like pain or dribbling are indications for further investigation, but usually urine microscopy and culture are the only investigations that are required. Children under 7 can be reassured that at least one of their classmates has the same problem, and that improvement should occur over the next few months. In older children, behavioural measures such as rewards for dry nights, 'bladder training' (which involves encouraging children with daytime enuresis to pass urine at lengthening intervals), and enuresis alarms (which set off a buzzer when the child wets the bed at night) are indicated. Vasopressin may be effective in resistant cases.

ENCOPRESIS

Encopresis is defined as the passage of normal stools in inappropriate places. By 4 years only 3 per cent of children show signs of faecal incontinence once per week or more, and by 10 to 11 years this figure has reduced to less than 1 per cent. Most of these children are probably showing soiling secondary to constipation, and only a minority have encopresis, Encopresis is three times more common in boys than in girls, and has several causes including coercive and rigid patterns of potty training, emotional disorders, conduct disorders (in which soiling may be used for aggressive purposes), and adverse events. Constipation, and occasionally anal fissures, are important precipitating and maintaining factors. Assessment should include a physical examination and careful charting of the circumstances and frequency of encopresis.

Treatment

Parents should be advised not to punish the child for soiling, but rather to encourage appropriate toilet habits, such as sitting on the toilet after every meal. This process, known as *shaping*, should be charted and a reward system should be devised (usually a star chart). It may also be necessary to treat associated psychiatric disorders. Bulking agents and oral laxatives may be helpful.

Psychotic disorders

Schizophrenia is very uncommon among pre-pubertal children, but there is a rapid increase in prevalence during adolescence. Diagnosis can be very difficult because the onset is often insidious and occurs in adolescents who were pre-morbidly withdrawn and odd. Differentiation from bipolar disorder is important but may be difficult. Psychotic adolescents usually require in-patient assessment and treatment; management being similar to that in young adults.

Anorexia nervosa

Most cases of anorexia nervosa have an onset between 14 and 19 years. The clinical picture is similar to that found in adult cases, as is treatment, except that there is a greater emphasis on family interventions. Young people should generally be treated as out-patients, with their consent, and in age-appropriate services. The prognosis of adolescent cases is often better than that for adults, but pre-pubertal cases may have a poor outcome.

School attendance problems

Although not a psychiatric syndrome as such, poor school attendance is common, and is associated with a number of adverse outcomes. The most common form is truancy, which may be defined as *not going to school while concealing the absence from parents*. Truancy is often a symptom of conduct disorder, and is therefore associated with factors like large family size, inconsistent parenting, and reading problems. It should be distinguished from school refusal, which may be defined as *remaining at home, unwilling to attend school*. School refusal is usually a symptom of emotional disorder, especially separation anxiety, and is frequently accompanied by depression. Complaints of illness are often used to secure staying at home. Parents are aware of the non-attendance, conduct problems are uncommon, and educational attainment is generally within the normal range. Management of poor school attendance depends on the cause, but in all cases an effort should be made to return the child rapidly to school. Close liaison with the school and the educational welfare service is important.

MANAGEMENT

Engagement, clarification and reassurance

Most child psychiatric problems do not present to medical services, and even fewer are referred to specialists. In general practice, the chance to ventilate concern and seek guidance and clarification is very important for parents, while considering a referral to a mental health service is generally a major step for them. Using diagnostic labels may help to validate a parent's experience and provide access to service, but others will feel stigmatized by them. For those that are referred to specialist services, a range of treatments are available and complex cases will usually receive help from several members of the multi-disciplinary team, working to a coordinated care plan.

Psychotherapies

Various strategies are available for providing support, for resolving problems in relationships, and for reducing stress. Allowing a child to talk and explain his feelings, to an empathic, supportive therapist may often be helpful. There is a growing body of research support for cognitive-behaviour therapy for depression, OCD, and eating disorders in adolescents. This uses cognitive restructuring (challenging faulty beliefs), behavioural tasks, and development of social skills. For adolescents, groups of various sorts are used, such as social skills groups and creative therapy groups.

FAMILY THERAPY

This entails working with all the family who live together, to identify family patterns that may contribute to the genesis or maintenance of a child's problem. In addition it aims to identify family resources that can be utilized to bring about positive change. This is particularly relevant where behavioural change is required, for example in family meal planning in anorexia nervosa. Traditionally all family members are involved, but 'separated' forms in which parents are seen separately from the child have been shown to be effective when there are high levels of hostility or critical comments directed to the child.

BEHAVIOUR THERAPIES

Various forms have been used to alter behaviour by eliminating unwanted and encouraging desired behaviours – especially in the treatment of phobic conditions, encopresis, and conduct disorders.

Drug treatments and diet

Drugs should be used carefully in child psychiatry, respecting the lack of understanding of their effects on the immature brain and the developing child. However when used appropriately, in suitable doses, drugs can be very effective, though rarely prescribed alone without other intervention. Prescribing needs to take account of the different pharmacodynamics and pharmacokinetics of children; they are not just small adults.

The major classes are stimulants such as methylphenidate for ADHD, selective serotonin reuptake inhibitor (SSRI) antidepressants for adolescent depression, and antipsychotics for psychoses. The relationship between food allergies or intolerances and behaviour disorders is controversial. Where parents believe there is a link, children may benefit from the 'few foods' diet in which they are started on a restricted diet and foods are added one by one, with careful attention to monitoring behaviour.

Day-hospital attendance

Day-hospital attendance is useful to allow detailed observation for the assessment of complex cases. It can provide more intensive therapeutic input, possibly within a group setting, and creative therapies. It can also provide relief and support to the family and school.

In-patient admission

In-patient admission to a paediatric ward or to a specialist child psychiatry unit extends the options for assessment and treatment. Admission is often considered for young people who put themselves at risk through self-harm, though in-patient units often have difficulty extinguishing this behaviour. Conditions such as psychoses and anorexia nervosa that require intensive treatment and rehabilitation, and in which the young person is socially isolated, often result in admission.

Reception into care

Reception into care may be needed for children who are at risk of significant harm in the community. The law relating to children and families is enshrined in the *Children Act 1989*. The main principles of the Act are that the welfare of children is paramount, that parents have certain responsibilities, and that local authorities have a duty to promote the welfare of children in need. The majority of children in care are placed in foster homes rather than institutions. Young people in care are vulnerable to further adversities, particularly educational failure, while those leaving care show very high rates of mental health problems.

FURTHER READING

Goodman, R. and Scott, S. (2005) *Child Psychiatry*, 2nd edition. Oxford: Blackwell.
Gowers, S. (Ed.) (2005) *Seminars in Child and Adolescent Psychiatry*, 2nd edition. London: Gaskell.
Graham, P., Turk, J. and Verhulst, F. (1999) *Child Psychiatry: A Developmental Approach*, 3rd edition. Oxford: Oxford University Press.

21 SEXUAL AND REPRODUCTIVE DISORDERS

This chapter is concerned with human sexual development throughout the life cycle. We therefore start with gender identity disorders, since these take their onset in the pre-school child, and pass on to consider homosexuality since it appears that events in childhood and adolescence are of some aetiological importance in both of these conditions.

The second part of the chapter considers the common sexual problems of adult life, with emphasis on their aetiology and assessment. The section on paraphilias is short, since these seldom request medical treatment.

The third part of the chapter considers disorders related to reproduction, once more arranged in sequence from menstrual disorders, through pregnancy to the puerperium, and ending with disorders relating to the menopause.

A summary of psychiatric classification of sexual disorders is included at the end of the chapter, as is suggested further reading.

GENDER IDENTITY DISORDERS

A person's *gender identity* refers to their awareness of being male or female, and *gender role* refers to the public expression of such an identity in clothing and behaviour. Externally a person's gender may be defined in terms of chromosome complement, anatomy of their internal sexual organs or gonads, or external genitalia and secondary sexual characteristics, which can be ambiguous, for example in androgen insensitivity or adrenal hyperplasia. Particularly in the latter cases the assignment of an incorrect gender at birth can be crucial to a person's developing sense of themselves.

A person's gender identity does not presuppose any particular sexual orientation, and they may be attracted to males, females, both or neither. In fact some people prefer to live in a neutral gender role.

Gender identity disorders also include some types of **transvestism**. This is where people dress as members of the opposite sex. In **dual role transvestism**, the person spends time in both gender roles. This is distinct from **fetishistic transvestism**, which is where the person is sexually aroused by dressing as the opposite sex, and this is classified differently under 'disorders of sexual preference' rather than gender identity disorders.

The aetiology of gender identity disorders is not fully understood. Most people with such disorders are anatomically, hormonally, and genetically indistinguishable from other members of their biological gender. It has been suggested that prenatal endocrine influences on the developing brain may be important, and it can be shown that if androgens are given to a pregnant rhesus monkey her female infant will behave as a male. However, hormonal abnormalities have not been demonstrated in humans.

Patterns of early rearing are likely to be important: the *'assigned sex for rearing'* refers to being called 'John', dressed as a boy and given a toy aeroplane; or called 'Jane', dressed as a girl and given a cuddly doll. However, once more, the parents of transsexual patients usually deny that they brought the child up in an unusual way. The available evidence suggests that the gender-related behaviours acquired in the pre-school child are critically important in determining later satisfaction with gender role: any deviant patterns learned before going to school tend to be reinforced rather than disturbed by experience at the infant's school.

Minor degrees of *gender dysphoria* are relatively common in the developing school-age child. It seems clear that a developing child needs a satisfactory role-model with whom he or she can identify if an appropriate gender identity is to be developed.

Transsexualism

EPIDEMIOLOGY

Males outnumber females by at about three to one in most societies. The prevalence in England is 1:34,000 men and 1:108,000 women, and similar figures are found in other European countries.

FEATURES

This disorder is a subgroup classified in ICD-10 within gender identity disorder. It is characterized by the person's persistent sense of discomfort and inappropriateness about their anatomic sex, together with a wish to be rid of their genitals and to live as a member of the opposite sex. These feelings take their origin in childhood. The patient wishes to be a member of the other sex and dresses in clothes of the desired sex without sexual arousal, but with a feeling of relief. The patients greatly dislike their genitalia, and request surgical removal of them. The idea of 'really' being a member of the other sex is an example of an **over-valued idea**.

Sometimes previously normal patients can acquire all the features of the syndrome during a psychotic illness, most usually schizophrenia. There is a strong association with depressive illness, and suicidal ideas and self-mutilation are common. Many people who suffer with this disorder however do not show any evidence of any other mental illness or psychopathology, which contributes to their view that this is a normal variation rather than a psychiatric disorder.

TREATMENT

The first gender reassignment surgery in Europe was done in the 1920s, and interest in this mode of treatment grew in the next decade with some high profile cases. The first text on the subject was written in 1966 by Harry Benjamin, the 'father of transsexualism', who laid out a set of diagnostic criteria. From the late 1960s the importance of treating transsexualism in a multi-disciplinary team began to be recognized, with management involving psychiatrists, endocrinologists, and surgeons. Patients who present to doctors requesting hormone treatment or sex change operations, should be referred to a specialist clinic.

Following rigorous psychiatric assessment, patients must undergo the 2-year 'real-life experience', where they are expected to live in the desired gender throughout all their social and professional life to ensure a clear commitment, and in order for them to discover some of the problems they may face. If this is successful, hormone treatment is commenced to promote relevant changes in secondary sexual characteristics. Men are treated with **anti-androgens**, and supra-physiological doses of **oestrogen**. It is essential that men commit to giving up smoking because of the ensuing health risks, including thrombosis. The physical changes produced by hormonal treatment are irreversible, hence the reason that this stage is delayed until a final decision has been made.

Following treatment people are described by their resulting sexual phenotype, thus men who are reassigned to be women are called trans-women, and vice versa.

Homosexuality

This is no longer classified as a mental disorder, but until surprisingly recently people regarded it as such, and tried with little success to treat it, usually unsuccessfully, with psychotherapy. It is a mistake to suppose that people are either homosexual or heterosexual, since many people are capable of either form of sexual activity. Figures from the USA suggest that approximately one-third of males have homosexual experience leading to orgasm at some time in their lives, most usually during adolescence, to be compared with about 6 per cent of women. Only about 3 per cent of men and 2 per cent of women have an exclusively homosexual experience.

Homosexual behaviour becomes much more common in conditions where the other sex is not available, such as prison; and it is common in those few societies where it is not stigmatized.

AETIOLOGY

Genetic factors are of some importance, since the MZ concordance for homosexuality is higher than the DZ concordance. Endocrine influences during pregnancy may determine gender behaviour in childhood, as mentioned above. The importance of *parental role-models* has also been emphasized: homosexual patients coming for treatment typically report disturbed relationships with the same-sex parent. A boy who has been unable to identify with a weak or absent father, and whose nascent sexuality has been influenced by an over-protective mother, may be expected to have difficulties in acquiring sexual feelings about women. At about puberty a developing child must bring three things together: their gender identity, the developing capacity for sexual responsiveness, and the ability to develop close interpersonal relationships. Thus effeminate boys are likely to develop a homosexual orientation at puberty, and those who are unconfident about their masculinity may be unattractive to the opposite sex, so that early attempts at striking up relationships are painful. The same boys may be more than usually attractive to males seeking 'unmasculine partners', so that the adolescent enters the rather less competitive homosexual world.

Similar arguments apply to the acquisition of female homosexual behaviour, although here additional factors might be fear or disgust at the sexual behaviour of men ('heterophobia'); deliberate avoidance of men as part of a feminist stance, and poor performance in heterosexual situations. There is also an increased incidence of homosexuality among women with a history of sexual abuse.

Until the emergence of HIV/AIDS in the early 1980s, there tended to be a high level of promiscuity in the male gay community, especially in large cosmopolitan centres, where some men had an enormous number of partners, often unidentified, and this made recurrent infections with sexually transmitted infections likely. Public health education on this issue has led to a change in behaviour for both homosexual and heterosexual individuals, promoting use of condoms, and regular sexual health checks. Lesbian women, it seems, do not present the same problem of frequent short-lived relationships as homosexual men and their forms of sexual behaviour do not put them at such high risk. It is important however in this group to promote regular sexual health checks, including cervical cytology, because of the commonly held erroneous belief that lesbian women are not at risk.

Although anxiety and depression have been reported frequently among homosexual men, there appears to be a truly increased prevalence only for those without a stable relationship. This inability to form lasting relationships may be indicative of interpersonal problems that go well beyond the patient's sexual orientation. This is more commonly the situation, but not exclusively, in individuals with a history of abuse or emotional neglect.

The relative frequency of sexual problems in homosexuals is the same as for heterosexual individuals, with men tending to report erectile and ejaculatory problems, and women tending to report a loss of sexual interest. It seems however that lesbian women are less likely to report problems than other women, and they are more likely to want to be managed by a therapist from within the lesbian community.

DISORDERS OF ADULT SEXUAL FUNCTIONING

The commonest forms of sexual disorders are those in which normal sexual activity is desired but not being achieved. **Primary sexual problems** are those that have been present since the onset of sexual activity, **secondary sexual problems** develop after a period of adequate sexual function.

Problems with sexual intercourse

Intercourse can be divided into three phases: *desire, arousal,* and *orgasm,* all under different innervation. Sexual interest is mainly under limbic control, arousal mainly under the

317

control of parasympathetic (cholinergic and peptidergic) systems, while orgasm is mainly under sympathetic (adrenergic) control. The various sexual problems that arise can most easily be classified under these three headings.

Both men and women can experience disorders of sexual desire. Problems with arousal lead in the male to erectile difficulties, and in the female to lack of lubrication and general sexual unresponsiveness. Difficulties in the orgasmic phase cause premature or retarded ejaculation in the male, and orgasmic dysfunction in the female.

EPIDEMIOLOGY

Few reliable statistics are available. The National Health and Social Life Survey in the United States found that 43 per cent of women and 31 per cent of men from a representative sample in the age group 18–59 complained of some sexual problems in the preceding 12 months. Many people may delay or avoid presentation because of embarrassment or a lack of awareness of available treatment.

Men presenters tend to be slightly older than women, both in mean and upper age limits of presentation. Presentation is also more common in social classes I and II, with a decrease towards the lowest presentation in social class V. In same-sex couples, men are more likely to complain of sexual dysfunction than women.

There is also a variation in the relative frequency of different disorders in men and women. The most common problem in men is **erectile dysfunction**, representing around two-thirds of male referrals. The next most common is **ejaculatory problems**. More commonly this is **premature ejaculation**. Erectile dysfunction can however predispose to premature ejaculation because of a desire to ejaculate quickly before the erection is lost, and also because anxiety is a potential aetiology in both disorders.

In women the most common presentation is **loss of desire** or impaired sexual interest. In one study 64 out of 105 women presented in this way compared to 12 out of 95 men in the study. When impaired sexual interest presents alone in women, there is commonly a co-existent relationship problem, however it is important to elucidate any problems with arousal or desire. The next most common problem in women is **vaginismus**, then **dyspareunia**. Vaginismus can also present as superficial dyspareunia.

AETIOLOGY

The aetiology of sexual problems can be either physical or psychological. It is always important to exclude physical causes of sexual problems so that they can be treated. This is because potentially serious conditions can present as sexual disorders, particularly cardiovascular disease in men, diabetes, and less commonly other endocrine disorders such as pituitary and thyroid problems. Recently there has been an increased awareness that erectile dysfunction in men can be a very sensitive early warning sign for small vessel disease, indicating that it is very important for doctors to enquire about sexual function when taking a history. Another important physical cause is potential side-effects of medication, and if this is not addressed, it can encourage lack of compliance. Very commonly, however, a sexual problem can have a combination of physical and psychological causes.

Sexual disorders can be very disruptive to people's relationships, and one study found more than 30 per cent of those referred were suffering from mild to moderate anxiety or depression. The same study found in a series of 200 couples that about a third had significant marital and relationship problems.

Male sexual problems

ERECTILE FAILURE

This may be primary or secondary.

Primary erectile difficulties arise because of inhibitions about sex, or difficulties experienced in early sexual encounters. There may rarely be a basic organic defect.

Secondary erectile problems may arise after occasional failures resulting from alcohol or fatigue, and this may lead to anxiety about the ability to perform, causing further failure and thus creating a vicious circle.

Organic factors may also be important, and it has been estimated that up to 85 per cent of men with erectile difficulties have some physical problems, although even where these are present anxiety about performance is likely to make things worse. **Diabetes** and **multiple sclerosis** sometimes present with erectile failure, and problems are likely to increase with age. There are definite physiological ageing changes affecting the strength of the erection and the ease with which it is obtained, and further impairment may result from *atherosclerotic narrowing* of penile arteries. Where there has been serious illness, for example a coronary, the patient may also be anxious about the adverse effects of the exertion needed in intercourse.

PREMATURE EJACULATION

This is common, affecting up to 6 per cent of all males at some time in their sexual lives. It often arises after initial sexual experiences in situations where intercourse has to be hurried, for example the back of a car or in the parental home, and is then perpetuated by the anxiety that it will recur. Occasionally it can occur after a period of normal control, perhaps after a traumatic experience of some kind.

RETARDED EJACULATION

This is very much less common. It often occurs after medication, especially with SSRIs and tricyclic antidepressants, but it may also occur in inhibited males who can usually masturbate normally to ejaculation.

RETROGRADE EJACULATION

This is ejaculation of semen upwards into the bladder instead of externally, and commonly follows prostatectomy, both transurethral and intra-abdominal.

Psychiatry in Medical Practice

PAINFUL EJACULATION

This is a rare complaint possibly resulting from infection and painful muscle spasm.

LACK OF INTEREST

This can occur as a primary complaint, often accompanied by general anxiety about sexual intercourse both between one individual and another and also at different times of life. Although psychological factors such as inhibitions from the past or relationship problems in the present are often important, organic factors may also be present. An increase in prolactin secretion, which may be a result of a cerebral tumour, or a side-effect of some medications, will cause loss of libido in both males and females. The ratio of testosterone to oestrogen in both sexes affects desire, with higher testosterone levels stimulating it.

Female sexual problems

LACK OF DRIVE

In the female this is often a result of inhibitions passed on from parents and society in general, or from unfortunate past experiences such as rape or incest. It may also be caused by increased prolactin levels in the blood, and by a diminished testosterone/oestrogen ratio as in the male. Many women experience different levels of desire at different phases of the menstrual cycle, and many lose interest in sex after childbirth for a time, probably because of a combination of factors. These may include changing hormonal patterns, dyspareunia after episiotomy, changes in the general marital relationship, and fear of further pregnancy.

LACK OF AROUSAL (GENERAL SEXUAL UNRESPONSIVENESS)

Arousal in the woman, as in the man, causes vasodilatation of the blood supply to the genital area. In the male this results in the cavernous sinuses of the penis filling with blood, and in the woman produces a cuff of dilated blood vessels encircling the lower part of the vagina. Some of the fluid from these vessels goes as a transudate into the vagina, producing the lubrication. A woman may not particularly desire sex but if adequately stimulated by a sensitive partner may be able to respond, lubricate and reach orgasm. Inability to respond may be due to inhibitions from learned attitudes or past experiences, or to adverse conditions in the present, including difficulties in the marital relationship. Any kind of anxiety connected with the situation, for example intercourse in the parental home or anxiety about the baby, may affect her ability to relax and respond. Inadequate stimulation from an inexperienced lover is often a cause of early difficulties. Lack of arousal will, in all these situations, cause dyspareunia (see below) because of lack of lubrication and this can easily produce a vicious circle leading to avoidance of all sexual encounters. This commonly occurs after childbirth.

320

Arousal in the female may also be affected, as in the male, by drugs and neurological and vascular disease, and in post-menopausal women lubrication may be diminished because of lowered oestrogen levels.

DYSPAREUNIA

Pain during intercourse from any cause will inhibit arousal and may be caused by *vaginal infections*, *pelvic inflammatory disease*, *endometriosis*, *episiotomy*, and by *operations affecting the cervix*, which may prevent the elevation of the uterus out of the pelvis that occurs in normal intercourse, leading to buffeting of the cervix by the penis.

ORGASMIC DYSFUNCTION

About 10 per cent of women never experience orgasm from any form of stimulation. About one-third of the rest reach orgasm in most acts of intercourse, and most of the rest will respond to clitoral stimulation only. A small group respond to breast stimulation or even fantasy alone.

A few women lack the normal bulbo-cavernosus reflex (stimulation of the glans clitoris causing reflex spasm of the perineal muscles) and may be physiologically unable to reach orgasm. Many of the 10 per cent however, may never have been adequately stimulated by their partners and have been too inhibited to masturbate themselves. Some women fear the momentary loss of control experienced during orgasm and are unable to 'relax and let it happen'.

VAGINISMUS

This is a spasm of the part of the pelvic musculature surrounding the lower part of the vagina, making penetration difficult or impossible. It may be primary or secondary. Primary vaginismus may rarely be a result of a small or even absent vagina or a very strong hymen, but is almost always psychological, resulting from phobic anxiety about penetration. These women may respond normally to arousal and be orgasmic with clitoral stimulation but cannot let anything, even their own finger or a vaginal tampon into the vagina. Secondary vaginismus may arise after painful vaginal lesions of all kinds.

Aetiological factors in sexual dysfunctions

PREDISPOSING

Psychological – Inhibited upbringing in relation to sexual matters, inadequate sexual education and traumatic early sexual experience such as incest or sexual assault.

Physical – These are rare causes of primary sexual problems, but anatomical problems such as hypospadias or Peronier's disease, or hormonal problems, may present in this way. Physically disabled people may have sexual problems, which can usually be overcome with a sympathetic partner.

PRECIPITATING

The first attempts at sexual intercourse form the precipitating factor in primary problems. Childbirth, infidelity, or other relationship problems commonly precipitate secondary problems. The onset of physical or depressive illness also does so, as can a sexual problem developing in the partner.

Physical illness may precipitate sexual problems directly – as with diabetes – or as secondary complications. Following myocardial infarction, impotence and ejaculatory difficulties are common; loss of interest may result from depression or from the unfounded fear that sexual activity will cause further infarction.

Other physical illnesses that may cause sexual dysfunction are: renal dialysis, abdominal surgery leading to ostomies, mastectomy, neurological conditions that cause spinal cord damage, or peripheral neuropathy.

Hysterectomy often leads to an improvement in sexual functioning because of relief of menorrhagia, but if this symptom has been used as a convenient excuse not to have intercourse a more overt problem may present after the operation. Vaginal shrinkage following the operation may cause pain and ensuing sexual dysfunction.

Both psychological and physical factors may occur together. About half of diabetic males develop impotence, especially the older men. But in many, erections occur early in the morning and with masturbation, so the mechanism cannot be entirely physical.

MAINTAINING FACTORS

These are often important. Anxiety occurring with sexual arousal leads to vaginismus and impotence, which often cause pain and shame. This can threaten the relationship so one or both partners may be afraid to attempt further sexual activity. If they do try, they are anxious in anticipation, which exacerbates the difficulty, further failure ensues and the problem is perpetuated. Poor communication between partners about sex, inadequate information about it, and conflicts in the general relationship all maintain sexual problems.

Assessment of sexual dysfunction

Although sexual dysfunction may require specialist treatment every doctor should be able to recognize and briefly assess such problems.

1. The sexual problem may be *presented directly* by the patient or the partner. Often it presents indirectly to the gynaecology, family planning, or infertility clinics. Depression, anxiety or general problems in the relationship may also be presented when the patient is ashamed or embarrassed to describe the sexual problem directly.

2. The *exact nature of the problem and its duration should be assessed.* Is it the patient who experiences the difficulty or is it the partner? Is it primary or secondary? Which phase of sexual activity is affected? Can masturbation or sex with another partner occur satisfactorily? (If it can, organic causes need not be considered!) During such questioning the doctor will become aware of the patient's attitude to and knowledge about sex. A history indicative of *psychiatric or physical illness* in either partner must be sought as this could be responsible for a change in the sexual relationship. Similarly a drug history is required.

3. The patient must be *physically examined* to investigate the possibility of physical causes for the problem. It is especially important to examine the secondary sexual characteristics and the cardiovascular system, and to do a neurological examination of the lower limbs. Impotence may be the first sign of diabetes, so examine the urine and be prepared to examine the Valsalva response.

4. *The partner must be seen* so that a history of the problem and the partner's attitude to it may be assessed. When the two partners are seen together the doctor observes their ability to discuss sex, whether one partner blames the other, and their attitude towards treatment. It is essential to see each partner alone on at least one occasion so that the doctor can explore the possibility that one partner has had an extra-marital affair. The upbringing and previous sexual experience of each partner are also evaluated individually. The couple's general relationship with one another should be assessed as well as their sexual relationship.

5. The expectations of, and preparedness to engage in, treatment must be assessed before it is commenced.

Treatment of sexual disorders

GENERAL MEASURES

Clarification of the problem and a full discussion of the sexual relationship will help the couple to talk about their difficulty more freely and this alone may lead to resolution of the problem. Improvement of the general relationship may be required before any improvement in the sexual relationship could be expected. However, this is not a medical problem.

Education and advice – A great deal can be done to help these patients by sex education, relieving anxiety, and helping to overcome inhibitions by giving them permission to enjoy their sexuality. Increasing communication between the couple is also important. All trained professionals can give simple counselling on these lines and this may be all that is needed for the couple to sort out their own problems. Where more help is required specialist treatment needs to be directed towards increasing the positive stimuli to make the reverberating circuit fire off to orgasm where this is possible.

If there are fears of pregnancy, then contraceptive advice is needed. Sometimes fear of infertility interferes with normal sexual function and such fears must be dealt with before more specific treatment is attempted.

Reassurance that physical illness will not be exacerbated by sexual intercourse may allow the couple to resume their previous satisfactory relationship. Specific advice may be appropriate – such as taking a beta-blocker before intercourse for the angina patient. Any underlying psychiatric or physical illness must be treated. Although antidepressants can cause impotence, their appropriate use to treat depressive illness may lead to greatly improved sexual functioning.

Physical treatment – Administration of testosterone has been shown to be useful where there is definite impairment of gonadal function. It has also been shown to increase libido even where testosterone levels are normal, but will not then improve function. Penile prosthetic surgery has been used in cases of neuropathy. Injection of vasoactive drugs such as papaverine directly into the corpus cavernosum of the penis causes pharmacologically induced erections. Patients can inject themselves at home but require careful instruction in the technique because of the risk of drug-induced priapism. Mechanical aids to erection, consisting of a vacuum pump with a penile constrictor ring, are preferred by some patients. These methods can be used to overcome the performance anxiety and loss of confidence associated with psychological impotence, but they are more commonly used when organic factors are present, as in diabetes mellitus.

SPECIFIC PSYCHOLOGICAL TREATMENT

Specialist treatment is usually the province of sexual dysfunction clinics but may be performed by any suitably trained professional. After individual and joint assessment, the couple are seen together for a number of sessions, with the understanding that between each session they will be required to do certain exercises together.

The treatment is based on a behavioural model. It is assumed that sexual arousal leads to anxiety and the new response of relaxation must be learned instead. Since the anxiety is usually greatest with penetration, the treatment programme begins with an absolute ban on attempts at full intercourse for the first few weeks. This means that instead of experiencing frustrating failed attempts the couple can enjoy mutual pleasurable stimulation. Initially this is solely non-genital stimulation; later genital stimulation is introduced, provided that increasing sexual arousal can be achieved while both partners remain relaxed. This must be practised over several weeks and discussed fully both with the therapist and with each other before steps toward full intercourse are taken. Specific techniques are used for premature ejaculation, vaginismus, and orgasmic failure (see Further reading).

As well as the behavioural techniques, counselling and education are usually required. Commonly resentment or embarrassment has developed between the partners and this must be faced and dealt with during sessions. If the problem has been labelled as that of one partner alone, both must recognize their role in the development and treatment of it. Suitable literature is available to guide the couple through sex therapy and to increase their understanding of normal sexual functioning.

Psychotherapy may be appropriate, either in the form of marital therapy if the couple's general relationship requires help, or individual psychotherapy if one partner is found to have problems of their own that will be helped with this form of treatment.

OUTCOME

Treatment of patients attending sexual dysfunctioning clinics leads to a satisfactory outcome in approximately two-thirds of cases. The outcome is best with vaginismus and premature ejaculation (often primary problems). The outcome of treatment depends on the quality of the couple's general relationship and their motivation for treatment.

Paraphilias

In these disorders sexual arousal is repeatedly obtained from non-human objects, or with humans, but involving suffering or humiliation or non-consenting partners.

FETISHISM

In fetishism a piece of clothing or part of the body, such as hair or feet, is used as a means of obtaining sexual arousal and orgasm. It is essentially a male perversion and there are many grades from using the fetish (often an item of female clothing) as an adjunct to normal sexual intercourse to using it as a sole means of gaining arousal.

PAEDOPHILIA

Paedophilia is the act or fantasy of engaging in sexual activity with young children as a repeatedly preferred method of achieving sexual arousal. Paedophilic acts usually take the form of immature sex play with coitus or violence only occurring rarely. Paedophilia often involves a child previously known to the man, and may be incest.

Aetiology

In adolescents, paedophilia may be an exaggerated form of immature sexual activity. Among older men, marital and social difficulties or social isolation are common and alcohol may be involved in releasing the behaviour. Medical involvement may be required to assess the man or aid the child and their family. The former may be a request from a court.

Treatment

Forensic services offer treatment programmes for these people, which usually involve the use of cognitive-behavioural techniques, and may be based on a group psychotherapy approach. This generally involves improving pro-social behaviour, including assertiveness training and anger management. Pharmacological treatments have also been used increasingly in the last 20 years. These include anti-androgens, hormones such as medroxyprogesterone acetate, gonadotrophin releasing hormone agonists, and SSRIs.

SADOMASOCHISM

Sadomasochism is sexual gratification involving fantasy or acts of cruelty either to the person (masochism) or to another (sadism). The phenomenon may remain entirely confined to fantasy or may accompany coitus either as a general humiliation or as a highly specific ritual. Sadism is generally performed by men on females, other males, or animals.

BDSM (bondage dominance sadomasochism) is not however always associated with psychopathology, and people in the BDSM 'scene' are often otherwise 'respectable members of society'. The term BDSM not only describes the particular repertoire of sexual acts carried out, such as flogging and rope work, but another important feature is that relationship dynamics, often including those outside the sexual part of a relationship, are mediated by a dominant/submissive concept. Sexual activity is often carried out in particular clubs or groups, and thus has a strong social element. It usually involves a particular style of 'bondage' dress. Sexual activity between partners in this situation often does not correspond to a relationship outside that setting, and to an extent in that respect it has an overlap with the practice of swinging.

TRANSVESTISM

Transvestism occurs in both sexes and involves the persistent wearing of clothes of the opposite sex. This is initially for sexual excitement and the person becomes intensely frustrated if cross-dressing is prevented. There are different forms, with some men wearing female clothing in secret, others doing so overtly. If the purpose remains one of sexual arousal this is a kind of fetish; if the behaviour becomes continuous it may lead to a state resembling transsexualism. Both heterosexual and homosexual men and women cross-dress. It should probably be thought of as a minor form of gender dysphoria allied to deviant sexual practices.

Anxiety, depression, or marital problems may present to the doctor, often with the spouse, rather than the patient, coming to the doctor. These are treated in the usual way, but if the cross-dresser is resistant to change, the future of the marital relationship may be in doubt. Clarifying this issue with both partners will then need to be a first step in treatment.

EXHIBITIONISM

Exhibitionism is the repetitive act of exposing the genitals to an unsuspecting stranger for the purpose of achieving sexual arousal. The desire to shock the innocent party is strong. The man may masturbate but experience intense guilt later.

Depression is an important cause in the elderly, and the behaviour is occasionally accompanied by schizophrenia, organic brain damage, or mental handicap. Exhibitionism may be a short-lived episode in an otherwise normal person but persistent offenders tend to come from troubled family backgrounds, are immature, and under-achieve as adults.

The medical task is to detect treatable psychiatric illness if it is present, to try to prevent stigmatization of the occasional offender, and refer for *behaviour therapy* those who are well motivated to stop the behaviour. The anti-androgen, *cyproterone acetate*, is occasionally used for short periods in conjunction with other treatments.

In relation to court reports the doctor must remember that the majority of convicted exposers do not repeat the crime; it is the repeat offender who seems to be neither easily treatable nor deterred.

VOYEURISM

Voyeurism is sexual gratification through looking at people (usually strangers) who are naked, undressing, or engaging in sexual activity. The observer does not attempt to engage the person whom he has watched in sexual activity but masturbates afterwards.

REPRODUCTIVE DISORDERS

Premenstrual tension

EPIDEMIOLOGY

Estimates of prevalence range from one-third to three-quarters of all women of reproductive age, depending on the severity and duration of the symptoms included within the definition and their timing in relation to the menstrual cycle. The frequency is such that it is probably inappropriate to regard this condition as pathological, but the extreme distress experienced by some women results in medical consultation.

CLINICAL FEATURES

The commonest physical complaints include breast tenderness and feelings of abdominal distension, and mental symptoms include depressed mood, anxiety, and irritability. These occur for up to 10 days prior to a menstrual period and end 1 to 2 days afterwards.

DIAGNOSTIC CRITERIA

The physical symptoms are characteristic. All symptoms are limited to a maximum of 11 to 12 days of each cycle. The 'biological' symptoms of depression do not occur. The condition should be differentiated from the affective disorders, in which symptoms may be exacerbated premenstrually but are more persistent throughout the cycle. If a daily symptom diary is kept, this may reveal that the complaints are persistent or intermittent throughout the cycle, indicating the possibility of the somatic presentation of an affective disorder.

AETIOLOGY

Despite the evident link between the timing of these symptoms and the menstrual cycle, various aetiological theories concerning imbalance of ovarian or pituitary hormones have not been substantiated, although bloating and irritability are associated with progesterone, which of course is at its highest level in the second half of the menstrual cycle. Symptoms of premenstrual tension disappear in about two-thirds of women after hysterectomy (with intact ovaries), indicating that hormonal factors are perhaps not of critical importance.

TREATMENT

Sympathetic explanation and reassurance are probably the most important aspects of treatment. Psychosocial stress should be considered, and psychological techniques such as cognitive therapy and relaxation training may be helpful. Many different pharmacological agents including progesterone, bromocriptine, anxiolytics, vitamin B_6, antidepressants, and diuretics have all been advocated. There is little evidence that any of these has more than a placebo effect, and possible teratogenic effects should be considered. The possible exception to this is the SSRI group of antidepressants.

Disorders of pregnancy

EPIDEMIOLOGY

During the first trimester approximately 10 per cent of women experience a new episode of minor affective disorder. During the second trimester this rate falls and is probably similar to the frequency in the general population. There is evidence of an increase in affective disorders in the third trimester.

CLINICAL FEATURES

Any mental illness can have its onset during pregnancy, or may occur as a continuation of a pre-existing disorder. There does not appear to be any increased risk for illnesses characterized by psychotic symptoms, and the vast majority are affective disorders with a mixture of depressive and anxiety symptoms. However, thought content is likely to be focused on the pregnancy and its implications for the future, including the related social and psychological consequences.

AETIOLOGY

Affective disorders that have their onset during pregnancy are associated particularly with the experience of negative life events, such as bereavement, and chronic difficulties, particularly the lack of a confiding relationship. Other factors include a previous history of mental illness, marital conflict, and ambivalence about continuation with the pregnancy.

Onset during the first trimester is associated particularly with a previous history of termination of pregnancy and worries concerning the normality of the foetus.

INVESTIGATIONS

These will usually be limited to a search for evidence of particular aetiological factors that may play a part, and the assessment should include interviews with the partner and possibly other informants. Particular attention should be paid to past history and pre-morbid personality, previous termination of pregnancy, recent life events and current difficulties, the marital relationship, and available sources of support.

TREATMENT

Supportive psychotherapy and counselling may be valuable to women for whom there is evidence of particular psychological difficulties, especially those who have failed to adjust to previous termination. *Joint marital therapy* may be indicated where there is evidence of particular difficulties in the marriage, which may be highlighted by the pregnancy. Women who have material social difficulties and inadequate social support will need help, which should be available from local social services departments. It is particularly important to follow up patients into the puerperium, to assess the development of bonding between mother and child, monitor the mental state, identify any additional potential sources of support, and ensure a satisfactory level of child care.

COURSE AND PROGNOSIS

The outcome of affective disorders during pregnancy remains uncertain. Studies based on married women of higher socioeconomic status suggest that most recover during the first 3 months of the puerperium. Those based on less socially stable populations with lower socioeconomic status indicate a more chronic course, with continuation during the puerperium and possibly for longer. It has been suggested that there are particular risks for subsequent child care and bonding between mother and child, which may have long-term implications for child development.

Termination of pregnancy

In 2005 186,400 abortions were performed on women resident in England and Wales. The woman must have grounds for termination under the Abortion Act (1967), one of which relates to psychological distress, and this is the most common reason given. Before the Act psychiatrists were frequently involved in assessing women prior to termination, which was often carried out on grounds of suicidal risk due to depressive illness. Since the introduction of this Act recommendations for termination must be made by two registered medical practitioners, who are usually the general practitioner and gynae-cologist. Psychiatrists are involved mainly when there is a past history of serious mental illness or a particular need to assess the patient's likely response to termination.

Adverse psychological responses to abortion are rare. Although depression and anxiety are common during unwanted pregnancies, these usually resolve within a few weeks after termination. However there is some increase in the risk of postnatal depression in women with a history of termination, when past feelings of guilt may be re-evoked. By contrast, studies of women refused abortion show they are more likely to suffer depression later on, have an increased risk of suicide, have difficulty in adjusting to their unwanted children, and have children who are at greater risk of delinquency and difficulties at school.

Disorders of the puerperium

There is a well-recognized increase in the prevalence of mental illness following childbirth. Research has led to the classification of these disorders into three main groups, which are considered separately below, but there is still much uncertainty about the extent to which these are different conditions and also their relationship to disorders occurring at other times.

'MATERNITY BLUES'

Epidemiology

Between 50 per cent and 80 per cent of all women develop the 'maternity blues' during the first week following delivery, and this has been a consistent finding in different countries, cultures, and ethnic groups. It is therefore doubtful whether this condition should be considered pathological, but it undoubtedly causes significant distress and requires medical recognition. No consistent relationship has been found to social class, parity, hospital as compared with home delivery, or obstetric complications.

Clinical features

Symptoms tend to develop in a predictable sequence starting on the *first post-partum day* with feelings of exhaustion, anorexia, and complaints of poor concentration. Mild perplexity and disorientation may occur. Weeping occurs in approximately 50 per cent of all women on the first day. However, about 80 per cent of all women also experience elation on the first day and this appears to be a normal response to childbirth, and in a minority (8 per cent) this persists or increases in the subsequent 3 days and is accompanied by garrulousness, over-activity, and excitability.

Symptoms, which have their peak onset on the *third to fifth days*, include depressed mood, restlessness, and irritability. Labile mood with swings from depression to elation on the same day is characteristic of this condition. Weeping tends to be precipitated by minor events and in a substantial minority of cases depressive thought content includes low self-esteem, feelings of guilt, and pessimism concerning the future. Irritability and anger tend to be directed particularly towards the husband or to hospital staff and may lead to self-discharge from hospital.

Diagnostic criteria

'Maternity blues' invariably have their onset within the first week of parturition. The mood changes are characteristically brief and fluctuate rapidly, usually persisting for only a few hours at a time and at most for 1 to 2 days. For the majority there is sudden onset and sudden recovery, with duration usually lasting between 1 and 3 days, and never more than 2 weeks.

Differential diagnosis

The disorder must be differentiated from **post-natal depression**, which starts later, is more prolonged and includes more persistent affective changes; and from **puerperal psychosis**, which has its onset at around the same time as 'maternity blues' and may have similar prodromal symptoms but then progresses with the development of psychotic features. **Acute toxic states** are suggested by evidence of clouding of consciousness or disorientation, but are now uncommon where good obstetric care is available. Approximately 40 per cent of mothers experience either **lack of affection** or negative feelings towards their baby in the first few weeks or months of the puerperium but this is not necessarily related to 'maternity blues'. An association has been described with amniotomy and painful labour. Mothers are usually extremely distressed by their lack of feelings, and may experience feelings of guilt. They may derive considerable benefit from reassurance that this is a common experience, which rarely persists, and is not indicative of either mental illness or inadequacy as a mother.

Aetiology

A biological contribution to the aetiology is strongly suggested by the relatively specific timing of onset and duration, the labile mood, and the lack of a clear relationship to psychosocial or cultural factors. While there is a strong suspicion that the profound hormonal changes occurring at this time are implicated, most studies so far have failed to show any association between the presence or severity of 'maternity blues' and hormonal status.

In the first post-partum week there is a precipitate decrease in the circulating concentrations of oestrogens and progesterone. There are several sites in the CNS, including monoamine neurones and receptors, which are sensitive to these hormones. There is a tendency for episodes (particularly more severe episodes), to be associated with a past history of depressive illness, including post-natal depression. Affective symptoms in the third trimester of pregnancy tend to be associated with poor social adjustment, and family and marital difficulties, fear of labour, and anxious and depressed mood during pregnancy. However, there is no evidence that life events other than childbirth contribute to onset and little evidence that there is any increase in risk of mental disorders generally.

Treatment

It is important to recognize the nature of the condition so that the patient and her family can be reassured about the likely course and outcome. Considerable tact and understanding are required by medical and nursing staff in their approach to the patient. Monitoring of the mental state should continue to ensure that complete recovery takes place, and that no other mental disorder is developing.

Course and prognosis

By definition recovery invariably takes place within 2 weeks without specific treatment and if this does not occur the diagnosis should be reviewed.

POST-NATAL DEPRESSION

Epidemiology

Between 10 per cent and 20 per cent of women develop a depressive illness during the first 3 months following childbirth, and the incidence is therefore increased compared with the general population.

Clinical features

Generally symptoms develop after the patient has been discharged from hospital 2 weeks or more after parturition. The patient feels despondent, is tearful, and is distressed by feelings of inadequacy and inability to cope, particularly with the baby. There may be feelings of guilt, usually limited to self-reproach about not caring for the baby. The mood is often labile and depression tends to be worse in the evening. Commonly there is marked irritability, anorexia, fatigue, and feelings of exhaustion. Sleep disturbance is usually limited to initial insomnia. Almost always the patient exhibits excessive concern regarding the health of the baby and often shows hypochondriacal preoccupation with her own somatic symptoms.

Diagnostic criteria

The disorder is characterized by mixed symptoms of depression and anxiety, which have their onset in the puerperium and persist for a minimum of 2 weeks.

Differential diagnosis

It must be differentiated both from the 'maternity blues' and from puerperal psychosis, and also from other non-psychotic disorders that have their onset before or during the puerperium.

Aetiology

There is no evidence that biological factors play any major part in the cause of post-natal depression, despite some claims to the contrary. There is an increased frequency in primipara over the age of 30. There is also an association with a history of a disturbed relationship between the mother and her own parents during her childhood. As with non-puerperal depressed women, there is evidence that adverse life events interact with social and personality vulnerability factors to induce depressive illness in the post-natal period. Some studies have suggested that there is a relationship between anxiety during pregnancy and post-natal depression. For some women childbirth presents a maturational crisis, imposing a new psychological and physical burden and increased demands from others for dependency. Lack of sleep can also contribute to post-natal depression, and the health visitor can help the mother work out ways of getting enough back-up support so she can get adequate sleep.

Investigations

No specific investigations are required, apart from establishing the time of onset of the disorder in relation to the puerperium, and a careful assessment of the psychological and social significance to the patient of childbirth.

Treatment

Tricyclic antidepressants are occasionally required, based on the usual indications. Claims for the effectiveness of specific treatment with progesterone on its own or in combination with monoamine oxidase inhibitors have been made but are at present unsubstantiated. For the most part treatment should focus on supportive therapy of the patient and her family by the primary care team, who should be particularly aware of difficulties that may occur in the process of bonding. With training, health visitors can provide counselling that results in early recovery by most patients.

Course and prognosis

The majority of patients recover within 6 to 12 months, but if untreated one-half of patients have failed to improve 1 year after childbirth. Chronic affective disorders starting after childbirth are not uncommon, tend to include poor libido and hypochondriasis, and may remain unidentified for many years.

PUERPERAL PSYCHOSIS

Epidemiology

Between one and two women per thousand deliveries develop a new episode of illness characterized by psychotic symptoms. The majority of these have their onset within the first 2 weeks of parturition. There is an increased risk particularly for primiparous women (double that for multiparous women) and possibly after caesarean section. No definite relationship has been found with other obstetric factors, with social class, or with marital status.

Clinical features

Symptoms generally have their onset between 3 and 10 days after childbirth, although a small proportion start in the subsequent 2 weeks. Usually they develop rapidly over the course of a few days. Any of the syndromes of the functional psychoses may occur but there is a particular tendency to find mixed states, with both affective and schizophreniform symptoms, and marked fluctuations in the type and severity of symptoms during the course of the disorder. Depressive symptoms predominate in over half these episodes and manic symptoms in about a third. Often these are mixed with 'first rank' symptoms of schizophrenia. Perplexity occurs in the majority and a substantial minority are disorientated at some stage.

Diagnostic criteria

Any mental illness that includes psychotic symptoms and has its onset within 4 weeks after parturition is included in this category. It should be differentiated from episodes of illness having a previous onset but continuing into the puerperium, and from acute toxic states (delirium).

Aetiology

After an episode of puerperal psychosis there is an increased risk of psychoses at times other than the puerperium, and there is also an increased risk of psychotic illness generally in first-degree relatives. Episodes of mania (i.e. elevated mood with psychosis) precipitated in the immediate puerperium show a strong association with a family history of puerperal mania in female relatives. Thus there appears to be some general genetic and constitutional predisposition. There is no evidence of an excess of negative life events or difficulties during pregnancy. It is generally believed that these disorders are precipitated by the rapid and extreme changes in the hormonal state following parturition, but confirmation has proved elusive. Comparisons of psychotic puerperal women with non-psychotic puerperal women have shown the former to have higher levels of thyroxin and prolactin (and possibly oestrogen) and lower levels of luteinizing hormone and progesterone, but the significance of these findings is uncertain.

Investigations

Careful monitoring of the physical and mental state is required to rule out the possibility of an acute toxic state. Details of the patient's social circumstances and the available sources of support will be important in planning her treatment.

Treatment

It is usually necessary to admit the patient to a psychiatric unit and wherever possible this should be with her baby to a specialized mother and baby unit. Patients with a predominantly depressive syndrome in the puerperium tend to respond less well to antidepressant drugs than those with depressive illnesses at other times. Those with predominantly manic or depressive illnesses are usually started on a neuroleptic medication. Electroconvulsive treatment is particularly effective and therefore tends to be used earlier than in other depressive illnesses. Despite claims for the value of treatment with oestrogen and/or progesterone there is little evidence to support their efficacy. Expert nursing, including attention to nutrition and fluid balance, is important and this should ideally be carried out on a dedicated mother and baby unit, which will allow the mother supervised access to the baby, and the opportunity to take part in baby care when well enough. This will facilitate bonding. As her mental state improves she should take increasing responsibility for the baby's care. Her ability to do this will require careful assessment, which will determine the amount and nature of supervision needed once they are discharged from hospital.

Course and prognosis

With treatment virtually all patients improve or recover within 3 months. Of those patients who have further pregnancies about 30 per cent have a recurrence of puerperal psychoses. If the patient has a bipolar illness the risk in subsequent pregnancy is as high as 50 per cent. However the risk of recurrence is by no means limited to the puerperium, and about 40 per cent of all women who suffer a puerperal psychosis will have another episode of psychotic illness at some time.

INFANTICIDE

Depression in the puerperium carries a small but definite risk that the mother will kill her child. If this occurs within 12 months of the birth and there is evidence that 'the balance of her mind was disturbed' at the time, this act is described as 'infanticide' and dealt with in British law as manslaughter rather than murder. Approximately half the women who kill their children in the puerperium also commit suicide.

Therapeutic use of drugs during pregnancy and the puerperium

1. Drugs taken by women of child-bearing age may have a **teratogenic** effect if they become pregnant.
2. Drugs taken at the end of pregnancy may result in **withdrawal symptoms in the baby** following delivery.
3. Drugs taken during lactation may result in **toxicity in the breast-fed child**.

In view of these possible effects it is desirable to avoid the use of medication for the treatment of mental illness during pregnancy, and – if the mother wishes to breast-feed her child – during the puerperium. However, if there is a strong clinical indication for medication, this must be balanced against the risks, and it is probably best to advise against breast-feeding if psychotropic medication is given.

TRICYCLIC ANTIDEPRESSANTS

There is probably no evidence of a teratogenic effect when tricyclic antidepressants are taken in therapeutic doses. Withdrawal effects occur in neonates and if possible it is preferable to stop these drugs a few days before delivery is expected. Tricyclics are excreted in the milk only in very small quantities and, therefore, breast-feeding is not contra-indicated when the mother is being treated with these drugs. However, **the more sedating antidepressants are best avoided** as they can lead to respiratory depression and drowsiness.

SELECTIVE SEROTONIN RE-UPTAKE INHIBITORS

Evidence is accumulating that use of SSRIs in pregnancy and the puerperium is not associated with any increase in congenital abnormalities. Most evidence is available for fluoxetene.

BENZODIAZEPINES

There have been reports of congenital malformations, particularly cleft lip and palate, in children born to women taking these drugs during pregnancy. Although the risk is probably small, the potential value of taking these drugs is unlikely to warrant their continuation during pregnancy and **they should be avoided**. Diazepam has been used for the treatment of pre-eclamptic toxaemia. This may result in toxicity in the neonate, causing the **'floppy infant' syndrome**, as well as withdrawal symptoms as a result of prior physical addiction, and both require specialized neonatal care. These drugs are excreted in milk and their use should be avoided in breast-feeding.

PHENOTHIAZINES AND BUTYROPHENONES

There is little evidence that these drugs have a teratogenic effect and it appears that toxic effects in the neonate are rare. When taken by the lactating mother these drugs are absorbed by the baby in very small quantities, and animal studies have shown there may be effects on the developing nervous system. **Avoidance is therefore recommended in breast-feeding**. Although best avoided during pregnancy, these drugs may be used if there is a strong clinical indication, such as in prophylaxis of previous puerperal psychosis.

LITHIUM

It is well established that lithium has a **teratogenic** effect, particularly related to foetal cardiac abnormalities. It should, therefore, be **gradually reduced then stopped prior to a planned pregnancy**, and contraception should be practised at other times. Until recent years use was more or less avoided in pregnancy, at least until the third trimester. In all circumstances the risks and benefits must be weighed in the balance, however where there is good clinical indication for its use, for example where there are difficulties with maintaining remission with other drugs, and previous illness has been associated with significant risk, then it can be used from the second trimester, after the foetal heart has developed. Because lithium has a narrow therapeutic range, above which there is significant risk of toxicity, careful monitoring must be taken to control the serum level of the drug. This is because lithium is water soluble, and there are big changes in salt and water balance during pregnancy because of the increased glomerular filtration rate, and big shifts that occur rapidly at delivery. Lithium passes into breast milk and this can result in toxicity. Although there is little evidence of any long-term effect, **breast-feeding should be avoided**.

ATYPICAL ANTIPSYCHOTICS

Sufficient data are now available on the use of some of these newer agents, in particular olanzapine, to suggest they are safe, however as emphasized in all cases above, risks and benefits must be evaluated.

MOOD STABILIZ|ING AGENTS

Anti-epileptic agents are used as mood stabilizers. **Sodium valproate should be avoided throughout pregnancy**, and has been shown to cause impairment in cognitive function in the developing foetus. **Phenytoin is associated with cleft lip and digital abnormalities, and carbemazipine should also be avoided**. Little information is available for lamotrigine, which should also therefore **not be given in pregnancy or while breast-feeding**.

Sterilization and hysterectomy

Recent prospective studies indicate that these procedures rarely contribute to the aetiology of mental illness. Sexual enjoyment is often enhanced by sterilization and regrets are uncommon. In a small proportion of cases there are prolonged difficulties in adjustment, including symptoms of anxiety and depression, and these are virtually limited to women in whom there is a past history of similar symptoms. Sometimes these procedures are embarked on as an unrealistic way of trying to deal with other problems, particularly in the marriage or in sexual adjustment. Therefore, a past history of mental illness or current interpersonal or social difficulties indicates a particular need for cautious assessment before surgery.

The menopause

There is no evidence that serious mental illness of any kind is commoner in women around the time of the menopause than at other times. The term 'involutional melancholia' was used in the past to describe severe depressive illness that was thought to be specifically linked to the menopause. The term is now obsolete because this form of the disorder is related to the effects of age on symptoms of depressive illness, rather than to the menopause.

EPIDEMIOLOGY AND CLINICAL FEATURES OF MENOPAUSAL SYMPTOMS

Symptoms commonly complained of by menopausal and post-menopausal women fall into two main groups. Complaints of **hot flushes and excessive sweating** are commonest 1 or 2 years after the cessation of periods, when they are experienced by up to 90 per cent of all women and then gradually dwindle in frequency over the next few years. These are caused by vaso-motor changes, are closely related to reduced ovarian activity, and respond to treatment with oestrogen.

In the year following the end of menstruation approximately one-third of women complain of symptoms including **irritability, anxiety, fatigue,** and **headaches** and this is approximately 10 per cent greater than the frequency in pre-menopausal and post-menopausal women. These symptoms do not differ in quality from affective symptoms occurring in women at other times, or in men.

AETIOLOGY

There is no evidence that the affective symptoms are related to reduced oestrogen production: they are primarily psychological in origin. To some extent they appear to be determined by the **meaning of the experience** of the menopause. The end of potentially reproductive life is mourned by many women and regarded as a sign of ageing. However, it is welcomed by others, particularly in those cultures where contraception is not practised.

It is also a time when many other changes commonly occur in a woman's life, including the loss of children who leave home and the death of parents. These changes require considerable adjustment and it is not surprising if symptoms of minor affective disorder are commoner at this stage of life, particularly in those individuals who generally have difficulty in making appropriate adjustments to change.

Careful assessment of the nature and duration of symptoms will help to determine the possible value of medication. Each patient will require an individual appraisal of their current social circumstances and their psychological response to recent events.

TREATMENT

Symptoms of affective disorder occurring at the menopause do not respond to oestrogen any better than to placebos. Both antidepressants and benzodiazepines have been found to relieve some symptoms better than placebos, but their use should be restricted to the usual indications for these drugs, and benzodiazepines should be avoided because of the significant risks of habituation and dependency. Psychosocial problems should be considered. Most patients will benefit from supportive psychotherapy.

CLASSIFICATION OF SEXUAL DISORDERS

Psychiatric disorders are classified in Britain and Europe according to the International Classification of Diseases – 10th Revision (ICD-10) as shown below.

ICD-10

F50–F59 Behavioural syndromes associated with physiological disturbances and physical factors

F52 *Sexual dysfunction not caused by organic disorder or disease*
F52.0 Lack or loss of sexual desire
F52.1 Sexual aversion, lack of sexual enjoyment
F52.2 Failure of genital response
F52.3 Orgasmic dysfunction
F52.4 Premature ejaculation
F52.6 Non-organic dyspareunia
F52.7 Excessive sexual drive
F52.8 Other sexual disorder not caused by organic dysfunction or disease
F52.9 Unspecified sexual disorder not caused by organic dysfunction or disease

F60–F69 Disorders of adult personality and behaviour

F64 *Gender identity disorders*
F64.0 Transsexualism
F64.1 Dual-role transvestism
F64.2 Gender identity disorder of childhood
F64.8 Other gender identity disorders
F64.9 Gender identity disorder unspecified

F65 *Disorders of sexual preference*
F65.0 Fetishism
F65.1 Fetishistic transvestism
F65.2 Exhibitionism
F65.3 Voyerism
F65.4 Paedophilia
F65.5 Sadomasochism
F65.6 Multiple disorders of sexual preference
F65.7 Other disorders of sexual preference
F65.8 Disorders of sexual preference unspecified
F66.0 Sexual maturation disorder
F66.1 Ego-dystonic sexual orientation
F66.2 Sexual relationship disorder
F66.8 Other psychosexual development disorders
F66.9 Psychosexual development disorder unspecified
  .x0 Heterosexuality
  .x2 Homosexuality

.x3   Bisexuality

.x4   Other, including pubertal

In order for the disorder to be pathological it:

- Must cause significant distress.
- Must not be due to a general medical condition.
- Must not be due to substance or alcohol misuse.
- Must impair ability to function in a sexual relationship.

FURTHER READING

Bancroft, J.H.J. (1983) *Human Sexuality and Its Problems*. Edinburgh: Churchill Livingstone.

Gath, D. and Cooper, P. (1982) Psychiatric aspects of hysterectomy and female sterilisation. In K. Granville-Grossman (Ed.), *Recent Advances in Psychiatry*, Volume 4. Edinburgh: Churchill Livingstone.

Gath, D., Osborn, M., Bungay, G. et al. (1987) Psychiatric disorder and gynaecological symptoms in middle aged women: A community survey. *British Medical Journal*, 294, 213–218.

Greene, J.G. (1984) *The Social and Psychological Origins of the Climacteric Syndrome*. Aldershot: Gower.

Hawton, K. (1982) Sexual problems in the general hospital. In F. Creed and J. Pfeffer (Eds), *Medicine and Psychiatry*. London: Pitman.

Hawton, K. (1985) *Sex Therapy. A Practical Guide*. Oxford: Oxford University Press.

Heiman, J.R. and LoPiccolo, J. (1999) *Becoming Orgasmic. A Sexual and Personal Growth Programme for Women*. London: Piatkus.

Melnik, T. and Abdo, C.H.N. (2005) Psychogenic erectile dysfunction: Comparative study of three therapeutic approaches. *Journal of Sex and Marital Therapy*, 31, 243–255.

Rosen, R.C. (2001) Psychogenic erectile dysfunction. Classification and management. *Urologic Clinics of North America*, 86, 2.

Singer Kaplan, H. (1989) *How to Overcome Premature Ejaculation* London: Brunner/Mazel.

Zilbergeld, B. (1999) *The New Male Sexuality. The Truth about Man, Sex and Pleasure*, Revised Edition. New York and Toronto: Bantam Books.

22   DISORDERS OF OLDER PEOPLE

Life expectancy is increasing throughout the world population. This means that more individuals survive into old age and as the number of births falls, the proportion of the population looked on as old increases. In the United Kingdom the population aged over 65 years has risen from 5 per cent to 15 per cent in less than a hundred years. Similar changes in the age structure of populations throughout the rest of the world are occurring at an even more dramatic rate so that an understanding of the special characteristics of older people, including their health/illness profiles and the way that they present, is increasingly important in medical practice. Women survive into late life more often than men and in the years beyond the age of 75 men are outnumbered by three to one. From 1985 to 2041 projections forecast that people in the UK over the age of 60 will increase from 21 per cent to 26 per cent while the rise in the over-85s will be from 6 per cent to 11 per cent (700,000 to 1,700,000). Illnesses and disability become more common in older people hence they are more likely to consult general practitioners, social services, and hospitals.

Change in normal psychological function is a necessary accompaniment of ageing and is reflected in everyday activities and social networks. On average older people are not involved in as wide a range of activities as young people, and this can be explained only in part by factors such as retirement, reduced income, upper age-limits, or failing health. Drive and ambition are often reduced, and enthusiasm for new ventures is limited. In healthy old age impulses and emotions are well controlled so that intemperate outbursts are uncommon. Specific skills and information acquired over a lifetime of experience are preserved, but the acquisition of new skills and adaptation to new situations is not so easy: they take time, but can be achieved. These normal changes of ageing bring with them a reputation for wisdom, a degree of suspiciousness of novel ideas, and a need for respect and time to achieve effective communication and to assimilate responses. There are limits to the total amount of change that an individual can tolerate, but more important is the rate at which change is presented.

Multi-generation households are rare in the UK. This means that the majority of older people live with other old people – marital partners, unmarried or divorced children, brothers and sisters or parents; or they live alone. This latter status is increasingly common for survivors, mostly women, into their eighties and beyond. Those who stay on in what has been the family home may be entirely happy, but sometimes find it

341

difficult to maintain if it lacks modern amenities. There is renewed interest in specialist 'sheltered' housing schemes that offer support and supervision, communal facilities that can be accessed when needed, and extra care at times of illness or other difficulty.

Many people find their retirement years very fulfilling, with adequate income, secure housing, and the time and opportunity to realize dreams that have been on hold through a lifetime dedicated to caring for others. Even so it can be a time of challenge and potential stress. This last may arise from illness experienced for the first time, loss or illness of a partner, parent, brother or sister, or disappointment or worry associated with children or grandchildren. Fear of robbery or violence may restrict what people feel able to do. Adverse social circumstances combined with failing physical health may produce pathologies of mental health and these same factors militate against quick recovery once a disorder has occurred.

AETIOLOGY

Background considerations

While retirement is often portrayed as tranquil and undemanding – rather like an extended holiday – it is in fact beset with stresses. Losses occur as a direct result of retirement: reduction of income, freedom from an imposed timetable, and loss of the territory of work and the challenges, company and status that were an integral part of the Monday to Friday routine. In their stead come new challenges: husbands and wives thrown into one another's company for longer periods than they have been accustomed to, and survival on a limited budget that cannot be supplemented by increased effort. Work has come to be viewed as a scarce commodity not to be shared with the old. Time in retirement has less intrinsic structure beyond the alternation of night and day, the sequence of the seasons, and the television schedules. Children and grandchildren may marry; grandchildren and great grandchildren may arrive. Even these happy events carry mixed messages. Inevitably, time brings further losses: bereavements, destruction of favourite haunts by redevelopment and, most significantly, loss of that sense of physical well-being that has hitherto been taken for granted. In its place for some comes reduced mobility, impairment of the senses of sight, hearing, taste and smell, and the possibility of pains associated with physical disease.

Physical health

The most consistent characteristic of psychiatric disorders in old age is their association with physical illness and disability. This applies across the range of psychiatric illness, including mood disorders and paranoid states as well as the dementias. Delirium (acute confusional state) often complicates or acts as a presenting feature of physical illness. Dementia becomes progressively more common with increasing age, is often associated with physical illness, and in some instances is a direct consequence of physical illness.

342

Medication and care-giving

Treatment prescribed for physical illness may also produce psychiatric symptoms, while the intrusive attention from nurses and other carers that may become necessary as a consequence of dependency may be received as further humiliations, be they provided at home, or in a hospital or nursing home.

Previous mental illness or family illness

Sometimes it is possible to uncover a history of illness in earlier life or a history of similar conditions in close relatives. Sometimes it seems relevant that the patient has known no model of successful ageing in his or her own family.

Personality

Certainly long-standing personality traits and coping strategies developed in earlier life are important in determining how an individual will respond to difficulties encountered in old age.

SYNDROMES COMMON IN OLD AGE

The dementias and delirium

(Please refer to Chapter 12, pp. 159–179)

Here are some additional points, relevant to old age:

1. The distinction between a **delirium** and a **dementia** may present difficulties, since the presence of the latter makes symptoms of confusion and disorientation more likely when intercurrent illness strikes. A history from a reliable informant is the key to a successful diagnosis, not infrequently an acute delirium may overlie a dementia syndrome (see p. 174).
2. Patients with **depressive illness** may appear confused and disorientated if they have impairments of vision or hearing as well; or if physical illness limits their ability to move. **Pseudo-dementia** is a term given to a functional disorder (usually depression) presenting with features of dementia. In extreme cases of rapid change, psychomotor agitation, and heightened arousal, a picture of **pseudo-delirium** may emerge.
3. Rarer conditions that should be distinguished from delirium include **dominant hemisphere cerebrovascular accidents** in which there is jargon aphasia but non-verbal tests are performed normally; and **transient global amnesias** related to bilateral temporal lesions.
4. The other point to grasp is that many demented patients manage perfectly well in a protected environment that makes few demands of them, but they develop symptoms of anxiety, disorientation, and suspicion when they are stressed by relocation

Psychiatry in Medical Practice

or the introduction of unfamiliar regimes or people. This is sometimes referred to as *'compensated'* (steady state – all is well in the routines of home) and *'decompensated'* (alarm – something very odd and unwelcome is going on) dementia. It is in this sense that *depression* or *anxiety* can release a syndrome symptomatically equivalent to subacute brain delirium in a previously apparently healthy old person: and thus depressive illness and anxiety states are included in the differential diagnosis of delirium. In addition *social and psychological stress* without evidence of an affective illness as such can also cause a person with dementia to decompensate and manifest a subacute delirium: such stresses include anything that suddenly disrupts the environment: a spouse dying or being admitted to hospital, moving to a new house, being admitted to hospital for some other reason, or going on holiday. Sometimes the cause seems to be loss of a familiar environment; sometimes it is too much stimulation from the environment. Thus a house with too much noise – perhaps dominated by the activities of teenage grandchildren – or a noisy ward with frightening machinery and frequent changes of staff, may overload the patient with too much input.

5. Depression can mimic dementia and the term *pseudo-dementia* was coined to describe patients who presented with cognitive impairment in the context of depressive symptoms. Studies using computed tomography (CT) scans have shown that such patients often have evidence of brain atrophy intermediate between normal age-matched controls and patients with dementia. Patients with depression and no associated brain abnormalities may also present with self-neglect and loss of interest, and may perform poorly on formal testing of cognitive function, often giving depressive 'don't know' answers to questions rather than providing an incorrect answer. The diagnosis of depression can be reached if patients are questioned about their mood, associated neurovegetative symptoms (e.g. diurnal mood variation, poor appetite, early morning wakening, poor concentration, anergia), and negative thoughts about the future and their own self-worth. Older people may not present with feelings of low mood but will admit to experiencing a loss of pleasure (anhedonia) and to giving up their interests over and above what might be normally expected for an older person. Such changes may be explained away by the patient as a natural reaction to growing old, or to limitations imposed by physical disability. An informed account of the situation from a relative or care-giver is invaluable in teasing apart the history.

Schizophrenia and allied states (see pp. 185–200)

CLINICAL FEATURES

Most patients who develop schizophrenia in early adult life will survive into old age. Some will have predominantly negative or defect symptoms with lack of initiative and drive, blunted emotions and lack of self-care (see p. 167), while others will present combinations of defect symptoms and florid symptoms – most usually persecutory delusions accompanied by hallucinations.

344

Some patients develop schizophrenia-like psychoses for the first time in old age, and because of their special features these illnesses have been called *persistent persecutory states of the elderly*. The principal abnormality consists of auditory hallucinations that are accompanied by delusions of persecution. Other patients develop persecutory psychoses with marked depressive features.

AETIOLOGY

Genetic factors are less important than in schizophrenias of earlier life. Persistent persecutory states are commoner in women, and patients tend to have previous life-styles and personalities characterized by emotional and sexual coldness. Social isolation, often exacerbated by failing vision, failing hearing, physical illness, or restricted mobility facilitate both the hallucinatory phenomena and the persecutory ideas.

TREATMENT

Formation of a reasonable therapeutic alliance is an essential, although often very difficult, first step. Hallucinations can usually be suppressed with antipsychotic medication: but compliance is always a major problem, and symptoms return when the medication is stopped. If the patient can be persuaded to persist with medication they often return to their former lives as competent, rather distant individuals. Life expectancy is not reduced, and treatment as an out-patient is usually possible. Old patients treated with antipsychotic medication for prolonged periods may experience apathy and reduced drive, or develop Parkinsonism or dyskinesia. Anti-parkinsonian treatment should be avoided if possible, and the patient maintained on the smallest dose of antipsychotic medicine that is effective in controlling their hallucinations.

Affective disorders

DEPRESSIVE ILLNESS: (see pp. 209–221)

Symptoms of anxiety and depression are found in 10 to 20 per cent of old people living at home, and even higher figures are found in those presenting for care to their general practitioner, to hospital out-patients, or to social services. Depressive illnesses are slightly less common than at earlier ages (although depressive symptoms may occur very commonly), and hypomania is comparatively rare.

Older patients are even more likely than younger patients to present with somatic symptoms when they are psychologically unwell (see Chapter 11). Those who will later be found to be suffering from a depressive illness will originally have sought help for complaints such as tiredness, weakness, palpitations, anorexia, constipation, breathlessness, and pains. It may be that physical pathology (for example, arthritis, a hemiparesis, or varicose veins) is indeed present and may account for some of these pains – but the symptomatology attributed to the physical disease is exaggerated by the mood disorder that itself may be hidden or denied.

Withdrawal from activities ('*Because I'm too old for them now and should give way to younger folk*') and **reluctance to leave the house** ('*I'm not so good on my feet now, and if I fell I'd be such a trouble to everyone*') may be presenting symptoms of a depressive illness, but the 'explanations' of the symptoms are easily accepted by relatives. Indeed, the 'understandability' of symptoms of depression and anxiety is a great hazard for the elderly, since detection and treatment are made less likely. There are therefore parallels with the depressive states secondary to malignant disease (see p. 216): in both cases, symptoms may respond to treatment, and they should therefore be regarded as morbid phenomena rather than as 'understandable' reactions to circumstance.

The risk of successful **suicide** increases with age and must always be borne in mind with depressed old people, especially if they live alone or are physically ill. Although some make suicidal threats for the effect that such threats have on others, it must be remembered that suicide becomes more common with advancing age. Thus any hint that an old patient is contemplating suicide must be taken seriously, and the doctor must ensure that adequate supervision is available and must provide active treatment. In practice, this will usually involve admission to hospital. Old people who have survived a suicide attempt should certainly be admitted to hospital – voluntarily if possible, but on a compulsory order if necessary.

PSYCHOTIC DEPRESSION (see p. 212)

In patients with psychotic depression, delusions of worthlessness, poverty, or nihilism occur at all ages, but delusions of infestation and cancer are also seen in the elderly. Psychomotor symptoms – either agitation or retardation – commonly accompany such delusions.

The differentiation of Parkinson's disease from psychotic depression can be difficult, since in both the patient may appear retarded: once more, correct assessment depends on careful history-taking.

DEPRESSIVE PSEUDO-DEMENTIA

This refers to the scenario wherein a depressed patient may be convinced that they are losing their memory (and often their mind) and performs poorly on tests of short-term memory during the mental state examination. This may lead to a diagnosis of dementia. The differentiation of *depressive pseudo-dementia* from degenerative dementias can be made by careful history-taking. In the former condition there will be a short time-scale of development, with anxious and depressive symptoms predominating from the outset, and there may also be a history of earlier depressive episodes. Even when the examination is confined to simple test material such as the Abbreviated Mental Test, the patient manages to communicate severe depression and self-doubt with his answers:

I don't know. I don't know. Oh, don't be bothering with me . . . it's all beyond me now.

In contrast, some demented patients produce inaccurate answers with confidence, sometimes amounting to confabulation.

MANIA (see p. 202)

This occurs in old people, but it is less common than in early adult life. Mixed states with both depressive and hypomanic features may bewilder both the patient and his relatives: the typical picture of earlier adult life (see p. 212) is unusual. Irritability, downright combativeness, and even paranoid sensitivity are more common than elation and a sense of well-being. There is a real risk that excessive activity combined with lack of both sleep and food may put life at risk by precipitating serious cardiac or respiratory problems. First onset of mania in older people may reflect a cerebral lesion and should be investigated thoroughly.

Alcoholism and drug dependence (see pp. 250–267)

Some of those dependent on alcohol in early adult life manage to survive into old age; and many more are now surviving into old age dependent on sleeping tablets and 'minor' tranquillizers. As such patients develop new pathology in their liver or brain, they may lose their tolerance for alcohol or other drugs, and are therefore at higher risk for organic brain syndromes and other psychiatric disorders.

Some old people – including surprising numbers of women – turn to drink or tranquillizers for the first time in old age. They have usually been prescribed such drugs for the symptomatic relief of symptoms of depression or anxiety, although in some dependence on the drug has been released by the disinhibition of dementia. These patients typically come to medical attention through complications that include confusion, falls, and self-neglect; or the problem is reported by embarrassed relatives or home helps who have been prevailed on to act as suppliers.

In theory treatment of those becoming dependent for the first time in old age should be straightforward, and should consist of withdrawal of the agent with appropriate treatment of the problem that has precipitated the dependence. However, in practice there are often real difficulties: partly because of the intractable nature of some of the associated social problems, but sometimes because of obstinacy on the part of the patient.

Learning disability (see pp. 287–296)

Life expectancy for individuals with a learning disability, even when associated with multiple disabilities or a recognized genetic abnormality, has increased dramatically during the past 30 years. Those handicapped individuals who survive into old age are typically cared for by sisters or brothers after their parents' death, though some will reside in specialist homes. They may present as depressed or as 'confused' when death or illness of a carer confronts them with their own limitations in coping ability. There are special considerations for individuals with Down's syndrome, where Alzheimer-like changes occur in most individuals who survive into their fifties or beyond.

Diogenes syndrome

A rare syndrome, Diogenes syndrome is typified by severe self-neglect (named after the Greek philosopher who lived in a barrel). Sufferers typically hoard belongings and rubbish, in particular newspapers, and may pose a hazard to neighbours. Frequently they have very poor self-care, neglect their diet, and are often reclusive. Some are found to be suffering from a frontal lobe dementia or paraphrenia. However, most will have no apparent psychiatric illness, but isolative traits in their personality.

INVESTIGATIONS

Home assessments

There are many advantages in making assessments in the patient's home. Not only is this convenient for the patient, but it provides an opportunity for the doctor to see the patient functioning in the environment in which the problems have been identified. Information about current stresses and potential supports is readily available, as well as a great deal of useful information concerning the patient's personal life. If the patient is to be admitted to hospital, it is possible to make arrangements with relatives about how care will be resumed outside hospital when the time comes. However, some elderly patients may prefer to be seen at the hospital.

Physical examination

In addition to the usual physical examination including weighing the patient and testing the urine, it is important to remember to test eye-sight (with spectacles), hearing (with any hearing aid), to inspect teeth (and dentures), feet, balance and coordination, and to carry out a rectal examination.

A full blood count, biochemical profile, and chest film should be carried out in every case, together with any further special investigations that are indicated by the particular circumstances of the case. It is now recommended that brain scans should be carried out to investigate the possibility of intra-cranial pathology, and to clarify diagnosis in all patients presenting with symptoms of dementia.

TREATMENT OF THE OLDER PATIENT

It is of the first importance to build a trusting relationship between members of the multi-disciplinary team on the one hand, and the patient and their family on the other. Psychological treatments are usually exploratory or supportive. Dependence on the therapist is unlikely to become intense, and can be sustained for relatively long periods while adjustment to new circumstances is achieved.

It is important that doses of psychotropic drugs are adjusted downwards, to take account of reduced body mass and reduced renal function in the elderly. High blood levels of drugs are easily attained, and may rise as the drug accumulates. The presence of other drugs, prescribed for other conditions, means that drug interactions may complicate the undesired effects of any psychotropic drugs that are prescribed. It is therefore important to make sure that all drugs being prescribed are really necessary, and that none are being prescribed in doses that are too high.

The problems described above should not lead to failure to prescribe necessary drugs: mental illness in old age causes much preventable suffering, and is also associated with premature death by suicide. It is important to work closely with primary care in the management of these patients, and to pay particular attention to physical as well as psychological problems.

Interview techniques with old people

When approaching an interview with an elderly patient it is important to *take account of their relative slowness*, the possibility that they will tire easily, and the greater likelihood that they will have difficulty with memory as well as problems with eye-sight, hearing, and mobility. Making sure that your face is at the same level as the patient, that your eyes and lips can be seen, and that you speak slowly and clearly take little trouble and are much appreciated – for it provides extra cues to supplement fading or unreliable hearing. However, do not assume that all elderly people are half-blind, half-deaf, and cognitively impaired!

Old people in particular have expectations about how a doctor will dress and behave: *a careful, polite approach is essential*. Repeated short interviews often achieve more than attempts to press on beyond the endurance of the patient. As in obstetric practice, two empty bladders are a good investment before you start.

Although you will encourage the patient to focus on their current problems as they give you the history, you should allow them to diverge from time to time to share a reminiscence with you – this shows an interest in them and their experiences, and will consolidate trust between you.

Since memory problems and confusion are common in elderly patients, it is unwise to rely only on information from the patient, and you should always be sure to *talk to a relative as well*. It is not unusual for an elderly patient to be quite unaware of problems that others have noticed, and they may even deny that abnormalities reported by others have actually occurred.

Mental status examination in elderly patients

As with any other patient, this starts with *careful observation* and recording of the patient's appearance, behaviour, and spontaneous speech. If you are carrying out an assessment in the patient's home remember to include the situation in which the patient is living. Thus there may be evidence of longstanding self-neglect or failure to cope; or multiple locks and hostile messages may indicate a paranoid disorder.

There are occasions when this is all that can be achieved as more formal testing may be beyond the patient's ability. On these occasions be sure to obtain a history from a relative, and return to an assessment of the patient's cognitive state as soon as the patient's physical condition allows.

Examination of cognitive function is especially important as delirium and dementia syndromes are common. However, there are traps for the unwary. It is easy to elicit lack of awareness of current events and deficits in new learning in an old patient who is depressed, anxious, feeling physically unwell, in pain, or even just feeling uncomfortable in strange surroundings. You may conclude that the patient is demented or confused, when what is really wrong is that your test procedures were too fast, too long, too complex, or just badly presented. Short, simple tests that encourage the patient to do well with early items are better accepted and provide more worthwhile information. A number of question and answer tests have been developed that require the retrieval of knowledge acquired in the distant past, and also require accurate recall of more recently acquired information

FURTHER READING

Blythe, R. (1981) *The View of Winter*. Harmondsworth: Penguin Books.

Burns, A., Gallagley, A. and Byrne, J. (2004) Delirium. *Journal of Neurology, Neurosurgery, and Psychiatry*, 75, 362–367.

Burns, A., Lawlor, B. and Craig, S. (2004) *Assessment Scales in Old Age Psychiatry*. London: Martin Dunitz.

Burns, A., O'Brien, J. and Ames, D. (2005) *Dementia*, 3rd edition. London: Edward Arnold.

Burns, A., Purandare, N. and Craig, S. (2002) *Depression, Confusion and Dementia in Older People: A Practical Guide*. London: Royal Society of Medicine.

Copeland, J.. Abou-Saleh, M. and Blazer, D. (2002) *Principles and Practice of Geriatric Psychiatry*, 2nd edition. Chichester: John Wiley and Sons.

Jacoby, R. and Oppenheimer, C. (2002) *Psychiatry in the Elderly*, 3rd edition. Oxford: Oxford University Press.

PART 4

SERVICES, ETHICS AND THE LAW

23   SERVICES FOR PEOPLE WITH MENTAL HEALTH PROBLEMS

Until the last part of the twentieth century, the focus of services for people with mental illness was in a number of large mental hospitals or 'asylums', which were usually built outside towns and cities and sometimes had more than a thousand in-patients. Such large hospitals for the treatment of mental illness still exist in some parts of the world, but in many countries mental health care has undergone a revolution during the last 30 years with the closure of such large institutions and the development of 'care in the community'.

During the same period it has become clear from large-scale epidemiological studies, that the majority of people with mental health problems are seen and treated in primary care settings, by their family doctor. In the UK more than 90 per cent of people with mental health problems are treated in this way and never come into contact with specialist services for mental illness.

Most NHS mental health services in England and Wales are provided by organizations called Mental Health Trusts (some primary care-based services may be run by the local Primary Care Trust), and in Scotland by Primary Care Trusts. These organizations have close links with social services provided by local government. People with mental health problems (usually referred to in specialist mental health services as '**service-users**' rather than 'patients') play a more important role in providing feedback to the NHS on how services should be provided than in general medical care.

There is increasing recognition of the importance of good interagency working between mental health, social services, and the primary care team to ensure that all aspects of care (particularly physical as well as psychological and social) are properly addressed in a multi-axial care plan.

MENTAL HEALTH AND ILLNESS IN PRIMARY CARE

The commonest mental disorders seen by general practitioners are anxiety and depression (see Chapter 15). Mental health problems are implicated in one in four primary care consultations in the UK, making mental health consultations second only to those for respiratory infection, and depression is the third most common reason for consultation in UK general practice.

The **primary care team** play an important part in detecting and managing common mental disorders and in ensuring good physical health care for people with severe and enduring mental health problems. There is a need for close liaison between the GP, the primary care team, and specialist services both regarding individual patients to ensure high quality care, but also to have a dialogue about service provision and developments that are inidicated.

General practitioners play a key role in diagnosis and treatment, and in decision-making about referral to other professionals. GPs vary a great deal in their attitudes towards people with mental illness and their ability to detect emotional problems in their patients. Good interviewing skills, of the types discussed in Chapter 2, are essential to detect and manage emotional problems, particularly in the short space of time that is available in the GP consultation (about 10 minutes in developed countries). Only about 40 per cent of GPs in the UK have done any further training in psychiatry beyond their experience at medical school.

Practice nurses and **nurse practitioners** work alongside GPs and also have an important mental health role. Some of them have had specific training in mental health, but again there is considerable variation. Practice nurses play an important part in reviewing people with chronic physical illness in primary care, such as diabetes, asthma, and cardiovascular disease, and so may be the first to recognize depression in patients with chronic illness in which depression is more common.

Health visitors are registered general nurses with a further qualification in health visiting. They play a key role in the recognition of post-natal depression, and some have received specific training in counselling to help them in managing this particularly common form of depression. They are also sometimes involved in the care of the elderly where they may be the first to detect that a person has mental illness.

Community nurses are general nurses who visit and treat a large number of people in the community, many of them elderly, who require physical health care at home. They are often the first to recognize the presence of mental illnesses such as depression or dementia.

Some primary care teams also have a **counsellor** who is a mental health professional specifically trained to offer a form of brief psychological therapy called non-directive counselling. Counsellors may be based in the practice or visit the practice from a base in mental health services, along with other mental health workers such as **community mental health nurses**, **graduate mental health workers**, and **psychiatrists** (see below).

COMMUNITY MENTAL HEALTH SERVICES

When a GP refers a patient on to another service because they consider that person needs more intensive care than can be provided in primary care, they can send the patient to a wide range of different agencies depending on the nature of the problem.

Voluntary agencies

There is a wide range of local agencies in most communities that offer support for people with all types of mental health problems from depression and addiction to 'hearing voices'. The best-known community voluntary agency in the UK for people with mental health problems is MIND (the National Association of Mental Health or SAMH in Scotland) others such as *Relate* and *Cruse* provide highly professional help for people with marital problems and bereavement respectively. Many of these agencies are run by people who suffer from, or are recovering from, a particular type of problem, such as *Alcoholics Anonymous*, which organizes groups for people with alcohol dependence across the world, or the *Eating Disorders Association*, which runs a telephone advice line as well as local groups to support people with eating disorders.Some aim to focus on particular groups of people who tend not to visit doctors when they have a mental health problem – for example young people, and people from some ethnic minority groups. Many provide useful written information for people with mental health problems.

Primary care mental health services

An increasing number of places in the UK have specifically primary care-based mental health teams, run by the local primary care trust, which are a first point of referral for GPs for support and help with their patients, who are seen in the primary care clinic. Such teams are usually composed of **community mental health nurses** (mental health nurses with specific experience and training in working outside hospitals), counsellors, and a new type of worker called a **graduate mental health worker**, who is (usually) a psychology graduate with a 1-year specialized training in providing brief psychological treatment, based on self-help and cognitive-behaviour therapy, in primary care. Some teams also have **clinical psychologists**, who are psychology graduates with a further postgraduate training in how to provide specific psychological treatments such as cognitive-behaviour therapy. Some mental health nurses are also trained in how to provide psychological treatments such as cognitive and behaviour therapy.

Community mental health teams (CMHTs)

These are the main points of referral for people with more severe mental health problems, such as psychotic illness, or people who are at risk of suicide. Each team usually takes referrals from a specific geographical location or 'patch', or works with a specific list of GP practices. The teams are multi-disciplinary and usually consist of **community mental health nurses** (sometimes still called CPNs – community psychiatric nurses), **social workers**, a **psychologist**, an **occupational therapist** and a **consultant (general) psychiatrist**, with his or her junior staff of doctors. CMHTs are usually provided by the local mental health trust, which provides specialist mental health services to the community, and they are generally based in a house or a purpose-built clinic or centre that is located within the area that they serve. These buildings (community mental health centres) are often used as a resource centre for other activities for people with severe mental health problems, such as group activities organized by local voluntary agencies.

Most consultants will run their out-patient clinic at the community base, rather than at a hospital, and some will run clinics based in the primary care clinic, particularly in rural areas where it may be difficult for patients to travel. The other members of the team may see the patient at their own home or at the community base.

Many places also have one or more specialist teams based in the community who particularly provide care for people with severe mental health problems (psychosis, severe depression, personality disorders):

- **Assertive outreach teams** are multi-disciplinary teams that provide particularly intensive support to patients with psychotic disorders who are at high risk of relapse and re-admission to hospital.
- **Early intervention services** specialize in offering help to people in the early stages of psychotic illness, with the aim of providing early diagnosis and treatment.
- **Crisis resolution teams** intervene when people with mental health problems are in crisis, and provide intensive support, usually into the evenings and at weekends as well as during normal working hours. They may also be linked with **home treatment teams** who provide treatment for people in their own homes in order to prevent hospital admission, and provide support for carers.

There may also be one or more specialist residential units for people with mental illness in the community that provide care outside a hospital setting. **Crisis houses** provide brief periods of care for people who are acutely disturbed and are an alternative to in-patient hospital admission. **Rehabilitation** units provide supported accommodation for people with severe mental disorders who have recently left hospital, but are not yet able to live independently in the community, and there will be a range of **hostels** and **supported accommodation** that provide housing to enable people with long-term mental illness to live in the community. Many of these are run by voluntary agencies such as MIND or Making Space (a voluntary agency that specializes in helping people with schizophrenia).

AT THE HOSPITAL

The psychiatric unit

Most psychiatric in-patient units in the UK are now based on the same site as the general hospital, although this is not the case in many parts of the world, where people requiring in-patient psychiatric care may still be admitted into large mental hospitals. There are many advantages to psychiatric care being provided on the same site as other medical services. Admission is potentially less stigmatizing than it might be to a 'mental' hospital, the general hospital is usually nearer to the patient's home (and easier for their family to visit), and medical services are conveniently located nearby for consultation if required, given that physical morbidity, such as cardiovascular disease and diabetes, is more common in people with severe mental disorders. The general hospital can also benefit from the proximity of mental health expertise as mental disorder is common in people with physical health problems (see Chapter 11) and people with mental disorders regularly present at the emergency department.

The psychiatric in-patient unit provides in-patient care for people with serious mental disorders who require admission to hospital, because it has not been possible to provide effective treatment in the community, or because they are at risk to themselves, or to others. A multi-disciplinary team again provides care, but psychiatric nurses play a lead role in the provision of in-patient care. Today, nurses are rarely in uniform (except sometimes in units for older people where there is a practical reason for wearing a uniform), and for most students, this is the major difference between a psychiatric ward and an ordinary medical ward, along with the discovery that patients are generally out of bed, dressed and occupied during the day, and 'ward-rounds' do not involve actually going around the ward but take the form of a multi-disciplinary team meeting. Patients are sometimes invited into this meeting, but as it can be difficult and unpleasant for them to be faced by a large group of professionals, they are usually reviewed before or after the 'round' by the consultant and the immediate team members who are directly involved in the care of that patient. Wards may be mixed, but more in-patient services are now being provided on a single-sex basis, which is more comfortable for female patients who may find the presence of acutely disturbed male patients rather threatening.

In the past, most small psychiatric units operated an 'open-door' policy allowing patients to come and go unless they were detained under the Mental Health Act (see p. 364). However more units are now locked to prevent people coming in or going out at will without observation by and permission from staff.

Most units have a small **psychiatric intensive care unit** (PICU), which provides more intensive one-to-one care for people who are acutely disturbed, and this unit is locked. Many units will also have a **day hospital** for patients to attend on a daily basis for care. Other specialist in-patient wards might include a ward for **older people**, a special unit for mothers with neonatal psychiatric illness where they can be admitted alongside their babies, and in-patient services for **drug and alcohol** problems for detoxification and withdrawal, although most substance-misuse services are situated out in the community.

The general hospital

Accident and emergency: Many people presenting with acute mental illness will first come to the emergency department, where they can be seen by the mental health team. Most departments now have a community mental health nurse who works on site during the day, and a duty psychiatrist will be available to carry out assessments at other times. Some larger hospitals have specific teams who provide assessments for people who present with **self-harm** (by taking an overdose or injuring themselves). In smaller units a **liaison psychiatrist** working with a psychiatric nurse and possibly also a social worker will provide this service. They will see people in the emergency department and also on the medical wards if they have been admitted. Liaison psychiatrists provide psychiatric assessments, when required, on any of the units in the general hospital. They will commonly see people with psychological reactions to physical illness such as cancer, post-natal mental illness (in the maternity unit), and substance misuse as well as self-harm.

Specialist services

Most districts also have a range of specialist services that provide care for specific groups of people. Some of these teams, which are multi-disciplinary and usually include psychiatrists, nurses, social workers and psychologists, may provide care to several districts or to a whole region if the care they provide is particularly specialized.

Specialist teams and services include:

- **Drug and alcohol services**: These teams work closely with voluntary agencies in the community, which also provide care and advice to people with substance-misuse problems. Community alcohol teams work closely with GPs to provide home detoxification and withdrawal from alcohol.
- **Services for older people**: These teams work very closely with GPs and residential homes for the elderly in the community.
- **Child and adolescent services**: These provide multi-disciplinary care to children and young people, usually up to the age at which they leave school. There may also be an in-patient unit for young people with more severe mental illness such as psychosis.
- **Psychological therapies**: A range of psychological therapies including cognitive-behaviour therapy and psychodynamic psychotherapy (see Chapter 8) are provided by psychology services and psychotherapy departments. Some services also provide more specialized care for particular groups of people, for example with eating disorders and sexual problems.
- **Forensic services**: These provide care to people who have mental health problems and exhibit anti-social and/or criminal behaviour. Most regions of the UK have one or more medium secure units that provide secure care and hospital accommodation for this group of patients, and also treat people with mental health problems who are identified in and transferred from the prison service. Care for people with mental illness who are considered to be dangerous is provided in one of the four special hospitals in the UK.

24   ETHICAL DILEMMAS AND LEGAL ASPECTS

ETHICAL ISSUES IN PSYCHIATRY

The *Four Principles model* is one of the most widely used frameworks in consideration of ethical problems:

1. **Respect for autonomy**: Respecting the decision-making capacities of autonomous persons; enabling individuals to make reasoned informed choices.
2. **Beneficence**: Balancing the benefits of treatment against the risks and costs; the healthcare professional should act in a way that benefits the patient.
3. **Non-maleficence**: The healthcare professional should not harm the patient. All treatment involves some harm, even if minimal, but the harm should not be disproportionate to the benefits of treatment.
4. **Justice**: Distributing benefits, risks and costs fairly; the notion that patients in similar positions should be treated in a similar manner.

Consideration of ethical issues in everyday practice requires being able to understand the other person's point of view, even if this view differs considerably from your own. Such a scenario is not uncommon in psychiatry where a patient may not only have differing views about what *treatment* they want, but *what they believe the problem to be*. 'Autonomy' means that people 'have a say' in not only what happens to them but how their problems are to be understood. Psychiatry has been at the forefront in medicine in not only taking into account but also promoting the growth of the 'service user' and 'carer' movements. Differences between how doctors and patients (and their carers) may view the nature of, and care required for, psychiatric problems are potentially much more diverse than in physical medicine. Conflicts can particularly occur when patients seem to lack insight into the nature of their problems.

It is quite impossible to provide an answer to all ethical dilemmas that will be faced in practice. The framework for discussion in *Box 24.1* will be helpful in thinking through a particular case, and there is often no simple answer. Good communication skills are essential for understanding multiple perspectives of the problem, and the insights provided by the multi-disciplinary team are particularly valuable. Some basic principles can however be described.

Box 24.1 A framework for thinking through an ethical problem

What are the relevant clinical and other facts?

Who is responsible for making the decision? When does the decision have to be made? Who should be involved? What are the procedural rules, e.g. need for confidentiality?

List the available options considering:

What does the patient want to happen?
Does the patient have the capacity to make the decision? (see pp. 363, 367)
If the patient does not have the capacity, what is in their 'best interests'?
What are the views of the broader multi-disciplinary team?
What are the views of the patient's family?
What are the foreseeable consequences of each option?
Do you need to get another professional opinion?

What do official guidelines/protocols/policy/the law/the Mental Health Act say about each of these options?

If in doubt *ask for advice*: e.g. Get expert advice on the law, the Mental Health Act, or where necessary consult your medical defence union.

For each realistic option, identify the arguments in favour and against.

Choose an option based on your judgement of the relative merits of these arguments considering:

How does this case compare with other cases? What have others done in the past when faced when similar situations?
Are the arguments absolutely valid?
What are the foreseeable consequences of the options?

Identify the strongest counter-argument to the option you have chosen.

Can you rebut this argument? How?

Make a decision.

Review this decision in the light of what actually happens, and learn from it.

Confidentiality

Doctors have an ethical duty to keep patient information confidential. The sharing of patient-identifiable information is, by definition, disclosure. The duty of confidentiality arises from grounds both of respect for autonomy and because of the benefits that derive from keeping such information private. Without assurances about confidentiality patients may be reluctant to give doctors the information they need in order to provide good care. Patients have a right to expect that doctors will keep confidential any personal information that they acquire during the course of professional duties, unless consent to disclose is given, or there is a statutory obligation on the doctor to disclose the information. Generally, therefore, psychiatrists must not disclose any clinical information about a patient to others, without that patient's consent. However, the duty of confidentiality also exists within a wider social context in which doctors have other moral and legal obligations that may conflict with their duty of confidentiality. These conflicts set limits to medical confidentiality. As a consequence, doctors have a further duty to inform their patients that in exceptional defined circumstances (usually harm to others) the duty of confidentiality may be overridden even in the face of a patient's refusal of consent to disclose. There would be no duty to inform a patient about the disclosure in exceptional circumstances if doing so would prejudice the reason for the disclosure (e.g. it might prejudice a police investigation if you inform the patient that you have made the disclosure to the police).

If a patient tells you something that indicates they pose a threat to the health and safety of others, for example that they intend to murder somebody, then this is a reason to breach confidentiality. Indeed, in the UK health professionals are legally obliged to report instances where the safety of children is potentially at risk.

In terms of **sharing information with others** it would not usually be acceptable for the patient to ask that you do not write a letter to their GP providing him with your views on diagnosis and treatment, but there may be some discussion about exactly what details are provided. There is a principle here that the doctor *'needs to know'* about what is happening for the patient's own benefit from treatment. In the National Health Service patients now have the option of receiving copies of correspondence that is sent to their GP.

TALKING TO RELATIVES

Family members may want to talk to you, share their concerns with you, or find out from you what is happening to their relative. As a general rule, members of a family should not be seen without the permission of the patient, and ideally that interview should take place in the presence of the patient, although this is not always possible. There will however be times when a family member wants to convey some information and the patient refuses permission for such contact. In this situation possible ways might be for the information to be provided in a letter, or for another member of the multidisciplinary team to meet with the family member and agree to convey, but not divulge, information at the same time as providing support to the family.

If a person with significant mental illness is living with their family, but refuses to allow you to talk to them, this can create problems. It is important to discuss with the patient the reasons why their family will need to be involved. If there is a situation of risk, then you will need to consider carefully whether, when, and how the family should be made aware of this.

This is an issue where there may be differences in practice between different cultures. In some communities the group is more powerful than the individual and may invade the privacy of the individual, especially in relation to women, the poor and illiterate, and those who are dependent on their families. Such factors need to be considered in managing the expectations of families who have migrated into western cultures.

Never agree to talk to a relative on the premise that you will keep such a meeting a secret.

Conflict of interest

It is not ethical to be involved in the clinical care of patients where you have a conflict of interest. No doctor should, unless it is an emergency, treat a family member, a friend, or a person working under one's responsibility. This can be a particular problem in general practice where GPs and their families may be registered as patients with their colleagues. If, for example, one of the GPs becomes depressed because of problems in the clinic with his colleague, who is also his registered medical practitioner, this can lead to problems not only in terms of conflict of interest, but also confidentiality. Further problems might arise in disorders where family relationships can be particularly difficult – for example anorexia. It would be very difficult to treat a colleague's teenage daughter for anorexia nervosa and at the same time maintain the correct degree of professional distance and confidentiality with a parent if they were also a work colleague and business partner.

Consent to treatment

Before you can touch anyone, you need to have a lawful justification, otherwise it is an assault. This applies to all medical treatments, including those for mental health problems. Consent to medical treatment is one such justification and must usually be obtained before any treatment is given. Consent can only be meaningful if a full explanation of the treatment has been given.

You should provide all the information that the patient needs in order to enable them to make a decision. This will include what the treatment is, what it will achieve, any likely adverse effects, what will happen if the treatment is not given, and what alternatives there are. You should encourage the patient to ask questions and answer them fully.

WHO IS ABLE TO CONSENT TO TREATMENT?

If the patient is over 18, only they can consent to their medical treatment. There are exceptional circumstances, such as being detained under the Mental Health Act 1983, when treatment can be given to adults who are not consenting (see p. 365).

If the patient is under 18, the law is more complicated. It may be that the patient can consent on their behalf, but this does not necessarily mean they have the same right to refuse. Others, such as parents, guardians, the local authority, or the court, may be able to consent on their behalf.

WHAT IF THE PATIENT DOES NOT WANT THE TREATMENT THAT IS BEING PROPOSED?

If the patient is an adult, and has the capacity to consent, they are quite entitled to refuse any kind of treatment for physical or mental health problems (although this may not apply if they are detained under certain sections of the Mental Health Act). Patients can ask for a second opinion to discuss the treatment proposed.

WHAT DOES 'CAPACITY' MEAN?

Generally, the law presumes a person is able to make a decision for himself. If it is thought that he might be unable to decide on a particular issue, for example whether to have a certain treatment or not, the law uses a test for this ability, which is in three parts:

- Is the person able to understand and remember information about the treatment?
- Does he believe that what he is being told is true?
- Can he weigh up the pros and cons of accepting or refusing the treatment, and make a decision based on that?

If a person fails any of these tests, then they will be 'incapacitated' and cannot give valid consent. The law then allows the treatment to be given, if it is in the best interests of the patient, according to the principle of 'necessity'. That means the treatment must be necessary to ensure health and welfare or prevent deterioration, and also that other doctors would agree that the proposed treatment was the correct one.

The consultant in charge of the person's care makes the decisions about a person's capacity and treatment. Good practice requires them to discuss the issues with other professionals involved in the patient's care, with their family, and with close friends, so that all relevant information can be obtained.

Euthanasia and assisted suicide

Euthanasia and assisted suicide have become hot topics of debate in recent years and it is now legal in some countries. In the view of many (but not all) doctors, deliberately ending life is unethical. Psychiatrists have to be aware that the views of a patient with serious (or terminal) physical illness who is seeking euthanasia may, as in the case of people who are actively suicidal, be distorted by mental illness such as depression. Doctors have to be extremely cautious with respect to wishes for death expressed by patients because of unbearable suffering. The clinical questions to ask are not only can the suffering be better relieved, but also is the patient suffering from depression? Effective treatment may reverse the apparent decision the patient has made that death is the only solution.

LEGAL ASPECTS OF PSYCHIATRY

The Mental Health Act (1983)

Until the 1959 Mental Health Act almost all psychiatric in-patients were compulsorily detained. Since then the proportion has fallen progressively, so that now most patients are informal, with the same rights and freedoms as any other hospital patients. Even for those who are compulsorily detained, there are restrictions on the powers of psychiatrists to treat them without their consent. The 1983 Mental Health Act is like most Acts of Parliament in that it is a lengthy and forbidding document, and like other Acts its paragraphs are numbered. This leads to potentially confusing references to 'Section 37' or the 'Sectioning' for compulsory detention. It is preferable and more intelligible to refer to each section by name: to a 'Treatment Order' (rather than Section 3), to a 'Hospital Order' (rather than Section 37), and so on.

There are complex and varying conditions for the making and renewal of each detention order: an 'Assessment Order' (Section 2) and a 'Treatment Order' (Section 3) are used most often, and so examples will be given in what follows.

ASSESSMENT ORDER ('SECTION 2')

An Assessment Order requires two medical recommendations, one from a qualified psychiatrist (approved under Section 12 of the Act) and one from another doctor, who may be the patient's general practitioner. The consent of the nearest relative – or an approved local authority social worker – is also needed (except for orders made by the courts or the Home Office). This kind of admission is used when a patient:

1. Is suffering from a mental disorder (the type need not be specified).
2. Is unwilling to be admitted to hospital.
3. Needs to be admitted *either for his own health OR safety, or for the protection of others.*

The wording 'health *or* safety' is important, since it means that if the patient has an illness that is a threat to health they may be detained. This allows the doctor a certain amount of latitude – compulsory powers are not confined to suicidal patients, or those whose clinical state is a threat to others.

Although the admission is for assessment, this can be followed by treatment. It lasts up to 28 days, and the patient may appeal within the first 14 days to a Mental Health Review Tribunal (MHRT). This is a small informal court with three members: a legally qualified president, an independent psychiatrist (in practice this means from another health district), and a lay person. The Tribunal has the power to discharge the patient from the order, so that he could then decide to leave or to remain as a voluntary patient.

ADMISSION FOR ASSESSMENT *IN CASES OF EMERGENCY* ('SECTION 4')

It is possible to detain a patient for 72 hours with one approved doctor and the nearest relative or approved social worker (ASW), but the doctor must confirm both of the following:

1. It is of 'urgent necessity' for the patient to be admitted and detained under Section 2.
2. Waiting for a second doctor to confirm the need for an admission under Section 2 would cause 'undesirable delay'.

TREATMENT ORDER ('SECTION 3')

If the patient needs to be kept in for longer than 28 days a 'Treatment Order' can then be made, detaining them for up to 6 months. Because this order deprives the patient of liberty for much longer, there are more stringent requirements:

1. The patient's mental disorder must be specified as either *mental illness, severe mental impairment, mental impairment,* or *psychopathy,* and details of the disorder must also be given.
2. It must be *of a nature or degree that makes it appropriate for them to receive treatment in a hospital.*
3. Treatment cannot be provided unless they are detained.
4. In the case of the milder disorders (mental impairment and psychopathy) treatment must be likely to 'alleviate or prevent a deterioration of their condition'.

HOLDING ORDERS ('SECTION 5')

These apply to patients in hospital. They may be detained for up to 8 hours by the nurse in charge of a ward to enable the patient to be examined by a psychiatrist.

HOSPITAL ORDERS ('SECTION 37')

These orders are made by magistrates if patients have appeared before a court. They can be made whether or not the person has been convicted of an offence, and can last for up to 6 months, renewable for a further 6 months, then yearly.

A Hospital Order requires evidence from two doctors that:

1. The offender is suffering from one of the specified categories of mental disorder of a nature and degree that makes detention for medical treatment appropriate.
2. If suffering from a psychopathic disorder or mental impairment, such treatment is likely to 'alleviate or prevent a deterioration' of their condition.
3. Taking into account all the relevant circumstances a Hospital Order is most appropriate.

These orders can be discharged by the responsible medical officer (RMO), the hospital managers or by a mental health review tribunal (MHRT).

Reform of the Mental Health Act (1983)

Proposals to amend the MHA have been made repeatedly since 1987, principally to increase powers to compel patients who do not meet the criteria for compulsory admission, but are felt by clinicians to be at risk of future relapse, to take medication while outside hospital. An early Draft Bill (2002) was opposed by a 'Mental Health Alliance', which united all the major professional and service user groups, who regarded the Bill as shifting the role of mental health services away from treatment and towards authoritarian control. The government responded with a revised Draft Mental Health Bill, published in September 2004.

The main differences between this proposal and the MHA (1983) are:

- It will be possible to require patients to accept care plans, including medication, outside hospital (though medication will only be given forcibly in clinical settings). Guardianship and Supervised Discharge will be abolished.
- The current distinction between assessment (Section 2) and treatment (Section 3) will be replaced with a single form of compulsory care plan, which could include hospital or community assessment or treatment as appropriate.
- All use of compulsory powers will be reviewed by a tribunal or court after 28 days, without requiring the patient to appeal.
- Services will be required to produce a care plan within 5 days of applying compulsory powers.
- The currently defined role of 'nearest relative' will be replaced, and patients will be able to nominate their own choice of relative and to have access to independent advocacy.
- Carers will have statutory rights to be consulted.
- Current roles such as ASW will be replaced with roles based on competence rather than professional background.

This Draft Bill was again strongly criticized by the Mental Health Alliance, and in July 2005 the government responded by accepting a number of these criticisms, most importantly accepting that:

- Guiding principles should be included in the Bill.
- As in the MHA 1983, compulsory treatment should not be given to people with a sole diagnosis of dependency on drugs and alcohol.

Patients' rights should be strengthened in a number of ways in this proposed new Bill, including giving greater weight to advance decisions and statements.

The Mental Capacity Act 2005

The Mental Capacity Act 2005 outlines who can take decisions for people who are not able to make their own decisions (i.e. they do not have **capacity**). It outlines when and how they should do this. A person has capacity if they can assess the situation sufficiently well to make a decision and can then communicate it to others. A person has a right to make a bad or eccentric decision. Many mental disorders could interfere with the capacity of someone to make decisions. These may be lasting conditions such as dementia, or conditions from which a person can recover and regain capacity such as severe depressive episodes. Doctors and social workers are called to make determinations of capacity.

The Act sets out rules under which advance decisions to refuse treatment can be made by patients when they have capacity, to apply in readiness for a clinical situation when they do not have capacity. If these refer to the refusal of treatments that may save lives then the **advanced directive** must be in writing, signed, and witnessed. For instance a patient may sign an advanced directive while asymptomatic and having capacity by means of which they can refuse electroconvulsive therapy (ECT) when they are in severe depression and lacking the capacity to consent. The Act also allows a person to appoint an attorney (**Lasting Power of Attorney**) to act on their behalf if they lose capacity at a later date. The attorney can make decisions about the health, welfare, or finances on behalf of the person lacking capacity. The Act requires that an **Independent Mental Capacity Advocate** speaks on behalf of the person who lacks capacity. These advocates can challenge the decisions of decision-makers including senior doctors. The Act sets up new procedures for research in people who lack capacity. A person found guilty of neglecting or ill-treating a person who lacks capacity can be imprisoned for up to 5 years.

Testamentary capacity

Any doctor may be asked to assess testamentary capacity, meaning the ability to make a valid will. A patient's general practitioner is much more likely to be asked to do this than a psychiatrist. If a patient is seriously ill, or even dying, he may decide to make a will, and may ask the doctor attending him to witness it. If the doctor does this he is said to have 'attested the will', and should have considered the patient to be of *'sound disposing mind'*. If the will is subsequently contested, he may have to answer questions in court about the patient's mental state.

Anyone over the age of 18 who is not 'of unsound mind' can make a will. Mild dementia would be unlikely to affect a simple will, although it might invalidate a complex one. However, someone who is confused, forgetful or even deluded may be able to draw up a will with legal assistance.

Having a *'sound disposing mind'* involves:

1. Knowing what property you own.
2. Knowing who has claims on it: you should know the names of your nearest relatives.
3. Being able to form a judgement on the relative strengths of these claims, without undue distortion because of mental abnormality.

FURTHER READING

Green, S. and Bloch, S. (2006) *An Anthology of Psychiatric Ethics.* Oxford: Oxford University Press.
National Institute of Health and Clinical Excellence (2004) *Self-harm: The Short-term Physical and Psychological Management and Secondary Prevention of Self-harm in Primary and Secondary Care,* available at: http://www.nice.org.uk/download.aspx?o=cg016niceguideline

National Institute of Health and Clinical Excellence (2005) *Violence: The Short-term Management of Disturbed/Violent Behaviour in Psychiatric In-patient Settings and Emergency Departments*, available at: http://www.nice.org.uk/download.aspx?o=cg016niceguideline

Royal College of Psychiatrists (2006) (Council Report 133) *Good Psychiatric Practice: Confidentiality and Information Sharing*, available at: http://www.rcpsych.ac.uk/files/pdfversion/cr133.pdf

UK Clinical Ethics Network, available at: http://www.ethics-network.org.uk/index.htm

GLOSSARY

Acute dystonia consists of muscle spasms, often painful and alarming in appearance, which may have their onset within the first week of starting a neuroleptic drug. They may include spasms of the tongue, neck, back, and extrinsic ocular muscles (oculogyric crisis). They respond rapidly to anticholinergic anti-Parkinsonian drugs.

Agitation is a state of increased motility that accompanies tension and is seen in some depressed patients. It may take the form of poorly organized but purposeful activities such as cleaning, in which the patient starts the same activity frequently, becomes distracted, starts an alternative activity, and so on. There may be repetitive hand wringing leading to excoriation of skin, or head rubbing resulting in hair loss. Behaviour may be importunate. For example, a patient may knock at a door, start to ask a question, break off and walk away, only to repeat this behaviour each time the door is closed. The inexperienced commonly fail to recognize that such behaviour may be caused by agitation and use meaningless terms such as 'attention-seeking' or 'hysterical' to describe the patient. The degree of agitation is not directly related to the severity of subjective anxiety, and a retarded patient may also describe inner feelings of great tension.

Akathisia is a state of increased motility accompanied by a subjective feeling of restlessness and is an extrapyramidal effect of neuroleptic drugs.

Akinesis is a reduction in motor activity particularly affecting muscles of facial expression, and accessory movements such as arm swinging when walking. It is a feature of Parkinsonism and is commonly drug-induced. Thus there is a particular risk of failing to differentiate this treatment side-effect from depressive retardation and of consequent inappropriate treatment.

Ambivalence. Refers to vacillation of motivation. Also used to mean vacillation between complying and refusing when asked to do something.

Approximate answers or 'answering past the point'. Replies to questions that are almost (but not) correct and imply a knowledge of the correct answer, for example 'How many legs has a sheep?' 'Five'.

Automatism. A simple or complex motor act, often inappropriate to the circumstances (for example, undressing in a supermarket) carried out while apparently unaware of the environment and without conscious motivation. Associated with organic cerebral disorders, particularly epilepsy, and with hysteria.

Glossary

Blunting of affect is a disorder that may be seen in schizophrenia, particularly in those with a chronic disorder. The usual modulation of mood is lost, and the patient lacks warmth, but does not convey the lowering of affect seen in severely depressed patients.

Catatonic symptoms. A collective term for a variety of motor behaviours, including ambivalence, negativism, posturing, and waxy flexibility.

Compulsions are closely related to obsessions, but are repetitive acts rather than thoughts. They may be simple actions, such as repeated checking, for example to see whether a door is locked before going to bed, or there may be complex rituals involving sequences of actions, each of which the subject feels compelled to repeat for a 'magical' number of times. For example, a patient may feel compelled to wash his hands seven times to avoid contamination, then he thinks this must be repeated in case he touched the sink, which might have been contaminated, and so on. Sometimes, as with obsessions, there is an attempt to resist compulsive actions. However, some patients practise compulsive acts in order to relieve the distress caused by an obsessional thought. For example, compulsive hand washing may be welcomed and practised to avoid the obsessional idea of contamination. The patient knows the actions are his own and based on his own will, even though they distress him and he may struggle to avoid them. In this respect they differ from passivity phenomena from which they must be distinguished.

Depersonalization is an unpleasant perception of change in mental functions or body image. The patient may no longer experience usual feelings towards others. Parts of his body may look unfamiliar, although correctly identified as his own. The experience may be accompanied by **derealization**, in which the external world seems altered and unfamiliar: the experience is unpleasant. Both can occur as isolated symptoms – especially due to fatigue – but they commonly accompany affective illnesses, or any other mental illness higher in the hierarchy.

Depressive delusions. Delusions of guilt, self-blame, poverty, infestation, and infection are associated with depression and reflect the low self-esteem and hopelessness for the future that are characteristic of that mood. Of course such ideas occur commonly in depressed patients without necessarily being delusional in quality. Nihilistic delusions are extreme variants in which the patient believes that he is losing his physical or mental functions due to disease, or that he is already dead. For example, a depressed patient insisted that his head was shrinking, that his forehead was growing smaller so that he no longer had a place to wear his glasses, and that this state would soon be incompatible with life.

Fugue. A disturbance of behaviour characterized by wandering, without conscious motivation, in a state of altered or diminished consciousness; subsequently there may be amnesia for the event. Associated with organic (including epileptic) and hysterical states.

Grandiose delusions include beliefs that the patient has special powers, is chosen by God, or has been sent to save the world. For example, following laminectomy a greengrocer believed he was in hospital because he was a famous neurosurgeon, was there to operate on the other patients, and that the staff were there to assist him. He strutted about the ward issuing imperious commands and held his hands as though 'scrubbed up'. Such beliefs are particularly likely to occur in manic patients, but are also found in schizophrenics and those with organic cerebral disorders.

Hysterical amnesia is differentiated from other memory defects by the characteristic loss of personal information, both recent and long term. For example, the patient is unable to remember his name and address, whether he has family, and fails to recognize close relatives. By contrast, he appears to have no difficulty in recognizing, naming, and using equally familiar objects, such as food and drink. Such profound and selective memory loss does not occur in other disorders.

Incongruous affect is a display of affect that is inappropriate to the patient's subjective mood state. For example, a patient may smile to himself briefly when describing a recent bereavement. Never assume that this is inappropriate, based on your own expectation of what the patient's mood should be. Ask the patient why he smiles. He may say he feels sad and does not know why he smiles, in which case this is probably an example of incongruous affect. However, he may say he was remembering an amusing incident at the funeral or thinking of the legacy he expects to receive. Inappropriate affect is a characteristic of schizophrenia.

Labile mood is when fluctuations occur in response to circumstances, but show rapid and excessive variation with loss of control. It is strongly suggestive of organic brain disease and may be a feature of dementia, but can also occur in histrionic personalities and in some manic-depressive illnesses.

Mannerisms. All people have certain mannerisms, which are habitual and meaningless movements, such as stroking the face or hair or clearing the throat, which tend to increase when they are tense. They imitate purposeful movements and can be brought under voluntary control.

Mutism is total absence of speech. It may occur as a feature of stupor in depressive illness, schizophrenia, or organic brain disease. Occasionally it may be a hysterical symptom. **Elective mutism** is seen mainly in disturbed children and is characterized by mutism that occurs in some settings but not in others. For example, the child may speak normally at home, but is mute at school.

Negativism. The response to a request that is the opposite to what is required. Sometimes also used to mean failure to carry out a task.

Obsessions are repetitive thoughts that the subject feels are forced into his conscious mind against his wishes; that is, he feels compelled to have them. The nature of these thoughts is unpleasant and, therefore, he tries to resist having them. Both the thoughts and the attempt at resistance are associated with anxiety. An essential feature is that the patient knows these are his own thoughts; that is, they originate in his own mind, even though their content is contrary to his own wishes. For example, the patient may find the idea forced into his thinking that his hands are contaminated by faeces, that he has failed to wash his hands properly, and that he may poison others for whom he is preparing food. It is also important to note that the idea is not a delusion: the patient is not convinced that his hands are contaminated, but fears that they might be and is unable to put this fear from his mind, although he may know intellectually that it is 'foolish'.

Over-activity becomes a problem when the actions are either inappropriate or not completed. Manic patients may display considerable energy, start many activities, but fail to complete them. **Loss of inhibition** may also lead them to inappropriate activities, such as spending sprees or sexual excesses.

Panic attacks are attacks of acute anxiety with a sudden onset, which may last short periods of time, or may be prolonged over several hours, typically resolving slowly. There are both somatic and psychological manifestations of anxiety. The former include tachycardia, palpitations, sweating, and tremor; the latter include fears that one is about to die, go mad, or has some serious illness – such as a heart attack.

Passivity. Delusions of passivity are included in the phenomena that characterize schizophrenia, which appear to be based on a breakdown of 'ego-boundaries'; that is, the normal awareness of the boundaries between ourselves and other people in the world outside ourselves. Included are beliefs that one's body is under the control of other people or forces, that other people control one's thoughts, are able to place thoughts into or remove them from one's mind, can read each thought as it goes through one's mind, or that the thoughts in one's mind do not belong to oneself. These beliefs are extremely concrete; that is, that a thought can actually be taken out of one person's mind and placed in another mind. The subject may feel physically controlled, like a marionette. It is easy to identify such beliefs incorrectly by asking inaccurate questions.

Perplexity. A mood state of bewilderment, with uncertainty about the nature of immediate experience of the environment. The subject usually appears puzzled.

Phobias are fears of specific objects or situations that are not generally regarded as dangerous, such as spiders, mice, heights, or crowded or enclosed places. The phobic person will tend to avoid the feared situations, but will not always do so. It is crucial to the definition of a phobia that the subject is aware that the fear is irrational, because the object of fear is not dangerous. Thus it must be differentiated from a delusion. For example, an agoraphobic patient may be housebound, but will know that there is nothing harmful outside the house. A patient with persecutory delusions may also fear to go out, but this is because he believes there is danger, for example a gunman waiting to kill him, and that it is, therefore, a sensible precaution to remain in the house.

Posturing. Used to refer to abnormal body posture. Manneristic posture is a stilted exaggeration of normal posture. Stereotyped posture is non-adaptive, rigidly maintained, and often uncomfortable.

Pressure of speech describes the rapid outpouring of ideas that is characteristic of mania. This is accompanied by an increase in the quantity of speech and often in the volume. It may be difficult to interrupt, to ask questions, or to direct a conversation successfully with a patient who shows this disorder. The continuity of thinking is often, but not necessarily, also affected.

Reference. Ideas (or delusions) of reference involve beliefs that events in the environment have special meaning for the subject and refer particularly to him. For example, the newsreader on television mentions an epidemic of fever, and the patient knows that this is a message specially intended for him rather than others and that it is a warning to guard himself against infection; the patient hears laughter from a nearby room and is sure that people are laughing at him; a stranger on a bus is overheard saying 'He's gay' and the patient knows he is referring to him. Ideas of reference occur in a wide range of disorders, including depression, mania, and schizophrenia, and have little diagnostic specificity.

Retardation of movement involves delay in initiating movement, slowness in subsequent performance of the movement and also a reduction in the total quantity of movement. It is usually accompanied by retardation of speech (see next entry) and is most commonly seen in depressive illness.

Retardation of speech is often associated with retardation of movement. It is characterized by delay in the initiation of speech, for example in response to a simple question, as well as by a slow rate of speech production. The volume of speech may be so low as to make it difficult to hear what is said. The quantity of speech may be greatly reduced. Retardation is usually symptomatic of depressive illness. Depressed patients who show retardation of speech do not usually experience slowness of thinking, but often describe their thoughts as being in a state of turmoil. The examination of the mental state of a retarded patient calls for great tolerance and patience on the part of the interviewer.

Secondary delusions. This refers to delusions that are secondary to some other abnormality, such as a hallucination. If you hear voices of spies planning to kill you, you may develop the belief that such plans exist! Other examples of secondary delusions would be those that can be understood in terms of abnormal emotion, or those that can be attributed to coarse brain disease, such as a cerebral tumour.

Stereotypies. These are utterances or movements that are monotonously repeated, non-goal-directed, executed in a uniform way, and have no obvious significance for the subject, for example rocking to and fro on a chair, endlessly repeating the same oath, or the same barking noises.

Stupor is characterized by total immobility, except for following movements of the eyes, and mutism. (Confirm by moving the patient's head yourself and seeing whether he moves his eyes to continue to fixate points in the visual field.) It can occur in depressive illness, in which it appears to be an extreme form of retardation. However, it can also be found as a catatonic feature of schizophrenia or due to organic cerebral disorders.

Tardive dyskinesia is a syndrome that may include many different rhythmic or jerking movements and tremors: these may be multiple, affecting most of the body, and are then disfiguring and extremely distressing. Most commonly they have their onset several months after the start of neuroleptic drugs. They are liable to become worse initially when the drug is stopped, and there is at present no reliable treatment.

Thought block is experienced by the patient as an interruption in the flow of thinking, so that thoughts are totally absent for a period of a few seconds. It is common in anxious people – for example, students during vivas. In psychotic illness the patient may suddenly go silent, for example in mid-sentence, look blank, and then continue on the same or a different theme. It is important to ask the patient what he noticed during this interlude, and what he was thinking about. Often it emerges that he was distracted by other thoughts, sounds, and so on, rather than experiencing total absence of thoughts, in which case thought block did not occur. This phenomenon must also be differentiated from petit mal epilepsy. Thought block occurs in some schizophrenics and is often associated with secondary delusions of interference.

Thought broadcasting. The delusion that one's private thoughts are being made known to others, perhaps throughout the world.

Thought echo. The experience of thoughts being repeated or echoed with very little interval between the original and the echo.

Tics are sudden involuntary twitchings of muscle groups, often mimicking expressive movements and particularly involving the face, for example frowning or 'screwing up' the eyes. They occur commonly in children at times of tension and may persist into or emerge during adult life.

Tremor at rest is a common feature of anxiety. Static tremor may also occur in Parkinsonism. All tremors, both static and intentioned (due to cerebellar disorders), are exacerbated by anxiety, and tremor in an anxious patient may, therefore, be due to an organic cerebral state in addition to the anxiety.

Twilight state. Conscious awareness is narrowed down to a few ideas and attitudes that dominate the subject's mind.

Volition is the state of energy and drive that directs our purposeful activity. Loss of volition is, therefore, a state of inertia in which a person fails to carry out necessary or usually enjoyable activities although the ability to carry them out is in other respects preserved. It is often difficult to assess during an interview.

Waxy flexibility. On moving parts of the patient's body into a new posture, the examiner notes a plastic resistance, and the posture may subsequently be maintained.

PROBLEM BASED LEARNING QUESTIONS

Problem based learning question 1

A 19-year-old student is in his first year at university. He seemed to enjoy university but in his second term he has become withdrawn, morose, not caring for himself, not attending tutorials and lectures, and not completing his course work.

1. Name four mental health problems that he might have. (4 marks)

His GP at the university medical centre was asked to assess him and thought he might be depressed.

2. Name eight symptoms that would help the GP to make a diagnosis of a depressive episode. (4 marks)
3. Name four treatment options that the GP has. (4 marks)

The following week a fellow student brings the student who had initially been depressed to the GP's surgery. He has been up all night singing at the top of his voice, shouting and claiming he is the Messiah, and blessing the other students. He has bought lots of pieces of art and jewellery.

4. Name a mental health problem he could now have. (2 marks)
5. Name six symptoms that the GP might ask about to find out what is wrong with the student. (6 marks)

Problem based learning question 2

A 27-year-old woman who has been married 1 year has become increasingly preoccupied and stays in her house most of the time. She keeps looking out of the window at the street outside and will not let anyone into the house except her husband. On the few occasions she has gone out of the house she has seemed scared and suspicious. She has accused the neighbours of spying on her.

Problem based learning questions

1. Name four mental health problems that she might have. (4 marks)

She says to her husband that he must get rid of the television because her thoughts are being broadcast on it against her will. She can hear two of the neighbours plotting to kill her wherever she goes in the house and wherever she goes outside the house, even several miles away.

2. What disorder do these symptoms suggest she might have? (2 marks)

The previous symptoms go away but she shows little interest in things, says very little and takes little care of herself or the house. There is no evidence that her local GP can find of a medical problem and the husband is sure his wife is not drinking or taking drugs.

3. What two conditions do these symptoms indicate? (4 marks)

The voices return and she becomes suspicious again of the neighbours. Her self-care is poor. Her GP refers the patient to see a psychiatrist at the local out-patient clinic.

4. What risks may this patient pose based on the symptoms that are already presented? (2 marks)
5. Name four different types of management that the psychiatrist might pursue. (4 marks)
6. Name four features that will either improve or worsen her prognosis. (4 marks)

Problem based learning question 3

A 22-year-old man has been brought into the local accident and emergency unit (emergency room) by ambulance. He complains of chest pain and thinks he may be having a heart attack. He has no history of previous medical problems. He has these attacks each time he goes out of the house to a crowded place. He is flushed, sweaty, breathing very fast, and he is very frightened that he is going to die any minute. He also complains of tingling in his fingers and lips. His blood pressure is slightly raised at 140/90 mmHg. His ECG shows a normal sinus tachycardia. His temperature and random blood sugar are normal.

1. What is the most likely (most common) cause for these symptoms? (2 marks)
2. Name six other symptoms or abnormal signs he might have. (6 marks)

His blood urea and electrolytes show a raised bicarbonate level. A concerned junior doctor had taken some arterial blood gases. The results show a low carbon dioxide and a high oxygen level.

3. What biochemical explanation do you have for these results and what is their cause? (2 marks)

Gradually the person recovers. He is concerned and wants to know precisely how he felt chest pain, had fast breathing, a thumping heart, and sweated so profusely.

4. How would you explain these symptoms to him? What two systems in the body other than the central nervous system are likely to be involved? (4 marks)

He reveals that he gets similar symptoms if he goes on his own into very crowded or open spaces, like supermarkets or parks, goes on public transport, or into lifts. He only goes to these places with a friend and if he can go by car.

5. What condition is he most likely to have? (2 marks)

On the advice of the accident and emergency department he goes to see his family doctor.

6. Name four effective treatments that the family doctor or a mental health specialist could offer. (4 marks)

Problem based learning question 4

A 50-year-old man appears very distressed at the first morning appointment with his family doctor. He is agitated and complaining of seeing small animals rushing across the room out of the corner of his eye. He can't sleep and he has been retching, vomiting at least three times. His hands are really shaky and he has spilled coffee down his shirt already this morning. He is flushed, sweating profusely, and his pulse rate is 112 beats per minute. The symptoms have been present for a couple of days and they are getting worse and worse. He is a businessman involved in running night-clubs. He has no medical problems other than being treated on two occasions for a peptic ulcer and for several injuries after falls or assaults. He thought he had been drinking far too much alcohol recently in the line of his work so he stopped drinking for Lent. He has never felt worse.

1. What is a likely explanation for his symptoms? (2 marks)
2. What do you need to take a particular history about, given your suspicions? (2 marks)

His wife comes in to see you. She tells you that this morning he went unconscious and his whole body started shaking uncontrollably for a few minutes. He was drowsy and has only come round in the last 40 minutes.

3. What might this problem be and how does it fit with the symptoms that the patient told you about? (4 marks)

You notice that the patient came to see your partner (other doctor) in the practice. The doctor ordered a full blood count and liver function tests.

Problem based learning questions

4. What abnormalities might be shown on these tests? (3 marks)

You are very concerned about this patient and explain to the couple that he needs urgent treatment.

5. What urgent treatment do you think he requires and why? (3 marks)

You see the same patient 2 weeks later. He wants some further help to stop the condition from happening again. He was frightened by it. He thinks he should stop drinking.

6. Name six features of his drinking that will indicate how severe a problem it is. (6 marks)

Problem based learning question 5

A doctor on a ward for the elderly was asked to assess an 81-year-old woman who was shouting out at night. She was also fighting with the nursing staff when they offered her personal care such as help with going to the toilet. She accused the nurses of interfering with her and shouted out 'Help I shouldn't be in jail'. Apparently in the day she slept much of the time. She had been admitted to the ward because she had a chest infection and cardiac failure. Her chest had got worse, and she had not behaved like this a few days ago when she was first admitted. The doctor found that she did not have any idea where she was, or the date, time, or even the year. She looked bewildered and frightened.

1. What is the most likely explanation of her mental state? (2 marks)
2. Name four cardinal features of the condition that lead you to this conclusion. (4 marks)

The nursing staff want you as the doctor to do something to help them to manage her. She is keeping the other patients awake and it is not their job to be repeatedly assaulted.

3. Name two actions that you could take to help the nursing staff to manage the patient. (4 marks)

You are called to the ward in the day 1 week later. She is much improved in terms of her behaviour and the nursing staff want her discharged home. Her daughter has arrived and insists that she has had memory problems for a long time. These are getting worse and now she is no longer capable of looking after herself. She accuses the hospital of neglecting their public duty if she is sent home and she can't stay with the daughter who does not have any room in her house. There are no other relatives in this country. You decide to take more of a history from the patient's daughter.

4. Name four symptoms that you might elicit to exclude dementia of Alzheimer's type. (4 marks)

378

The patient bursts into tears. You notice that she has a resting tremor and one of the sides of her face does not move as well as the other side.

5. Apart from dementia of Alzheimer type, name four other common conditions that might explain her memory loss. (4 marks)

The daughter is particularly concerned about her mother's ability to cook safely in the kitchen, and that she might get lost in the street.

6. Name two types of assessment that will help determine the extent to which these concerns will need to be addressed. (2 marks)

Problem based learning question 6

An 11-year-old boy has been referred to the community paediatrician by a school nurse with the permission of the boy's parents. He is in the second term at secondary school and unlike the other children he has not settled into the school. In fact he is disruptive, repeatedly leaving his seat in the classroom, and even climbing across tables in the classroom during class. He is always fidgeting. He butts into the games of the other children, can't wait his turn in any queue such as school lunchtime, and shouts out wrong answers in class before the teacher has finished the question. He never brings his games kit to school, always forgets his homework, and even goes to the wrong class room for his lessons. He won't listen and the teachers have lost patience with him. Other children call him names and have started to bully him. The community paediatrician thinks he may have attention deficit disorder.

1. Name six features of attention deficit disorder that this boy seems to show. (6 marks)

The community paediatrician orders an assessment by an educational psychologist.

2. Name two problems that the educational psychologist might find in relation to this boy's ability to learn in school. (2 marks)

A child psychiatrist has been asked to see the child.

3. Name four other conditions that the psychiatrist has decided to rule out apart from attention deficit disorder. (4 marks)

Discussion with the parents and the school has led the community paediatrician to propose a drug treatment for the 11-year-old boy's problems.

4. Name one drug that is used for the treatment of attention deficit disorder. (2 marks)

Problem based learning questions

This boy has an older brother aged 14 years whom the child psychiatrist has seen before. This boy was repeatedly in trouble at school for bullying other children and truanting. He was also in trouble with the police for holding up another child at knife point and stealing their mobile phone, and breaking into a derelict house and setting fire to it. The behaviour started when he was 9 years old and he now sleeps rough most of the time. He usually carries out this behaviour on his own.

5. Which childhood mental disorder does the 14-year-old brother seem to have? (2 marks)
6. Name four symptoms that indicate this diagnosis. (4 marks)

POSSIBLE ANSWERS TO PROBLEM BASED LEARNING QUESTIONS

Problem based learning question 1

1. Depression, schizophrenia, drug abuse, alcohol abuse, medical condition leading to depression or psychosis. (4 marks)
2. Depressed mood, loss of interest, change in sleep pattern, change in appetite, weight, or libido, loss of energy or motivation, fatigue, poor concentration, slowed down thinking, speech, or movement, agitation or restlessness, self-blame or worthlessness, guilt, hopelessness, thoughts of death, suicidal ideas or plans. (4 marks)
3. SSRI, SNRI and/or tricyclic antidepressants, watchful waiting and review, psychological treatments such as cognitive therapy or problem solving, referral to psychiatrist or community mental health team. (4 marks)
4. Mania, hypomania, antidepressant or drug-induced mania, medical cause for mania, schizophrenia. (2 marks)
5. Elated mood, irritable mood, decreased need for sleep, increased level of activity, increased level of energy, spending too much money, increased speed of speech, increased confidence and self-worth, grandiosity, delusions, hallucinations, passivity symptoms, persecutory ideas, consumption of drugs, medical problems. (6 marks)

Problem based learning question 2

1. Schizophrenia, depression, agoraphobia, drug abuse, alcohol abuse, medical condition leading to depression or psychosis. (4 marks)
2. Schizophrenia. Symptoms suggest thought broadcast and third-person auditory hallucinations. (2 marks)
3. Negative symptoms of schizophrenia, post-schizophrenia depression (depression is sufficient). (4 marks)
4. Risk of self-neglect (evidence of poor self-care already), risk of harm or aggression to the neighbours (persecutory ideas about neighbours were already expressed). (2 marks)
5. Neuroleptic medication (1 mark – do not give marks for different drug names), psychological treatment, involvement of community mental health team, early

intervention team, crisis team, psychiatric day hospital, psychiatric in-patient care, series of out-patient appointments. (4 marks)

6. Good or poor pre-morbid function (work, social), depressive symptoms, catatonic features, obsessional symptoms, insidious onset, long delay before treatment, poor response to drug treatment, long hospitalization. (4 marks)

Problem based learning question 3

1. Panic attack or hyperventilation. (2 marks)
2. Faintness, dizziness, or light headedness, palpitations, feeling hot or cold or chills, nausea, urinary frequency, loose bowels or diarrhoea, trembling or shaking, feeling short of breath, or feeling smothered or choking, feelings of unreality (derealization) or being detached from the self (depersonalization), fear of losing control or going crazy. (6 marks)
3. Respiratory alkalosis due to hyperventilation. (2 marks)
4. In anxiety, catecholamines (adrenaline or noradrenaline) are released into the blood. The autonomic nervous system contains noradrenaline. It is also overactive and this system connects to the heart, lungs, digestive system, urinary system, and skin. The symptoms are due to overactivity of these two systems in anxiety. (4 marks)
5. Agoraphobia. (2 marks)
6. Antidepressant drugs, anxiety management training, behaviour therapy or exposure, cognitive-behaviour therapy. (2 marks)

Problem based learning question 4

1. Alcohol withdrawal. (2 marks)
2. A drinking history. (2 marks)
3. He may have had a grand mal seizure, which is a feature of alcohol withdrawal. (4 marks)
4. Macrocytosis of red blood cells, raised γ-glutamyl transpeptidase (γ-GT), other abnormal liver function tests. (3 marks)
5. Alcohol detoxification with long-acting benzodiazepines or chlormethiazole, monitoring in hospital because of possible history of grand mal seizure. (3 marks)
6. Salience of alcohol consumption over other activities, increased tolerance to its effects, alcohol withdrawal on other occasions, alcohol taken in much larger quantities than intended, persistent desire or unsuccessful attempts to cut down drinking, continued drinking despite knowledge of the harm being caused, giving up other activities to drink, recurring failure to carry out major work or social obligations because of drinking, recurrent drinking when it is dangerous, legal problems due to drinking, repeated social or interpersonal problem such as fights because of drinking. (6 marks)

Problem based learning question 5

1. Delirium, or acute confusional state, or acute brain syndrome. (2 marks)
2. Reversed variation in level of alertness – drowsiness in the day and hypervigilant at night, disorientation in time and place, brief history of change in behaviour over a few days, underlying medical condition, reduced clarity of awareness of surroundings, paranoid ideation and perceptual misinterpretation. (4 marks)
3. Move the patient to a side room or a quieter and brighter part of the ward. Nursing staff repeatedly explain where she is and what they should do. Give small doses of neuroleptic or major tranquillizer medication. More effectively treat underlying medical condition. (4 marks)
4. Gradual decline in memory, executive function (such as planning, organizing, sequencing),with dysphasia, dyspraxia, dyscalculia or agnosia. (4 marks)
5. Multi-infarct or vascular dementia, Lewy body dementia, depressive episode, Parkinson's disease, alcohol dementia, amnestic syndrome. (4 marks)
6. Occupational therapy assessment (particularly kitchen assessment), neuropsychological assessment (such as Mini-Mental State Examination). (2 marks)

Problem based learning question 6

1. Any of the following: hyperactivity – fidgets, repeatedly leaving seat in classroom, inappropriate climbing, repeatedly talking; impulsivity – blurting out answers before questions are completed, difficulty waiting his turn, often interrupts or intrudes on others; inattention – difficulty sustaining attention on tasks, does not seem to listen when spoken to directly, often forgetful, often loses things, often fails to follow instructions, avoids engaging in tasks requiring sustained effort. (6 marks)
2. General learning difficulties, confirms attention deficit disorder, specific learning difficulty such as dyslexia. (2 marks)
3. Childhood depression, conduct disorder, childhood anxiety disorder, learning disorder, Asperger's disorder or autism, school refusal. (4 marks)
4. Methylphenidate, dexamphetamine, atomoxetine. (2 marks)
5. Conduct disorder. (2 marks)
6. Any of the following: bullying, fighting, use of a weapon to threaten, stealing while confronting a victim (mugging), setting fire to property (arson), breaking into homes, truanting from school, runs away from home, ignores parental control or restriction, age before 13, initiates anti-social behaviour. (4 marks)

INDEX

Psychiatry in Medical Practice